ADVANCES IN

Pharmacology and Chemotherapy

VOLUME 10

ADVISORY BOARD

ADVANCES IN

Pharmacology and Chemotherapy

EDITED BY

Silvio Garattini

Istituto di Ricerche Farmacologiche "Mario Negri" Milano, Italy

A. Goldin

National Cancer Institute Bethesda, Maryland

F. Hawking

Clinical Research Centre Harrow, Middlesex, England

I. J. Kopin

National Institute of Mental Health Bethesda, Maryland

Consulting Editor

R. J. Schnitzer

Mount Sinai School of Medicine New York, New York

VOLUME 10

ACADEMIC PRESS New York and London 1972

ACADEMIC PRESS, INC.
111 Fifth Avenue, New York, New York 10003

United Kingdom Edition published by
ACADEMIC PRESS, INC. (LONDON) LTD.
24/28 Oval Road, London NW1

LIBRARY OF CONGRESS CATALOG CARD NUMBER: 61-18298

PRINTED IN THE UNITED STATES OF AMERICA

CONTENTS

Effect of Drugs upon Axoplasmic Transport

William O. McClure

The Metabolism of the Tetrahydrocannabinols

Louis Lemberger

Biological Activities of Antilymphocytic Serum

Federico Spreafico

Selective Multiphase Cancer Therapy: Conceptual Aspects and Experimental Basis

Manfred von Ardenne

The Application of Anthelmintics in the Feedlot

John R. Egerton

CONTRIBUTORS TO THIS VOLUME

Numbers in parentheses indicate the pages on which the authors' contributions begin.

F. M. BERGER (105), *Wallace Laboratories, Division of Carter-Wallace, Inc., Cranbury, New Jersey*

JOHN R. EGERTON (381), *Merck Institute for Therapeutic Research, Rahway, New Jersey*

GERHARD R. F. KRUEGER (1), *Hematopathology Section, Laboratory of Pathology, National Cancer Institute, National Institutes of Health, Bethesda, Maryland*

LOUIS LEMBERGER (221), *Lilly Laboratory for Clinical Research, Marion County General Hospital, and Departments of Pharmacology and Medicine, Indiana University School of Medicine, Indianapolis, Indiana*

WILLIAM O. MCCLURE (185), *Department of Biochemistry, University of Illinois, Urbana, Illinois*

S. J. POWELL (91), *Amoebiasis Research Unit, Institute for Parasitology, and Department of Medicine, University of Natal, Durban, South Africa*

LOWELL O. RANDALL (119), *Department of Pharmacology, Research Division, Hoffmann-La Roche Inc., Nutley, New Jersey*

WILLIAM SCHALLEK (119), *Department of Pharmacology, Research Division, Hoffmann-La Roche Inc., Nutley, New Jersey*

WALTER SCHLOSSER (119), *Department of Pharmacology, Research Division, Hoffmann-La Roche Inc., Nutley, New Jersey*

FEDERICO SPREAFICO (257), *Istituto di Ricerche Farmacologiche, "Mario Negri," Milano, Italy*

MANFRED VON ARDENNE (339), *Forschungsinstitut Manfred von Ardenne, Dresden-Weisser Hirsch, Deutsche Demokratische Republik*

Morphology of Chemical Immunosuppression

GERHARD R. F. KRUEGER

Hematopathology Section, Laboratory of Pathology
National Cancer Institute, National Institutes of Health
Bethesda, Maryland

I. Introduction

In this chapter the author will try to correlate the results of three large fields of research, which, though originating at about the same time and developing at about the same rate, have advanced in a parallel and independent fashion. Referred to are the fields of immunology and serology, pharmacology and chemotherapy, and pathology. If one reads present-day textbooks on immunology, pathology, or chemotherapy, the information gained is somewhat unilateral despite obvious effects of one field on one or both of the others. The only exception may be the fast-growing subspecialty of transplantation research.

No complete study of immunology, chemotherapy, or immunopathology is provided in this chapter; the reader may refer to the many already available review articles (Miescher and Müller-Eberhard, 1968; Letterer, 1967; Gell and Coombs, 1968; Diener, 1970; Steffen, 1968; Morrison, 1960; Sellei *et al.*, 1970; Wilmans, 1964; Abramoff and LaVia, 1970; Mandel, 1959). Instead, the author will introduce a synthetic approach to the problem of immunosuppression and reintroduce at the same time the value of careful morphological investigations.

II. Molecular Biology and Morphology of Antibody Formation

Before concentrating on the main subject—the morphology of immunosuppression—a summarizing review needs to be given of the current knowledge on the normal immune response. Readers interested in detailed descriptions of this subject may refer to the "Biology of the Immune Response" by Abramoff and LaVia (1970), or for the morphology and pathology, to Letterer (1967), Cottier *et al.* (1969), and Turk (1970).

Violation of the integrity of the human or animal body by foreign substances of a certain nature is followed by a specific reaction of the injured body called an *immune reaction.* Foreign substances that are able to elicit an immune reaction are named *antigens*; if a known antigen in a given organism induces an immune reaction, this substance may be well called an *immunogen*; if it introduces tolerance, it may be called *tolerogen.* Both tolerance and immunity (i.e., allergy) can be caused by the same antigen at different dose levels, at different routes of administration, or at different ages of the recipient. The specific reaction of the affected individual toward the antigen is carried out by antibodies. Antibodies are proteins with a variable fraction of their molecule that, on induction, is synthesized in a way to fit specifically with a certain segment of the antigen. This antigenic segment is called the *specific determinant.* A few examples of various antigenic determinants are given in Table I, and an example of the composition of an antibody molecule is given in Fig. 1. The cellular and molecular events that are initiated by the entrance of an antigen into the living organism are summarized in Fig. 2.

TABLE I

SIZES OF VARIOUS ANTIGENIC DETERMINANTS

Antigen	Determinant	Size in most extended form (Å)	Molecular weight
Dextran	Isomaltohexaose	34 × 12 × 7	990
Silk fibroin	Gly [gly_3ala_3] tyr	27	632
	Dodecapeptide mixture	44	1000
$G_{60}A_{40}$, $G_{60}A_{30}T_{10}$ and $G_{42}L_{28}A_{30}$	Hexaglutamic acid	36 × 10 × 6	792
Polyalanyl bovine serum albumin	Pentaalanine	25 × 11 × 6.5	373
Polylysyl rabbit serum albumin	Penta- (or hexa-) lysine	27 × 17 × 6.5	659
Polylysyl phosphoryl bovine serum albumin	Pentalysine	27 × 17 × 6.5	659

From Kabat (1966), reprinted with the permission of the author and of Williams & Wilkins, Baltimore, Maryland.

Phagocytosis has been known since Metschnikoff (1892) as the first visible reaction of the host toward an administered antigen. Extensive studies of Nossal, Ada, and co-workers have shown that, in lymphoreticular tissues, antigenic materials are fixed by phagocytic sinus endothelial cells, by cortical and medullary histiocytes, and by dendritic reticulum cells of the follicle (Nossal *et al.*, 1964; Ada *et al.*, 1967; Lang and Ada, 1967; McDevitt, 1968). However, dendritic reticulum cells apparently do not phagocytize antigen but absorb it to their surface and so probably allow a close contact of antigenic determinant sites with immunoreactive lymphoid cells (Szakal and Hanna, 1968; Schoenberg *et al.*, 1964). Antigen may persist 2–6 weeks in these various phagocytes and dendritic reticulum cells after a single primary injection. Within phagocytes, complex antigens then are broken down to simple antigenic molecules (Gill and Cole, 1965). This step of antigen processing appears important for the development of a primary immune response, although it may not be essential for all antigens (Pribnow and Silverman, 1967; Frei *et al.*, 1965; Feldman and Gallily, 1967). From these phagocytes information for the synthesis of specific antibodies is passed to immunoreactive lymphoid cells via the transfer of ribonucleic acid (RNA) or RNA–antigen complexes (Pinchuck *et al.*, 1968; Fishman and Adler, 1963a,b; Friedman *et al.*, 1965; Askonas and Rhodes, 1965; Gottlieb *et al.*, 1967). Since both ribonuclease (RNase) and pronase can destroy the activity of RNA extracted from sensitized animals,

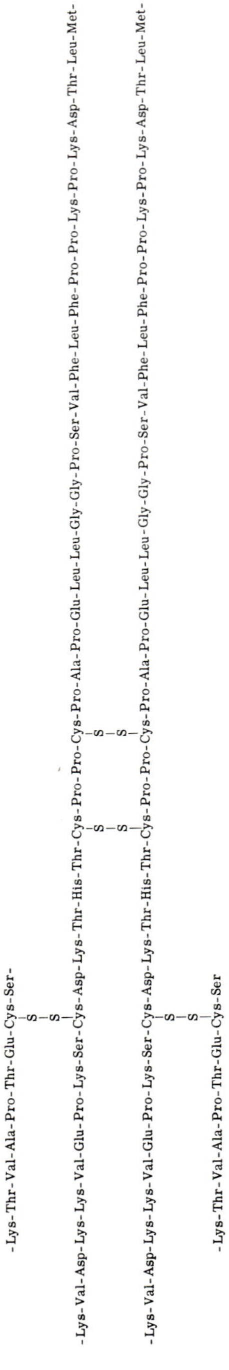
-Lys-Thr-Val-Ala-Pro-Thr-Glu-Cys-Ser-
S
S
-Lys-Val-Asp-Lys-Lys-Val-Glu-Pro-Lys-Ser-Cys-Asp-Lys-Thr-His-Thr-Cys-Pro-Pro-Cys-Pro-Ala-Pro-Glu-Leu-Leu-Gly-Gly-Pro-Ser-Val-Phe-Leu-Phe-Pro-Pro-Lys-Pro-Lys-Asp-Thr-Leu-Met-
S
S
S
S
-Lys-Val-Asp-Lys-Lys-Val-Glu-Pro-Lys-Ser-Cys-Asp-Lys-Thr-His-Thr-Cys-Pro-Pro-Cys-Pro-Ala-Pro-Glu-Leu-Leu-Gly-Gly-Pro-Ser-Val-Phe-Leu-Phe-Pro-Pro-Lys-Pro-Lys-Asp-Thr-Leu-Met-
S
S
-Lys-Thr-Val-Ala-Pro-Thr-Glu-Cys-Ser

FIG. 1. Example of the chemical composition of an antibody molecule (fragment). From Steiner and Porter (1967). Reprinted from *Biochemistry* **6**, 3957–3970. Copyright 1967 by the American Chemical Society. Reprinted by permission of the copyright owner.

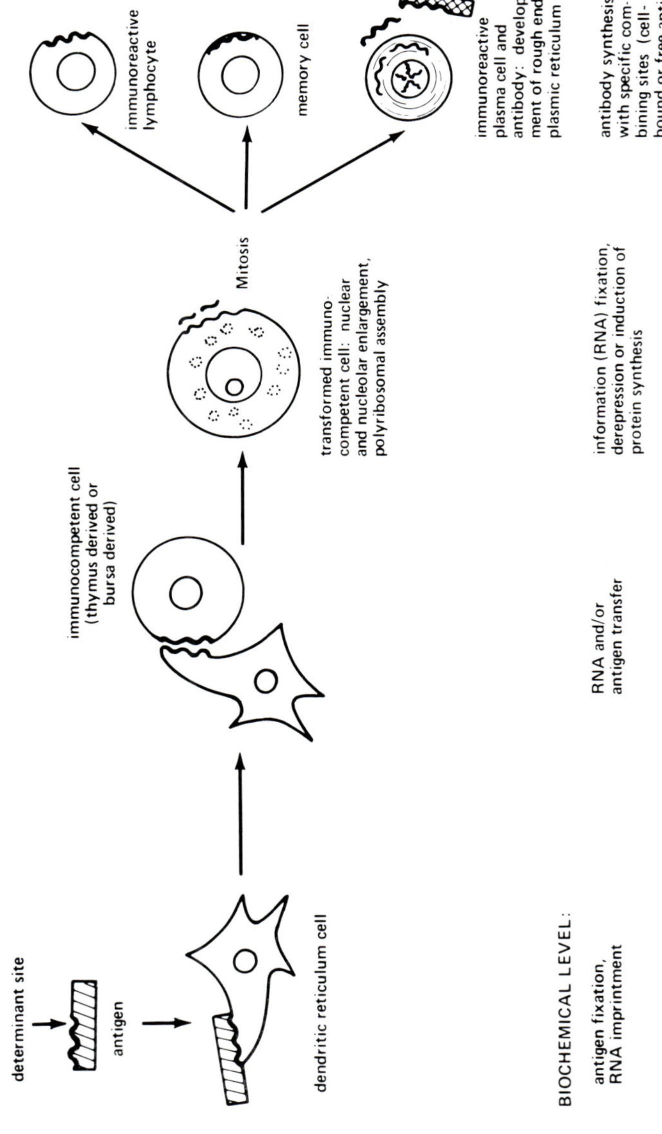

FIG. 2. Biology of antibody formation.

a complex of RNA and of antigen or antigen fragments may be essential for the induction of antibody synthesis.

Morphologically, activation of phagocytes after administration of antigents is manifested by their increase in size and by the increase in number of cytoplasmic granules which parallel the rise in acid phosphatase and β-glucuronidase activity. These granules are recognized as lysosomes by electron microscopy, and, in addition, ribosomes, polyribosomes, and mitochondria are increased in number. The larger size and the metabolic activation of phagocytes renders these cells more prominent in lymphoreticular tissues.

Following antigen fixation and processing in phagocytes is the induction period, during which lymphoid cells synthesize *de novo* ribosomal RNA (rRNA) (Abramoff and LaVia, 1970). Histologically, activation (or transformation) of lymphoid cells to small basophilic reticulum cells (immunoblasts) with prominent pyroninophilia is noted in the primary follicle and in the paracortical region of lymphoid tissues. These cells aggregate to

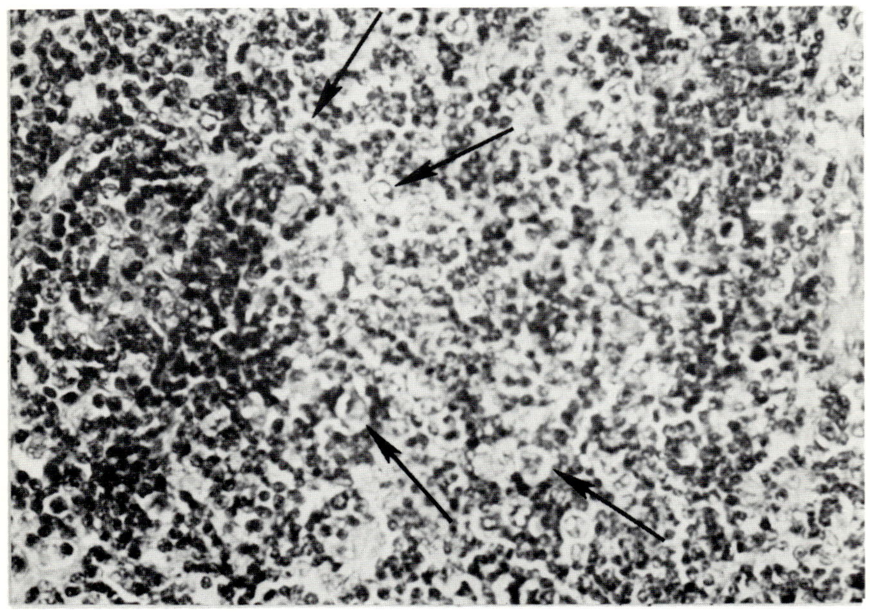

FIG. 3. Paracortical region of a mouse lymph node draining the site of injection of tubercle bacteria in adjuvant. Note increased number of activated reticulum cells, (immunoblasts arrows). H&E; magnification ×375.

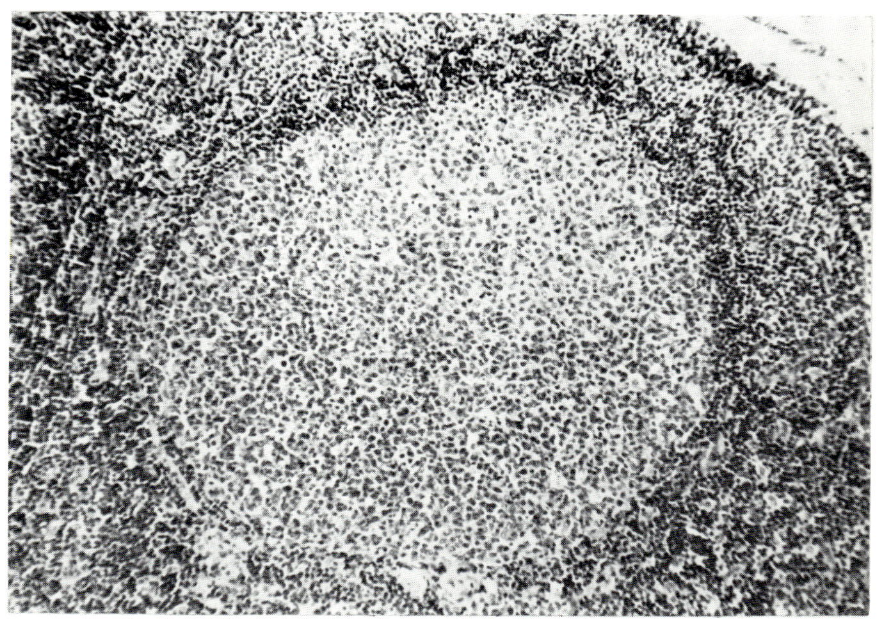

FIG. 4. Secondary follicle of a mouse lymph node draining the site of injection of bovine serum albumin. Note the division of the secondary follicle into the pale and the basophilic parts. H&E; magnification ×150.

form in the primary follicle a secondary follicle also called the *germinal center* (Figs. 3 and 4). This secondary follicle formation often is preceded by a transient dissociation of a preexistent secondary follicle (Congdon, 1962, 1964). Probably this dissociation is closely related to the period of induction, while reaggregation and *de novo* formation of secondary follicles represents the first step in antibody formation. Not in all cases of antigenic stimulation, however, is follicular dissociation obvious (Mariani *et al.*, 1971; Congdon, 1969). By electron microscopy, activated lymphoid cells, i.e., small basophilic reticulum cells, show increased numbers of polyribosomes but only a little rough endoplasmic reticulum. Their nuclei are enlarged and contain prominent nucleoli. Some authors subclassify these cells according to their cytological details into basophilic stems cells, germinoblasts, and germinocytes (Lennert, 1961; Mori and Lennert, 1969), although these may only represent variant states of activity of the same type of cell. Histochemically, cells in the secondary follicle characteristically contain a high concentration in 5′-nucleotidase (Braunstein *et al.*, 1958;

Lennert and Rinneberg, 1961), indicating that these cells are actively engaged in nucleic acid metabolism.

Following the induction period is the period of actual antibody synthesis which follows the general biochemical pathways of protein synthesis (Kabat, 1968; Mahler and Cordes, 1968): transcription of information for protein synthesis from deoxyribonucleic acid (DNA) to RNA, and translation of this information from RNA into the basic polypeptide chain. Each cell capable of antibody synthesis contains the DNA-encoded information for protein synthesis, and, according to the clonal selection theory of Jerne (Jerne, 1955) and Burnet (Burnet, 1959), may even contain the information for a single specific antibody. Antigenic stimulation is interpreted as selection and activation of these cells to produce their precoded antibody congruent to the inducing antigen. Another older theory, the instruction theory of Breinl and Haurowitz (1930) and Haurowitz (1965), also may be still valuable. According to this theory, only the information for protein synthesis is DNA encoded. The antigenic determinant, probably attached to RNA, serves as a template to modify nonspecific transcription and impose the synthesis of the specific group in the antibody molecule.

Amino acids are assembled to immunoglobulin chains at the site of polyribosomes, directed and assisted by messenger RNA (mRNA) and transfer RNA (tRNA) (Mahler and Cordes, 1968; Williamson and Askonas, 1967). It appears possible that the size of polyribosomal units is directly related to the size of the immunoglobulin chain (Kuff and Roberts, 1967). As in the synthesis of other proteins, polyribosomes involved in immunoglobulin synthesis appear membrane-bound, i.e., they are a component of rough endoplasmic reticulum (DePetris and Karlsbad, 1965; LaVia *et al.*, 1968). The release of antibody globulins from these membranes and from the cell is finally preceded by the addition of a carbohydrate group (Melchers and Knopf, 1969; Swenson and Kern, 1968).

Histological changes in lymphoreticular tissues during the period of antibody synthesis consist of fully developed secondary follicles, various numbers of pyroninophilic reticulum cells in the paracortical region, and differentiation of lymphoid cells to plasma cells in the medullary cords of lymph nodes (Fig. 5) (Ringertz and Adamson, 1950; Movat and Fernando, 1965; Krüger, 1967b; Krüger and Harris, 1970; Harris and Harris, 1956; Congdon and Makinodan, 1961). Histochemically, markedly elevated activities of glucose-6-phosphate dehydrogenase and alkaline phosphatase are noted in basophilic reticulum cells (immunoblasts) (Turk, 1967). Basophilic reticulum cells contain abundant aggregated cytoplasmic ribosomes, and plasma cellular differentiation in the medullary cords is paralleled by the marked increase in rough endoplasmic reticulum. Accordingly, intra-

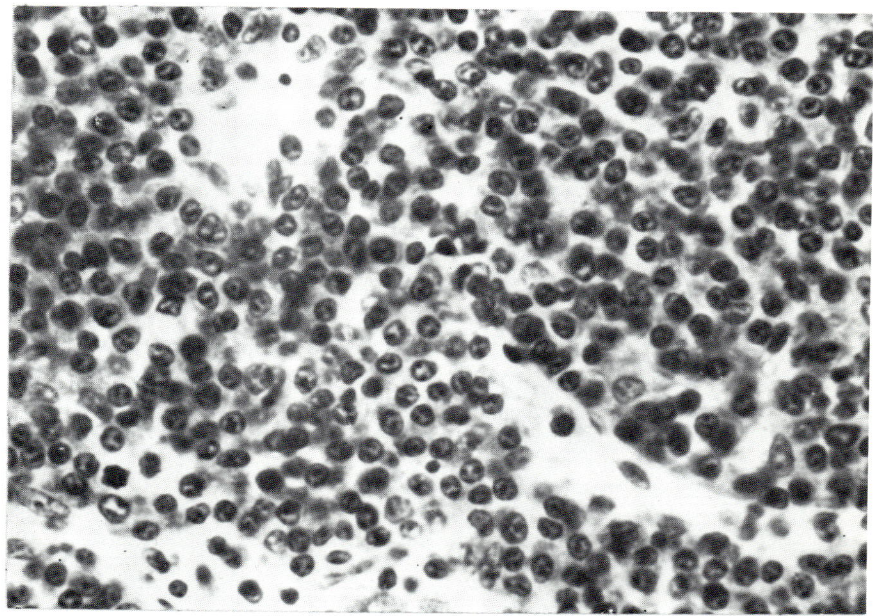

FIG. 5. Medullary cords of a mouse lymph node draining the injection site of bovine serum albumin. Note increased number in plasma cells. H&E; magnification ×675.

cellular antibody has been shown in basophilic reticulum cells of the secondary follicle (Pernis, 1967; Young and Friedman, 1967) and in cisternae lined by endoplasmic reticulum of plasma cells as well as their less well-differentiated precursors (DePetris and Karlsbad, 1965; Leduc *et al.*, 1968; Avrameas and Lespinats, 1967; DePetris *et al.*, 1963). Differentiation to antibody-producing cells usually is accompanied by cell proliferation in lymphoreticular tissues, the extent of which appears to depend upon the "strength" and on the dose of the antigen.

It is not yet well understood what the relationship is of the above-described mechanisms of antibody formation to the development of immune lymphocytes eliciting a cellular immune response. It appears that macrophages also play a role in cellular immunity (Dumonde, 1967) and that cell activation or transformation to pyroninophilic reticulum cells in the paracortical region of lymph nodes precedes the state of delayed hypersensitivity (Krüger and Harris, 1970; Oort and Turk, 1965). It has been suggested that immune lymphocytes may carry antibody-like substances

TABLE II

List of Immunosuppressants and Cancer Chemotherapeutic Agents

A. Hormones and antihormones
   1. Corticosteroids
   2. Corticosteroid antagonists (Metopirone, Mitotane)
   3. Estrogens and progesterone

B. Alkylating agents
   1. Nitrogen mustards
   2. Ethyleneimines
   3. Esters of alkylsulfonic acid
   4. Epoxides

C. Antimetabolites
   1. Pyrimidine and purine antagonists
   2. Folic acid antagonists
   3. Glutamine antagonists

D. Antibiotics
   1. Chloramphenicol
   2. Actinomycins
   3. Mitomycin C
   4. Daunomycin and adriamycin
   5. Mithramycin
   6. Bleomycin
   7. Puromycin
   8. Azotomycin
   9. Neocarzinostatin
   10. Streptonigrin

E. Enzymes
   1. L-Asparaginase
   2. Ribonuclease

F. Mitotic Inhibitors
   1. Colchicine and derivatives
   2. Podophyllin derivatives
   3. *Vinca rosea* alkaloids

G. Polyanions
   1. Pyran copolymers
   2. Polyinosinic acid–polycytidylic acid (poly I:C)

H. Miscellaneous Substances
   1. Methylhydrazine derivatives
   2. Mycophenolic acid
   3. BCNU [1,3-bis(2-chloroethyl)-1-nitrosourea]
   4. Newer alkylating agents

(Hashimoto *et al.*, 1965; Akiyama, 1965). If this theory is further proved, cellular immunity may be linked metabolically to humoral immunity.

III. Types of Chemicals Used for Immunosuppression

Several review articles about the chemistry and the pharmacology of immunosuppressants are available (Aisenberg, 1971; Berenbaum, 1967; Schwartz, 1967; Schwartz, 1968) so that here only brief mention is made of the major substances representing the different groups. Immunosuppression and cancer chemotherapy are widely overlapping fields so that the reader also may refer to monographs on the latter subject for information of immunosuppression (Brodsky and Kahn, 1967; Ochoa and Hirschberg, 1967; Schnitzer and Hawking, 1966; Burchenal, 1963; Goldin *et al.*, 1970; Timmis, 1967). Since drugs used for cancer chemotherapy often, if not always, combine carcinostatic with immunosuppressive effects, no clear-cut line can be drawn in this chapter between immunosuppressive and chemotherapeutic agents.

A list of cancer chemotherapeutic agents currently in use is given in Table II; these substances usually also exhibit immunosuppressive effects.

Schemes 1–6 summarize the chemical formulas of representative compounds from each group.

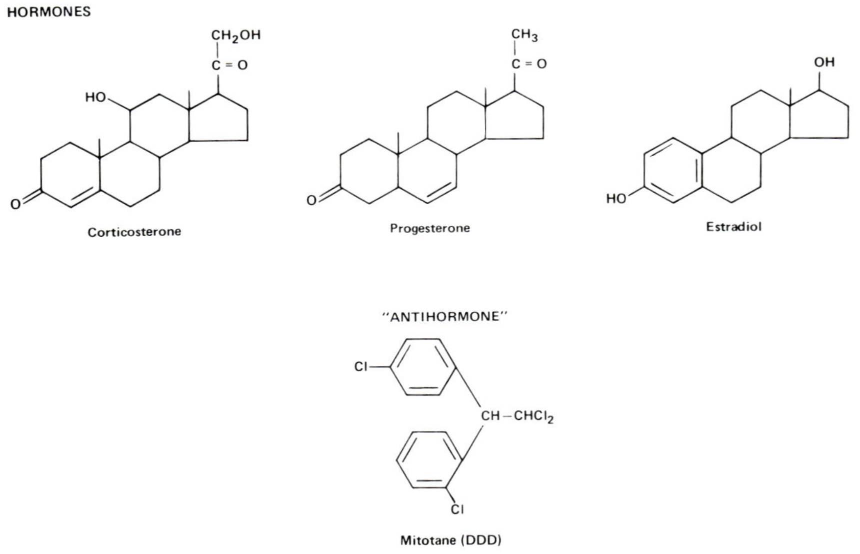
HORMONES
CH2OH
C=O
HO
O
Corticosterone
CH3
C=O
O
Progesterone
OH
HO
Estradiol
"ANTIHORMONE"
Cl
CH–CHCl2
Cl
Mitotane (DDD)

SCHEME I

ALKYLATING AGENTS

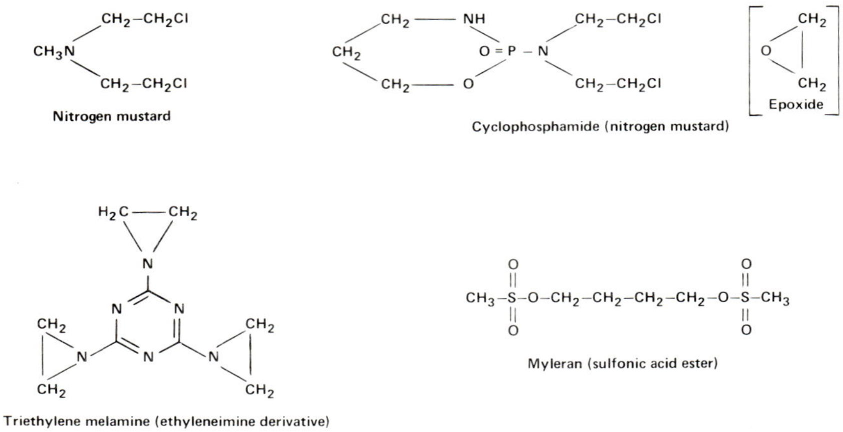

$CH_3N(CH_2-CH_2Cl)_2$

Nitrogen mustard

Cyclophosphamide (nitrogen mustard)

Epoxide

Triethylene melamine (ethyleneimine derivative)

$CH_3-SO_2-O-CH_2-CH_2-CH_2-CH_2-O-SO_2-CH_3$

Myleran (sulfonic acid ester)

SCHEME 2

PYRIMIDINE ANTAGONISTS

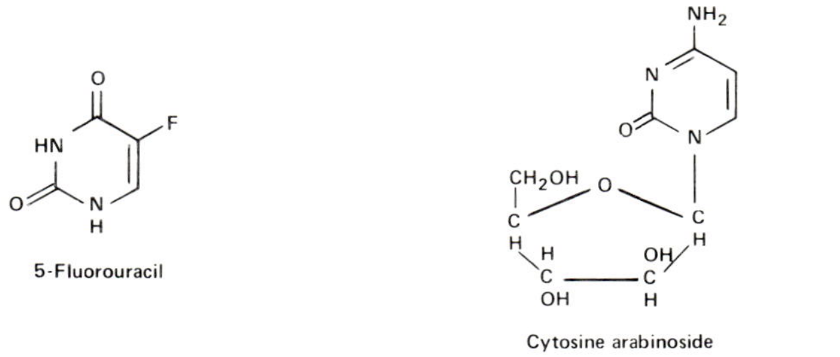

5-Fluorouracil

Cytosine arabinoside

PURINE ANTAGONISTS

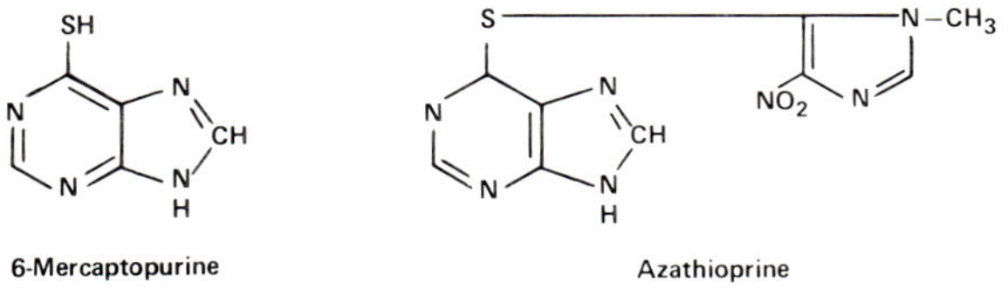

6-Mercaptopurine

Azathioprine

SCHEME 3

FOLIC ACID ANTAGONIST

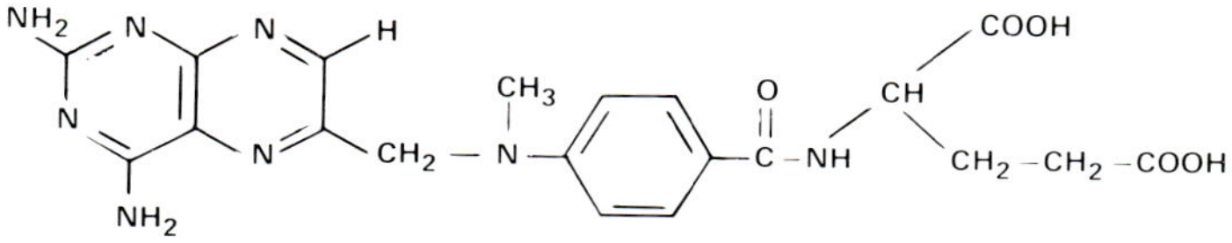

Methotrexate

GLUTAMINE ANTAGONIST

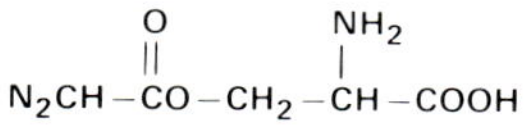

$$N_2CH-\overset{\overset{O}{\|}}{C}O-CH_2-\overset{\overset{NH_2}{|}}{C}H-COOH$$

Azaserine

SCHEME 4

ANTIBIOTICS

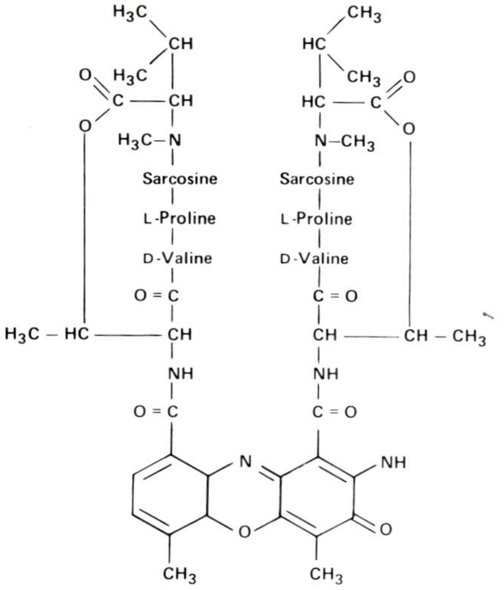

Actinomycin D

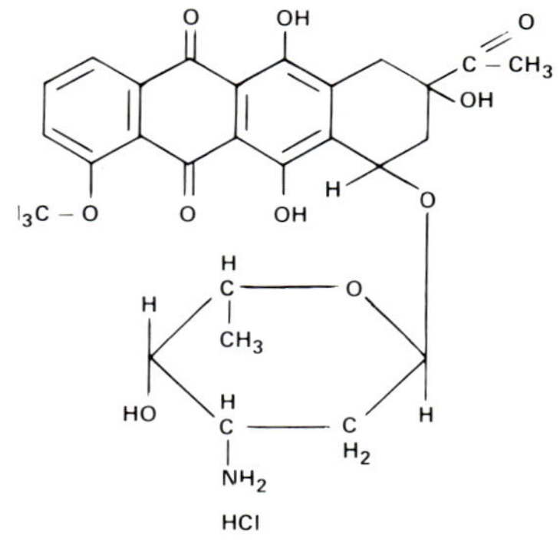

Daunomycin

SCHEME 5

MITOTIC INHIBITOR

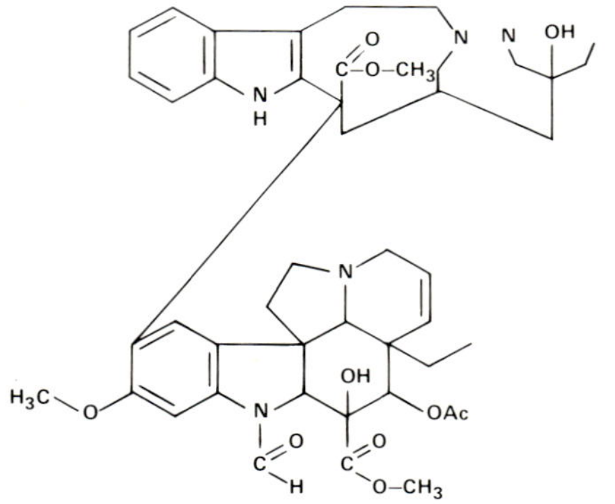

Vincristine

ANTIVIRAL SUBSTANCE

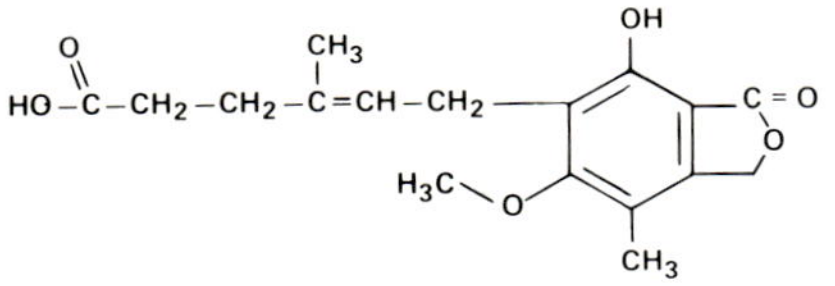

Mycophenolic acid

SCHEME 6

IV. Pathophysiology of Chemical Immunosuppression

For a detailed review of the pathophysiology of cancer chemotherapeutic agents refer to Mandel (1959), and of immunosuppressants to Berenbaum (1967).

A. Hormones and "Antihormones"

Corticosteroids possess a well-known lymphocytolytic activity, the mechanism of which is still not entirely understood (Feigelson and Feigelson, 1968; Gordon, 1955; Hansen, 1957). An immediate toxic effect on the lymphocyte was demonstrated (Dustmann and Stolpmann, 1968; Lundin and Schelin, 1966; Claesson and Ropke, 1969) as well as inhibition of protein synthesis of lymphocytes (Werthamer *et al.*, 1969; Hansen, 1957) and diminished mitotic activity (Gabourel and Arnow, 1962; Roberts *et al.*, 1952). Lymphoid tissues contain less RNA secondary to a rapid impairment of RNA synthesis after treatment with corticosteroids (Kass and Kendrick, 1952; Kidson, 1967); DNA synthesis is also inhibited (Brinck-Johnson and Dougherty, 1965; Pēna *et al.*, 1966). Activation of autolytic enzymes probably favors the immediate effect of corticosteroids on lymphocytes (Halkerston *et al.*, 1965). From all this it appears that antibody formation and production of immunoreactive lymphocytes is inhibited directly by corticosteroids. However, influence upon antibody synthesis has not yet been proved, nor whether the appearance and disappearance of antibodies is affected by corticosteroids (Baltch *et al.*, 1966; Fischel *et al.*, 1951). The immediate immunosuppressive action of corticosteroids, therefore, may mainly be limited to cellular immunity which explains its usefulness as an additive in the therapy of transplant rejection (Starzl *et al.*, 1963). Decreased phagocytosis (Spain *et al.*, 1950), secondary to an impaired mobility of phagocytes in cortisone-treated mammals, and the impaired development of an inflammatory response in addition interferes with the morphogenesis of immunologically induced cell and tissue damage (Travis and Sayers, 1965). Interestingly enough, also the opposite effect, the suppression of adrenal glucocorticoid synthesis, may interfere with the immunological reactivity as shown by the suppression of the graft-vs.-host reaction by Metopirone [2-methyl-1,2-dipyridyl(3^1)-1-oxopropane], a potent inhibitor of corticosteroid synthesis (Abe *et al.*, 1969; Abe and Nomura, 1970). This is of special interest since another depressor of adrenal cortical function, Mitotane [*o*,*p*′-DDD; 1,1-dichloro-2-(*o*-chlorophenyl)-2-(*p*-chlorophenyl)ethane] was introduced for treatment of adrenocortical carcinoma (Hutter and Kayhoe, 1966; Bergenstal *et al.*, 1960).

The atrophy of lymphoreticular tissues during pregnancy and malignant trophoblastic disease suggests that estrogens and progesterone have an effect on the immune reaction (Gregoire, 1946; Pepper, 1961; Nelson and Hall, 1967). It has been speculated that follicular hormones act as mitotic poisons (von Möllendorff, 1939; Lettré, 1943) and inhibit absorption by the cell of essential metabolites at the site of the cell membrane (Kuchler *et al.*, 1962). However, this effect apparently does not apply equally to all cells, since these hormones are able to stimulate granulopoiesis (Boll *et al.*, 1968). Depression of the homograft rejection with estrogens was successfully tried in experiments (Müller-Beissenhirtz *et al.*, 1971). It was effected, however, rather by interference with the morphogenesis of the transplant rejection than by interference with the immunocompetent tissues.

B. Alkylating Agents

It exceeds the scope of this chapter to discuss in detail the function of alkylating agents, since there are several hundred compounds in this group, and each of these compounds is polyfunctional, i.e., it may react with several of the biologically active groups in the cell. For a more extensive review the reader may refer, therefore, to Sellei *et al.* (1970), Mandel (1959), Whitelock (1958), and Ross (1962). Four main chemical groups exist: (*1*) nitrogen mustards; (*2*) ethyleneimines; (*3*) esters of alkylsulfonic acids; and (*4*) epoxides. Epoxides, however, have almost no clinical application. The general principle of the biological activity of alkylating agents depends upon the formation of a positively charged carbonium ion which binds to a negatively charged nucleophilic group of biologically important molecules; this is referred to as alkylation (Scheme 7). Among biologically active groups with which these agents may interfere are inorganic and organic anions, amino groups, sulfhydryl groups, and sulfide groups (Ross, 1958). Alkylating agents bind to guanine groups of DNA. This may lead to DNA–DNA, DNA–RNA, DNA–protein, RNA–

PRINCIPLE OF ALKYLATION

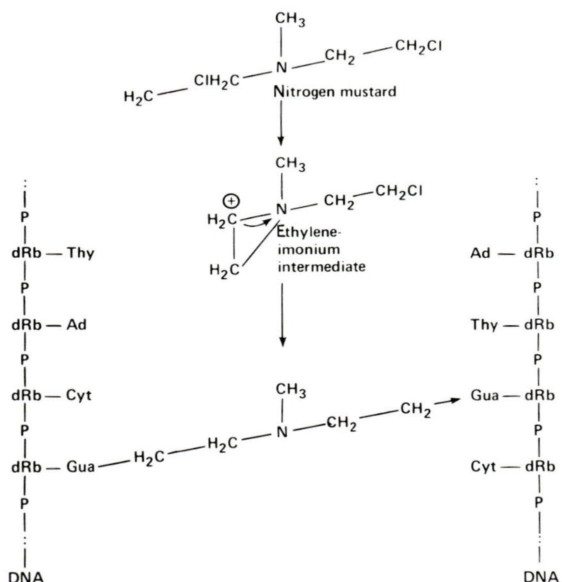

Crosslinkage of 2 DNA strands by nitrogen mustard

P:	phosphate	dRb:	desoxy-ribose
Ad:	adenine	Gua:	guanine
Cyt:	cytosine	Thy:	thymine

- - - : labile ribose-phosphate linkage susceptible to scission.

SCHEME 7

RNA, and RNA–protein cross-linking and, thus, may interfere with the replication of nucleic acids and the synthesis of proteins and enzymes (Press and Butler, 1952; Ross, 1962; Timmis *et al.*, 1959; Brookes and Lawley, 1961; Wheeler, 1962; Steele, 1962; Rutman *et al.*, 1961; Hölzel *et al.*, 1965; Liss and Palme, 1964). The process applies to bifunctional alkylating agents such as Myleran (busulfan). A blocking effect on cell division has also been described (Brewer *et al.*, 1961; Palme and Liss, 1964; Levis *et al.*, 1965). Immunosuppression, therefore, may be effected by alkylating agents in several ways: (*1*) by blocking and chemical changes including rupture of DNA and/or RNA, which serve as templates for the synthesis of antibody protein or of enzymes needed for the antibody synthesis; (*2*) by interference with cell division and proliferation which may affect both the increase of the pool of antibody-forming cells or of immunoreactive lymphocytes, and the proliferation of cells participating secondarily in the inflammatory response of delayed hypersensitivity reactions; and, finally (*3*) by immediate cell death. As described above, antibody synthesis is preceded by phagocytosis of the specifically sensitizing antigen. Among the normal cell types that ingest foreign materials, dendritic reticulum cells apparently have the special function of processing antigen in a way that enables them subsequently to induce antibody formation in immunocompetent cells (Ada *et al.*, 1967; McDevitt, 1968). Whereas immunoglobulin G (IgG) synthesis seems dependent upon the function of these cells, synthesis of immunoglobulin M (IgM) does not (Diener and Nossal, 1966). There are probably also differences between the induction of a primary and a secondary immune response in so far as macrophages appear rather essential in the primary but not in the secondary response (Feldman and Gallily, 1967). Antigen processing in phagocytes is accompanied by the development of protolysomes that combine with the phagosome to form a phagolysosome. In these structures, antigens are split into smaller fragments before antibody production (Garvey and Campbell, 1957). This step, preceding antibody formation, is not blocked by the alkylating agent, cyclophosphamide (Potel and Brock, 1965; Potel, 1970). Chlorambucil, nitrogen mustard, and benzimidazole derivatives, in contrast, have been shown to inhibit phagocytosis on the cellular level (Zschiesche and Augsten, 1970). These results indicate that the effects on phagocytosis of different members of the same group (i.e., of alkylating agents) are not consistent so that no comparative conclusions can yet be drawn when new drugs have to be evaluated. Zschiesche and Augsten (1970), however, feel that certain relationships between chemical structure and function do exist.

The next step in the process of antibody formation involves the transfer of information from the macrophage to the immunocompetent cell and the induction of synthesis of the antibody protein. The way this information induction acts needs still to be elucidated, but the participation of RNA, probably mRNA, appears proved by its sensitivity to RNase (Fishman and Adler, 1963b; H. Friedman, 1964). The inhibition of both induction and synthesis of antibody is probably the most prominent effect of alkylating agents. Cyclophosphamide decreased the incorporation of ^{14}C into DNA and RNA (Wheeler and Alexander, 1964) and so interferes immediately with the synthesis of nuclear acids, probably at the level of purine synthesis. This effect occurs at low dose levels so that cross-linking of nucleic acid strands, as mentioned above, probably plays a role here. Cross-linking, however, in addition blocks nucleic acid replication and also may cause its destruction. This action readily explains the blocking by alkylating agents of the induction of antibody synthesis which is in general the same as protein synthesis (Kabat, 1968).

Finally, the last step, the immediate synthesis of antibody globulin itself in immunocompetent cells, appears to be impaired by alkylating agents as mentioned before. Functions of enzymes and coenzymes, energy generation, and assembly of amino acids to polypeptide chains are hampered (Armborst and Maass, 1964; Dold *et al.*, 1962; Hilz *et al.*, 1962; Obrecht and Fusenig, 1965; Pütter, 1961; Bellelli, 1961; Hayashi *et al.*, 1964a,b; Limburg and Krahe, 1961; Lührs, 1961; Mielsch *et al.*, 1962; Takabatake, 1961). This interference of alkylating agents with the production of circulatory antibodies is clinically evident from an inhibition of the Arthus reaction (Bukantz *et al.*, 1949) and, experimentally, from many investigations demonstrating a depression of the primary antibody response to a variety of different antigens (Berenbaum and Brown, 1964; Amiel *et al.*, 1964a). Among the agents tested were HN2 (mechlorethamine), TEM (triethylenemelamine), L-phenylalanine mustard, and cyclophosphamide. Other authors, however, found no significant effect on the primary immune response of cyclophophamide or HN2 (Santos and Owens, 1964; Neidhardt, 1969a,b), or even a hightened antibody production after busulfan, for instance (Spitler and Fudenberg, 1970). In all these studies, the dose and the time of administration as related to antigenic stimulation are of major importance.

Aside from the effect of alkylating agents on antibody production itself, there is an immediate effect on cells which leads to inhibition of cell division and to cell destruction (Stefani and Schrek, 1964; Aisenberg, 1971; Cronkite and Chanana, 1968), thus causing an impairment of the cellular immune response on both levels—the generation of immunoreactive lymphocytes and the morphogenesis of the peripheral antigen–antibody reaction.

C. Antimetabolites

1. *Pyrimidine and Purine Antagonists*

These compounds represent a group of substances chemically analogous to uracil (2,6-dioxypyrimidine) or hypoxanthine (6-oxypurine). The latter ones are compounds essential for the biosynthesis of DNA and RNA. In purine and pyrimidine analogs, certain groups of the naturally occurring compounds are replaced by other chemical groups (see Table II). If these substances are then administered to the living organism, they interfere with the conversion of the natural purines and pyrimidines into the several biological active nucleic acid bases and also interfere via a competitive antagonism with the incorporation of natural bases into nucleic acids. For instance, 6-mercaptopurine inhibits the conversion of inosinic acid to xanthylic acid or adenylic acid (Abell *et al.*, 1965; Galton, 1956; Armborst and Maass, 1964; Fujikami *et al.*, 1962; Hölzel *et al.*, 1961). After conversion of 6-mercaptopurine to thioinosinic acid, it may also be incorporated into DNA or RNA itself, leading in this way to incorrect templates (Biesele, 1963; Brookes and Lawley, 1964). Further effects of this drug on enzymes and coenzymes have been discussed, and the reader may refer for further references to the review articles of Elion (1967) and Mandel (1959). Closely resembling 6-mercaptopurine is 6-thioguanine (Mandel, 1959). Azathioprine has the same chemical activity as 6-mercaptopurine and is most commonly used today for immunosuppressive therapy; azathioprine in broken down to 6-mercaptopurine (Bresnick, 1959; Elion *et al.*, 1962). Another purine analog, nitrosoguanine, is known to interfere with the cell cycle (Barranco and Humphrey, 1970). 8-Azaguanine is incorporated into RNA and DNA (Mandel and Carló, 1953; Matthews, 1958), and probably also inhibits protein synthesis (Malmgren *et al.*, 1952a). In a similar way as the purine analogs, the pyrimidine analogs 5-fluorouracil or 5-fluoro-2-deoxyuridine are incorporated into nucleic acids replacing uracil (Zubrod, 1961; Schneiderman, 1962; Nadler and Moore, 1964). 6-Iodo-2′-deoxy-uridine, 5-iodo-2-deoxycytidine, and 5-bromouracil are further compounds similar to natural pyridines and replace these in nuclear acids.

Finally, two substances deserve to be mentioned here which, despite lacking chemotherapeutic activity per se, enhance the action of other pyrimidine analogs. These are tetrahydrouridine, enhancing cytosine arabinoside (Neil and Moxley, 1970), and 5-cyanouracil, inhibiting the catabolism of 5-fluorouracil and 5-fluorodeoxyuridine (Gentry *et al.*, 1970).

Since antibody synthesis follows the general rules of protein synthesis, it is well understood from the above summarized biochemical actions of purine and pyrimidine analogs that these substances interfere with the antibody synthesis itself. The replication of the genetic code (DNA) or the template for protein assembly (RNA) may be blocked, available coding material destroyed (chromosome breakage), transcription and translation of information disturbed, and finally also the last step of assembly of amino acids to proteins blocked by interference with certain enzymes. Besides, production by cells of proteins for extracellular use (i.e., antibodies), production of proteins and of nucleic acids for the cells own use, i.e., for cell replication may be disturbed. The latter then may interfere with establishment of cellular immunity. Although both purine and pyrimidine analogs theoretically possess these abilities, the antipyrimidines, 5-fluorouracil and 5-bromodeoxyuridine, have proven ineffective *in vivo* for immunosuppression (Gabrielsen and Good, 1967). Recently, however, another pyrimidine analog, azacytidine, has been shown to suppress the synthesis of hemagglutinating antibodies and to interfere with the formation of hemolytic plaques (Vadlamudi *et al.*, 1970). The purine analogs, 6-mercaptopurine, 6-thioguanine, and azathioprine, have been shown to inhibit both the primary and the secondary humoral immune response (Schwartz *et al.*, 1958; Borel *et al.*, 1965; Frisch and Davies, 1962a,b; Frisch *et al.*, 1962; LaPlante *et al.*, 1962; Epstein and Maibach, 1965). 6-Mercaptopurine also is a potent inhibitor of cellular immune reactions (Borel and Schwartz, 1964; Obretenova, 1963), as is azathioprine, which today is in common use in human organ transplantation (Porter, 1967; Hume, 1966). The morphogenesis of the immune reaction, in addition, may be inhibited by suppression of the inflammatory reaction subsequent to antigen–antibody reaction as shown for 6-mercaptopurine (Page *et al.*, 1962). This is discussed further in Section V.

2. *Folic Acid Analogs*

Folic acid in its reduced state as tetrahydrofolic acid (THy) constitutes the base compound of several coenzymes necessary for the transfer of C_1 fragments. This transfer is essential for the synthesis of many biologically important substances, as for instance, serine, methionine, creatine, histidine, and the nucleic acid bases, inosid and uridine. Two substances, aminopterin and amethopterin, with a chemical constitution similar to folic acid have been shown to have carcinostatic and immunosuppressive activity. Folic acid analogs compete with folic acid for the enzyme dihydrofolate reductase which is bound primarily to the analog for which it has a greater affinity (Huennekens, 1963; Delmonte and Jukes, 1962; Werkheiser, 1963). This results in an inhibition of purine synthesis and leads to interference with DNA and cell replication. Besides, protein synthesis, i.e., antibody synthesis, may also by affected immediately (Webster and Johnson, 1955). For more detailed discussion of the biochemical action of these drugs the reader may refer to Petering (1952) and Bertino *et al.* (1967).

Besides aminopterin and amethopterin, the pyrimidine analog 2,4-diamino-5-chlorophenyl-6-ethylpyrimidine (Pyrimethamine, Daraprim) appears to act as a folic acid antagonist (Hamilton *et al.*, 1954). This drug, used for the treatment of malaria and toxoplasmosis, also has antineoplastic activity (Murphy *et al.*, 1954).

Among the folic acid analogs, amethopterin has been extensively tested for immunosuppressive effects and has proved valuable in inhibiting the cellular immune response (Prichard and Hayes, 1961; Friedman and Baron, 1961). The drug apparently affects the expression of delayed hypersensitivity rather than interfering with the development of a state of delayed hypersensitivity, since transfer by lymphoid cells of delayed hypersensitivity from amethopterin-treated animals to nonsensitized untreated animals is possible (R. M. Friedman, 1964a; Friedman and Buckler, 1963). Also, immunological memory was not affected by amethopterin (R. M. Friedman, 1964b). Humoral immunity, i.e., the production of circulating antibodies, was effectively suppressed by amethopterin if administered during the inductive phase (Santos and Owens, 1964; Brown and Berenbaum, 1964; Malmgren *et al.*, 1952b) and persistent tolerance toward homografts was achieved in experimental animals (Santos and Owens, 1966).

Recently, several new folic acid analogs of the 2,4-diaminoquinazoline group with a glutamyl or aspartyl moiety (deazaaminopterin, Quinaspar, and Methasquin) were tested experimentally. Despite an obvious cytostatic effect of these drugs on mouse leukemia, the development of a state of immunity against leukemic cells was not depressed (Shimoyama and Hutchison, 1970).

3. *Glutamine Analogs*

Two compounds of this group, *O*-diazoacetyl-L-serine (azaserine) and 6-diazo-5-oxo-L-norleucine (DON), have shown carcinostatic activity in experimental animals. The application to human tumors, however, is limited by toxic side effects and a less marked cytostatic effect (Reilly, 1958; Henderson *et al.*, 1957; Clarke *et al.*, 1957; Levenberg *et al.*, 1957). Azaserine and DON act as competitive antagonists for glutamine by binding irreversibly a specific enzyme necessary for glutamine-dependent steps in purine synthesis (Levenberg *et al.*, 1957; Herrmann *et al.*, 1959). Another drug which may act similarly is azotomycin (Carter, 1968c). Although both cellular and humoral immune reactions could possibly be affected by these drugs by interference with nucleic acid and protein synthesis, no pertinent information is yet available on this point.

D. Antibiotics

This group comprises carcinostatic compounds of different chemical constitution (Table II), most of which are extracted from different *Streptomyces* strains. A few of the list of antibiotics tested or used in clinical trials are actinomycin C and D (Hackmann, 1952; Busch, 1955), mitomycin C. (Hata *et al.*, 1956; Tasaka *et al.*, 1965), daunomycin and adriamycin (DiMarco *et al.*, 1964; Venditti *et al.*, 1966; Mathé, 1966; Bonadonna *et al.*, 1970; Tan *et al.*, 1970) mithramycin (Curreri and Ansfield, 1960; Kofman and Ream, 1963), bleomycin (Umezawa, 1965; Aso *et al.*, 1970), puromycin (Oleson *et al.*, 1955; Troy *et al.*, 1954), azotomycin (Carter, 1968c), Neocarzinostatin (Maeda and Meienhofer, 1970; Kumagai *et al.*, 1970), and streptonigrin (Kremer and Laszlo, 1967). In addition, antibiotics not used for tumor therapy are known to interfere with the immune response, as for instance chloramphenicol and cetophenicol (Freedman *et al.*, 1968; Weisberger *et al.*, 1964a,b). Also, streptozotocin shall be mentioned here. It apparently destroys primarily β cells of pancreatic islets and is tested, therefore, against islet cell carcinoma; its depressive effect on bone marrow suggests that it may act on lymphoreticular tissues as well (Samaan, 1970; Vogel *et al.*, 1970). The methods of action of compounds in this group are diverse and not always readily known. Several affect nucleic acids, as for instance actinomycin, which combines with DNA of the guanine–cytosine residue (Newton, 1965; Reich, 1963), bleomycin, which also binds to DNA through –SH groups and inhibits cell division (Fujita and Kimura, 1970), daunomycin and the closely related adriamycin, which also bind to DNA (Calendi *et al.*, 1965; DiMarco, 1967; DiMarco *et al.*, 1969), or neocarcinostatin, which inhibits DNA synthesis and mitosis (Bradner and Hutchison, 1966; Kumagai *et al.*, 1970). Puromycin binds to peptide groups at the side of the tRNA and inhibits protein synthesis (Darken, 1964). Mitomycin C and its *N*-methyl analog (porfiromycin) act as alkylating agents and probably bind at the guanine residue of DNA, causing cross-linkage between the double strand (Carter, 1968a,b; Goldberg, 1965). The antibiotic, azotomycin, has been mentioned already among the glutamine analogs because of the specific way in which it inhibits purine synthesis. Chloramphenicol and cetophenicol inhibit protein synthesis by binding to mRNA and suppressing the activity of peptide transferase (Weisberger *et al.*, 1964b; Weisberger, 1967).

In summary, all antibiotics, the method of action of which has been elucidated, may interfere with the humoral response either by immediate inhibition of antibody protein synthesis by interaction with mRNA or tRNA, or by alteration of the genetic code. Some of these drugs, as for instance, bleomycin, mitomycin C, and neocarcinostatin, also may depress cellular immunity by disturbances of cell proliferation. Actually proven so far are the immunosuppressive effects of chloramphenicol (Freedman *et al.*, 1968), actinomycins (Hoehn, 1965; Wust *et al.*, 1964), mitomycin C (Bloom *et al.*, 1964), and puromycin (Smiley *et al.*, 1964). In many, however, the *in vitro* effect is by far more significant than the *in vivo* effect, so that their clinical application as immunosuppressants is rather limited.

E. Enzymes

Two enzymes, L-asparaginase and RNase, are currently being investigated or used for their cancer chemotherapeutic and immunosuppressive effects. L-Asparaginase catalyzes the deamination of asparagine to aspartic acid and ammonia; aspartic acid then serves as one of the basic metabolites for the synthesis of purines and pyrimidines as well as serving for the synthesis of urea (Buchanan and Wilson, 1953; Reichard and Lagerkvist, 1953; Ratner and Petrack, 1953; Levenberg *et al.*, 1956; Sonne *et al.*, 1956; Hartman *et al.*, 1956). Ribonuclease catalyzes the hydrolysis of the 5′-ester linkage of nucleic acids leading to depolymerization of RNA to a core of polynucleotides and 3-phosphomononucleotides (Brown and Todd, 1952; Volkin and Cohn, 1953). Also, synthesis of polynucleotides from cytidylic acid has been observed (Heppel *et al.*, 1955) but not uniformly with all types of RNase (Hakim, 1957, 1960).

It appears probable from these activities, therefore, that both nucleic acid and protein synthesis are disturbed in tissues treated with L-asparaginase or RNase. Whereas administration of L-asparaginase may result in blocking DNA–RNA and protein synthesis, RNase rather catalyzes the breakdown of RNA. A decreased uptake of leucine-^{14}C and thymidine-^{14}C, in fact, was demonstrated during L-asparaginase treatment (Oerkermann and Hirschmann, 1970; Benvenisti *et al.*, 1970), suggesting a reduced synthesis of both proteins and DNA. Both enzymes, therefore, may theoretically interfere with humoral immune reactions, i.e., antibody synthesis and cellular immunity, in terms of cell replication, proliferation, and differentiation. L-Asparaginase, accordingly, was shown to inhibit blastic transformation of antigen-responsive cells (Eridani *et al.*, 1970; Astaldi *et al.*, 1969a), to block antibody synthesis presumably at the level of the precursor cell (Müller-Bérat, 1969), and to inhibit the graft-vs.-host reaction (Hobik, 1969b) which is primarily cellular in nature. Micu and co-workers (1970) assume that its action may even primarily affect cellular immunity.

Ribonuclease, also, is capable of suppressing both the primary and the secondary humoral immune response (Mowbray, 1967; Mowbray *et al.*, 1969) and of interfering with the development of cellular immunity, according to our own results (Krüger and Yun, unpublished data). Established immunological memory, however, cannot be abolished by RNase treatment (Levey and Medawar, 1966).

F. Mitotic Inhibitors

Several drugs which have antimitotic effects as well as carcinostatic activity have been mentioned earlier; these include alkylating agents, such as Myleran and the dibromohexitols. In addition, the colchicine derivative, deacetylmethylcolchicine (demecolcine, Colcemid), podophyllin derivatives, and the *Vinca rosea* alkaloids, vincristine and vinblastine, must be mentioned here as mitotic inhibitors (as such). The classification of these drugs as mitotic inhibitors, however, is somewhat subjective, since all of these show other activities besides interference with cell devision. However, Lettré and Lettré (1946) have defined the class of mitotic poisons which allows us to group these drugs separately. Colchicine and derivatives cause mitotic arrest in metaphase, secondary to a failure of spindle development (Lits, 1934).

Podophyllotoxin and derivatives supposedly act similarly to colchicine. *Vinca rosea* alkaloids bind to cytoplasmic precursors of the mitotic apparatus and produce mitotic arrest in metaphase (Johnson, 1968; Creasey, 1967; Cutts, 1961; Cardinali *et al.*, 1961; Journey *et al.*, 1968), but their effect on nucleic acid synthesis is not uniform and varies with the type of tissue and strain of animal investigated (Johnson *et al.*, 1963; Creasey and Markin, 1964; Richards and Beer, 1964); however, depressive effects on both DNA and RNA synthesis have been observed (Richards, 1968; Creasey, 1968; Rowland and Edwards, 1969).

Since cell proliferation in immunocompetent tissues is an integral part of the host response to antigenic stimulation, mitotic inhibitors theoretically may interfere with the immune response by inhibiting this cell proliferation. Besides, as for the *Vinca* alkaloids, the synthesis of template and messenger nucleic acids also may be disturbed. Practically, the inhibition of the immune response by vincristine and vinblastine, for instance, is not very obvious and often only achieved with lethal doses (Maguire and Stiers, 1963; Berenbaum and Brown, 1964). Others, however, demonstrated both the inhibition of the primary antibody response and of delayed hypersensitivity when these drugs were administered coincidently with the antigen (Aisenberg and Wilkes, 1964).

G. Polyanions

Recently, polyanions were introduced into experimental tumor therapy (Levy *et al.*, 1969; Regelson and Munson, 1970; Adamson *et al.*, 1969), and since they also show immunosuppressive activity these compounds must be mentioned here: (pyran copolymer and the synthetic polynucleolides, polyinosinic acid–polycytidylic acid (poly I:C). The mechanism of action is still to be elucidated, however. Beside an immediate action on cells (Isaacs, 1963), interference with protein synthesis (Levy *et al.*, 1969) or induction of interferon production is suggested (Rabson *et al.*, 1969). Immunologically, polyanions may alter antibody production and also decrease cellular immunity by blocking the action of phagocytes and, therefore, interfere with antigen processing during the induction phase of a state of hypersensitivity (Regelson and Munson, 1970; Regelson *et al.*, 1970).

H. Miscellaneous Substances

A few further substances remain to be mentioned for their immunosuppressive and antitumor activity: methylhydrazine and its derivative, procarbazine, are used for treatment of Hodgkin's disease (Mathé *et al.*, 1963; Hansen *et al.*, 1966), and their immunosuppressive activity is well documented in experimental animals (Amiel *et al.*, 1964). Although the mode of action is not quite apparent, effects similar to those of ionizing radiation are suggested.

1,3-Bis(2-chloroethyl)-1-nitrosourea (BCNU), a carbamide derivative used for treatment of various tumors (Schabel *et al.*, 1963; Clifford *et al.*, 1967), probably also is an immunosuppressant (Bonmassar *et al.*, 1962).

Two new alkylating agents, sulfonic acid esters of aminoglycols, have been recently introduced by Japanese scientists (Hirano *et al.*, 1970). They possess alkylating groups identical to Myleran and show strong immunosuppressive activities.

The potential antiviral chemotherapeutic agent, mycophenolic acid, has shown marked immunosuppressive activity (Mitsui *et al.*, 1970). It affects both the primary and the secondary immune response. The induction period of antibody formation is prolonged, and the formation of 7 S immunoglobulin is inhibited, leading to a sustained level of a 19 S immunoglobulins in the serum. Also the number of plaque-forming cells is reduced after administration of mycophenolic acid. Clinically, the development of anaphylatic shock is suppressed in experimental animals.

V. Morphological Changes during Immunosuppression

A. General Considerations

Despite the large amount of information that is available on the depressive effects of many drugs on the immune response, descriptions of the concomitant morphology of the immunocompetent tissues as well as of the site of antigen–antibody encounter are rare. This is regrettable since the exact morphological investigation of these tissues represents an easy and cheap tool that offers valuable information to supplement information that can be gained by measurement of the actual antibody formation. Also, this may be of utmost importance as will be pointed out later, since even quantitation of antibody production allows no conclusion to be drawn about cell proliferation in immunocompetent tissues.

Because of this lack in information about the morphology of immunosuppression, many of the data presented in this chapter are results of the author's own investigations in human and animal pathology, many of which are yet unpublished (and, therefore, constitute a tribute to the title of these volumes: "Advances in Pharmacology and Chemotherapy"). These results are complemented by whatever additional information is available from the literature.

From the current knowledge on the molecular biology of the immune response and on the mode of action of immunosuppressive drugs, as discussed in Sections II and IV, it appears reasonable to assume that, in immunocompetent tissues, proliferating cells and differentiated cells that synthesize immunoglobulins may be affected by immunosuppressants. The effect of different chemicals on these two compartments of cells, however, is not uniform. Instead, there are compounds that primarily interfere with cell proliferation and others that disturb the preparation for antibody synthesis or antibody protein synthesis itself. Accordingly, the expected metamorphosis of antibody-forming lymphoreticular tissues under the influence of these drugs is variable. Furthermore, the time factor is important in all these studies, since results from acute and chronic experiments are not entirely congruent. This must be stressed, since many determinations of the immunosuppressive effects of a new drug are done in short-term experiments. Before use of these drugs for long-term immunosuppression, as in the homograft situation, chronic experimental trials must be demanded.

Finally, investigations of the morphological effects of immunosuppressive agents should not be concentrated solely on immunocompetent tissue, since alterations in other tissues may affect the realization of an antigen–

antibody reaction and since toxic effects on nonimmunocompetent tissues may limit the use of effective immunosuppressants.

B. Antibody-Forming Tissues

1. *Hormones*

Most extensively investigated of all immunosuppressive agents for their morphological effects are the glucocorticosteroids. Intravenously administered tritium-labeled corticosteroids are concentrated rapidly in medium-sized periodic acid–schiff (PAS) positive lymphoid cells of lymphoreticular tissues as well as in mast cells (Csaba *et al.*, 1967). Whereas low doses are stimulatory on phagocytosis, high doses have depressive effects (Snell, 1960; Nicol and Bilbey, 1960). Morphologically, a reduced attachment of materials to be phagocytized on the cell membrane of phagocytes may be noted (Wiener *et al.*, 1967). This is followed by a marked acute depletion of lymphoreticular tissues of small and medium-sized lymphocytes (Dougherty, 1951; Dustmann and Stolpmann, 1968), rendering lymph nodes and thymus similar to their immature anlage (Masshoff and Gross, 1962; Ernström and Larsson, 1967). The lymphocyte depletion probably is caused both by an increased release of lymphocytes from lymphoreticular organs and an immediate destruction of these cells. The thymus and the short-lived small lymphocytes appear very sensitive to the action of corticosteroids, whereas the long-lived "memory cells" are less so (Ernström and Larsson, 1967; Miller and Cole, 1967). The depletion of lymphocytes of lymphoreticular organs is accompanied by a marked edema and by disappearance of mitotic figures in antigen-sensitized tissues. Lymphoid cells are especially sensitive to the effect of cortisone during the metaphase stage (Dougherty *et al.*, 1964). Subsequently, numerous macrophages containing nuclear debris (so called "germinal center macrophages" or "starry sky cells") are noted. Secondary follicles (germinal centers) are also reduced in antigen-stimulated and corticosteroid-treated lymphoreticular tissues (Cooper and Weller, 1969), and postcapillary venules may be less prominent (Krüger, 1968). On the cellular level, disintegration of the nuclear membrane of lymphoid cells is followed by chromatinolysis, cytoplasmic bleb formation, and cytoplasmic shedding (Dustmann and Stolpmann, 1968; Dougherty *et al.*, 1964). Damaged cells are phagocytized by histiocytes giving rise to the starry sky effect. There may be also a diminution of plasma cells. After cessation of steroid action, there is usually a rapid morphological recovery of lymphoreticular tissues. In mice, repopulation of lymph nodes with small lymphocytes starts by 24 hours after the last dose (Dustmann and Stolpmann, 1968). This pertains, however, to short-term experiments. Functional recovery probably is delayed when compared with morphological recovery, as indicated by an increase in Nigrosine-stained cells (dye exclusion test) over a period of 3 days after a single injection of cortisol (Claesson and Ropke, 1969).

Sustained action of corticosteroids on lymphoreticular organs over longer periods of time (months) may lead to a selective activation and even proliferation of reticulum cells and histiocytes. Since these cells are markedly resistant to the effect of steroid hormones, they are still able to synthesize DNA and RNA and probably constitute the pool of progenitor cells for later repopulation with lymphocytes. Under protracted influence of cortisone, reticulum cells acquire a more basophilic cytoplasm (activation) which is caused by ribosomal aggregation; the nuclei and nucleoli also enlarge. This probably represents a hypertrophic rather than a hyperplastic response, and no significant reactive cell proliferation or tumor formation in lymphoreticular tissues has been observed.

In vitro, corticosteroids inhibit the transformation of lymphocytes when stimulated with phytohemagglutinin (Stefani and Oester, 1967; Ono *et al.*, 1968).

Not all glucocorticoid compounds are equally effective on lymphoreticular tissues. It appears that an unsaturated A ring, a ketone at the 3 position, a hydroxyl or oxy group of 11 position, and a side chain (C_{21} compounds) are related to lymphocytolytic effectiveness (Dougherty *et al.*, 1964). The greatest thymolytic capacity is shown by cortisol, which is followed by cortisone, corticosterone, and 11-dehydrocorticosterone (arranged according to falling activity). Also, the lymphocytolytic effect of cortisone and 11-dehydrocorticosterone appears to be dependent upon the ability of lymphoid cells to reduce the 11-oxy group (Dougherty *et al.*, 1964).

The morphological effect of progesterone on lymphoreticular tissues is known from alterations in these tissues during pregnancy and from the pathology of malignant trophoblastic disease. The thymus and lymph nodes atrophy during pregnancy, secondary to a lymphocytolytic effect of estrogens and progesterone (Gregoire, 1946; Jolly and Lieure, 1930; Dougherty, 1952). Changes in malignant trophoblastic disease are similar and even more prominent (Nelson and Hall, 1967). Secondary follicles are usually absent. It is of practical interest, however, that in contrast to glucocorticosteroids, estrogens apparently do not inhibit cell proliferation. Instead, despite their lymphocytolytic effect, these drugs may even support proliferation of lymphoreticular cells as suggested by several experiments in which spontaneous and induced leukemia and lymphoma development was markedly enhanced by estrogen treatment and was decreased in female mice by castration (Gardner, 1950; Kirschbaum *et al.*, 1955; Gardner *et al.*, 1940; Silberberg and Silberberg, 1949). Testosterone, although not yet used for immunosuppression, has a well-documented lymphocytolytic activity and inhibits the development of the bursa Fabricii, probably by its antiproliferative effect (Aspinall *et al.*, 1961; Warner and Burnet, 1961).

The protective effect of the antihormone Metopirone on animals with homologous disease (Abe *et al.*, 1969; Abe and Nomura, 1970) is apparently not caused by lymphocytolysis, since Metopirone does not decrease significantly the number of circulating lymphocytes. In animals surviving acute homologous disease after Metopirone administration, a marked proliferation of reticulum cells is noted in lymphoreticular tissues. This proliferation is unorganized and may be somehow similar to incipient malignant neoplasia. However, it cannot be clearly decided whether reticulum cell proliferation is only secondary to chronic homologous disease or whether the proliferation is stimulated by Metopirone. The description of the morphological effect of Metopirone in normal control animals is regrettably incomplete and the mode of action of Metopirone in homologous disease is not clear; it may be, however, that it exerts a protective effect on the host's lymphoreticular tissues against the aggression of allogeneic lymphocytes.

The second antihormone mentioned earlier, *o,p'*-DDD (Mitotane), so far has not been investigated for immunosuppressive effects. No morphological changes in lymphoreticular tissues were observed after feeding of DDD to dogs (Nelson and Woodard, 1949). In my own review of 10 autopsies of patients with adrenocortical carcinoma who were treated with *o,p'*-DDD, atrophic lymph nodes were noted in 8. In 5 cases this atrophy was generalized, including all cell lines except for sinus endothelial cells and, therefore, was consistent with the picture seen in tumor patients and in experimental animals in late stages after tumor isotransplantation (Krüger, 1967a). In 3 cases, however, the lymph node atrophy clearly comprised the paracortical area, sparing the cortex and the medullary cords (Fig. 6a). Also large atypical lymphoid cells were noted (Fig. 6b). This effect was not observed in tumor cachexia, nor was it caused by excessive corticosteroid production and it, therefore, deserves further investigation. Finally, these investigations may prove to be quite important, since it has been shown that the widely used pesticide DDT [1,1,1-trichloro-2,2,-bis(*p*-chlorophenyl)ethane] may be converted by bacteria to DDD (Johnson *et al.*, 1967), and this substance in trace amounts possibly may be ingested with drinking water or seafood.

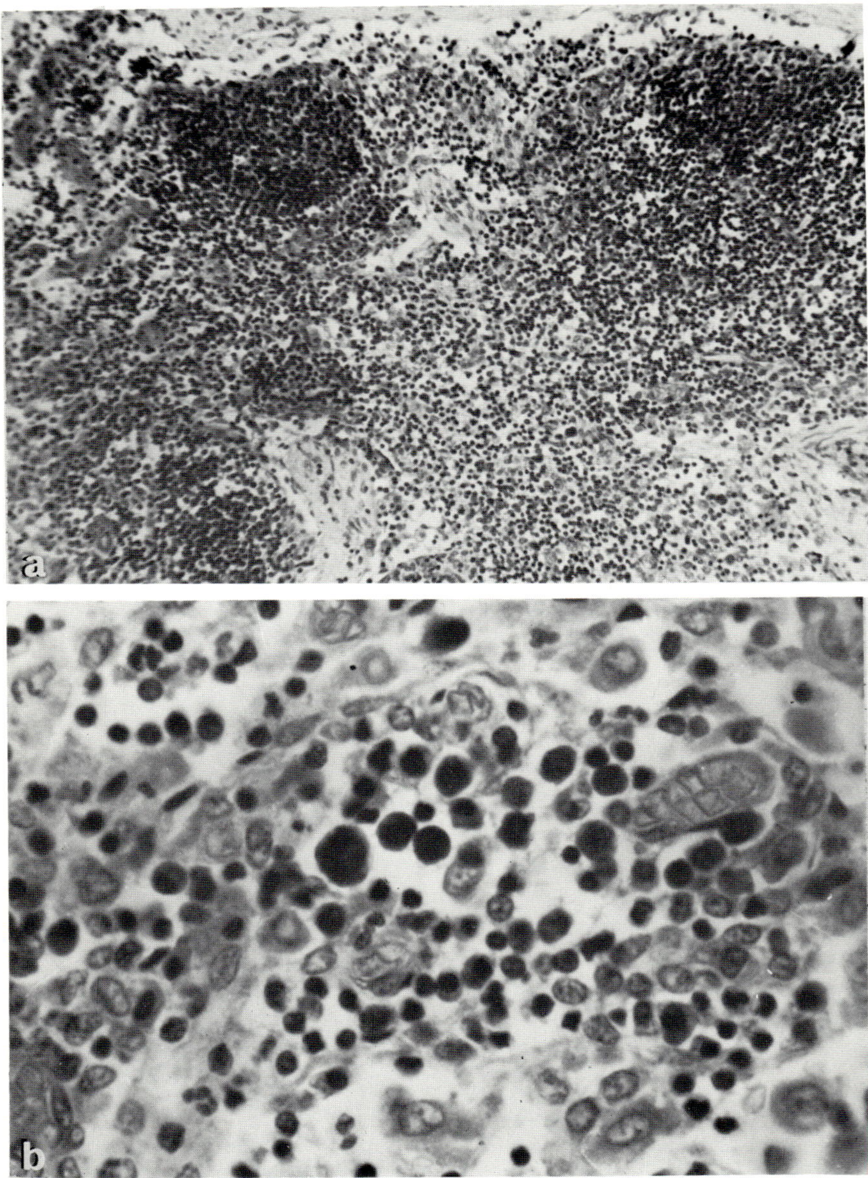

FIG. 6. Lymph nodes of a patients who received o,p'-DDD for carcinoma of the adrenal cortex. (a) Note moderate atrophy of paracortex and absence of secondary follicles. H&E; magnification ×150. (b) Note atypical lymphoid cells with hyperchromatic nuclei, pyknotic lymphoid cells, and sinus histiocytosis. H&E; magnification ×675.

2. *Alkylating Agents*

Although this group of agents includes potent immunosuppressive compounds, there are few and incomplete reports available as to their morphological effect on immunocompetent tissue. Most often the lymphocytopenic effect of alkylating agents is mentioned (Eckhardt *et al.*, 1965; Lane, 1967; Karnofsky, 1967). We have studied tissues obtained from complete autopsies of dogs and mice treated with cyclophosphamide and TEM. These dog studies included short-term experiments with administration of acutely toxic doses (100 mg/kg dog/day) of cyclophosphamide resulting in death in a few days and long-term experiments with chronic administration of cyclophosphamide and TEM (doses: TEM, 0.3 mg/kg mouse/day; cyclophosphamide, 45 mg/kg dog/day) varying from 1 to 10 years duration. The effects on lymphoreticular tissues varied markedly when normal animals or antigenically stimulated animals were treated with these two alkylating agents. Early changes of unstimulated animals treated with cyclophosphamide consisted in a moderate decrease in small lymphocytes in lymph nodes, thymus, and spleen and in a prominent swelling of

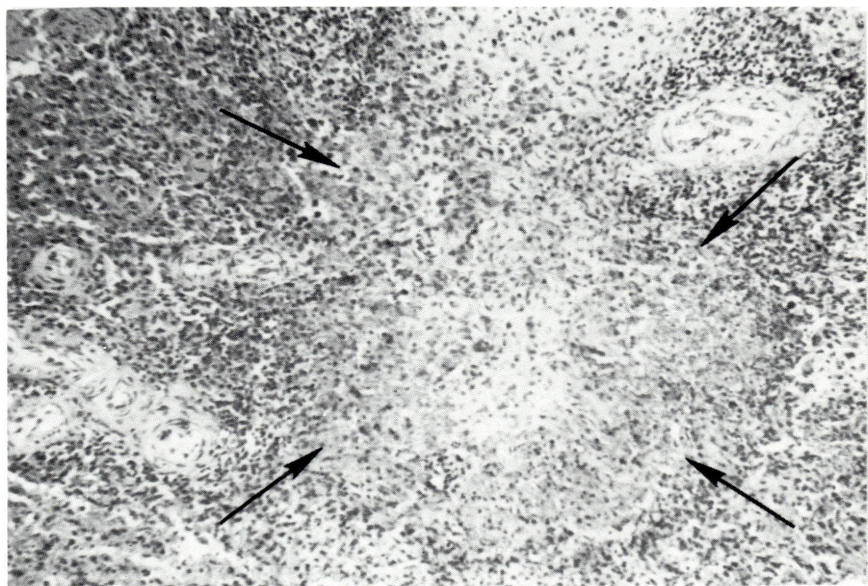

FIG. 7. Spleen of a dog treated with cyclophosphamide in preparation for bone marrow transplantation (100 mg/kg). Note extensive necrosis of preexisting secondary follicle (arrows). H&E; magnification ×150.

histiocytes in these organs. Antigenically stimulated animals showed a prominent acute necrosis of secondary follicles (germinal centers) in lymph nodes (Fig. 7); also splenic follicles became necrotic (Göing *et al.*, 1970). This effect occurred quite rapidly and was observed after only a few hours. It was described earlier also by Cameron and co-workers (1947). The morphological changes in human lymphoreticular tissues are similar although less prominent (Lane, 1967). The transformation of lymphocytes, i.e., the formation of blast cells or small basophilic reticulum cells that precedes antibody formation is suppressed (Astaldi *et al.*, 1969b; Turk, 1964b). These changes are completely reversible after discontinuation of the alkylating agent; however, atypical large histiocytes may be present for some time. Also, the speed and extent of functional recovery probably differs in individuals with or without thymic tissue (Aisenberg and Davis, 1968).

If the action of alkylating agents persists for a longer time (several days to a few weeks), severe lympyocytopenia of lymph nodes, spleen, and Peyer's patches leads to almost complete cortical and follicular atrophy. The paracortical zone is also depleted of nearly all cells, leaving behind

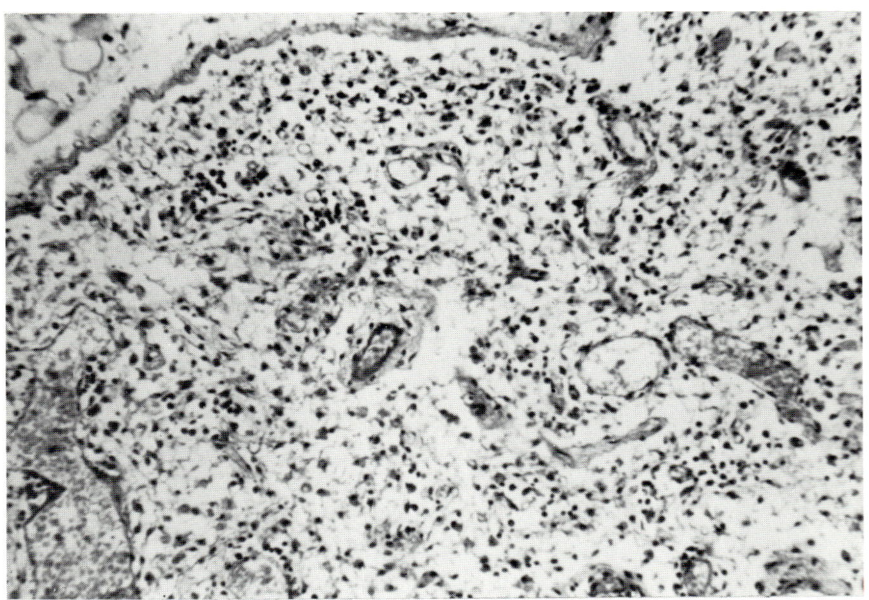

FIG. 8. Lymph node of a dog receiving 100 mg/kg cyclophosphamide in preparation for bone marrow transplantation. Note complete atrophy, leaving connective tissue network and occasional inactive-appearing round cells. H&E; magnification ×150.

only sinus histiocytes and prominent postcapillary venules as major structural components (Fig. 8). The presence of abundant sinus histiocytes concurs with the observation that, in carbon clearance studies in mice treated with alkylating agents, the number of phagocytes is not decreased (Zschiesche and Augsten, 1970). Often acute focal necroses and hemorrhages destroy large parts of the lymphoreticular tissues in high-dose cyclophosphamide-treated individuals. The loss of differentiated cells includes small lymphocytes in all areas, i.e., probably both long-lived and short-lived cells, despite the finding that long-lived cells apparently are more resistant to cyclophosphamide than short-lived cells (Miller and Cole, 1967). The few persistent reticulum cells or stem cells are quite atypical, anaplastic, polymorphous, and unclassifiable (Fig. 9a and b). Similar cells have been seen in chemotherapeutically treated human leukemias, reactive hyperplasias of lymphoreticular tissues, and in patients after bone marrow transplantation (Gross, 1964; Krüger *et al.*, 1971a). This has led to the term "polyblastic reticulosis" when these atypical cells are present in greater numbers. The occurrence of these bizarre large cells in cyclophosphamide-treated humans and animals may be secondary to blockage of this drug of cell division in the premitotic phase, but nucleic acid and protein synthesis continues to function (Schwartz, 1968). These changes differ somewhat from others obtained in rat experiments, where the medullary cords of lymph nodes were less atrophic, and depletion of plasma cells in these areas was less obvious (Miller and Cole, 1967). This however, may be a dose-related difference, and the number of plasma cells noted in the medullary cords of lymph nodes and in the spleen may depend on the interval between the last administration of cyclophosphamide and the day of collection of tissues for histological investigation, since a reactive plasmacytosis often follows discontinuation of treatment. Experimental animals and probably also humans showing the extensive acute atrophy of lymphoreticular tissues, with focal necroses and hemorrhage, usually die of septic infections, and no late changes secondary to therapy with alkylating agents are seen. Also, it is impossible to decide whether acute focal necroses are caused by the treatment itself or by sepsis, although bacterial or fungal colonies are usually not observed in these foci. Animals that have survived in long-term experiments have continued to show a marked decrease in number of small lymphocytes. The overall atrophy of lymph nodes and spleen, however, was less prominent; instead, a uniform population of reticulum cells was noted in these organs. Similar changes have also been described by others using tris(β-chloroethyl)amine in several animals (Gieldanowski *et al.*, 1969). There appeared to exist a positive relationship between the percentage of long-term survivors and antigenic

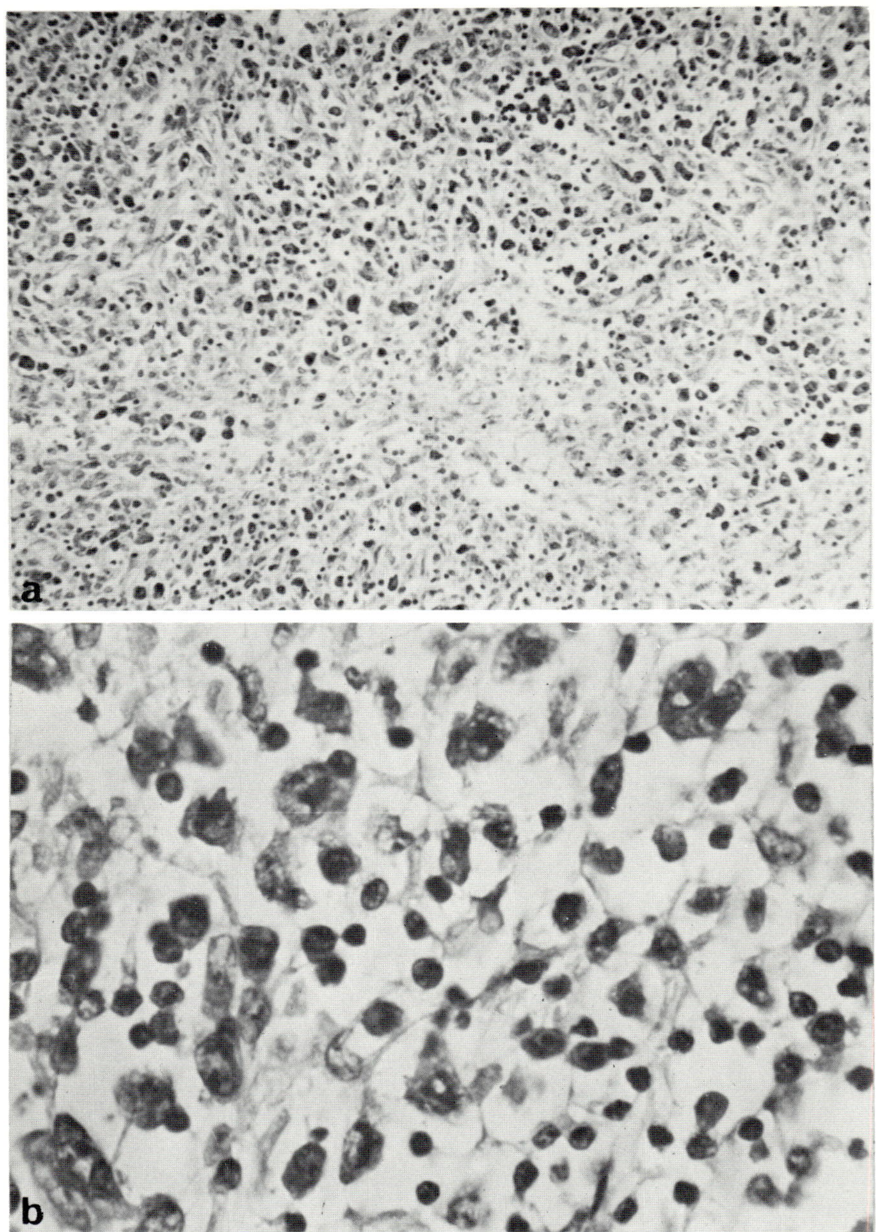

FIG. 9. (a) Lymph node of a patient treated with cyclophosphamide in preparation for bone marrow transplantation and with methotrexate posttransplantation. Note loose population of atypical unclassifiable cells and lymphoid cells representative of polyblastic reticulosis. H&E; magnification ×150. (b) Detail of Fig. 9a. ×675.

stimulation, i.e., mice on chemotherapy alone died faster and showed more severe signs of lymphoreticular atrophy than did mice on both chemotherapy and persistent antigenic stimulation. The latter ones often had focal reticulum cells proliferates in lymph nodes and spleens. This was also observed in a few human kidney transplant recipients on immunosuppressive chemotherapy (Krüger, 1970c) and in a dog that survived 10 years with a lung allotransplant (Fig. 10). The clinical significance of these lesions, as stressed in two publications (Krüger, 1970a; Krüger *et al.*, 1971b), will be discussed later.

Chronic treatment of mice with TEM in intermediate doses led to reactive reticulum cell hyperplasias, primarily in the paracortical region of lymph nodes. In the spleen, immature lymphoid cells and reticulum cells were noted to replace the follicles, and a marked hyperplasia of hemopoietic stem cells occurred in the red pulp (Fig. 11). Megakaryocytes appeared normal in number or slightly decreased. These changes were observed from the fifth week on after onset of treatment, and their extent was markedly increased when the animals were stimulated by antigenic substances at the

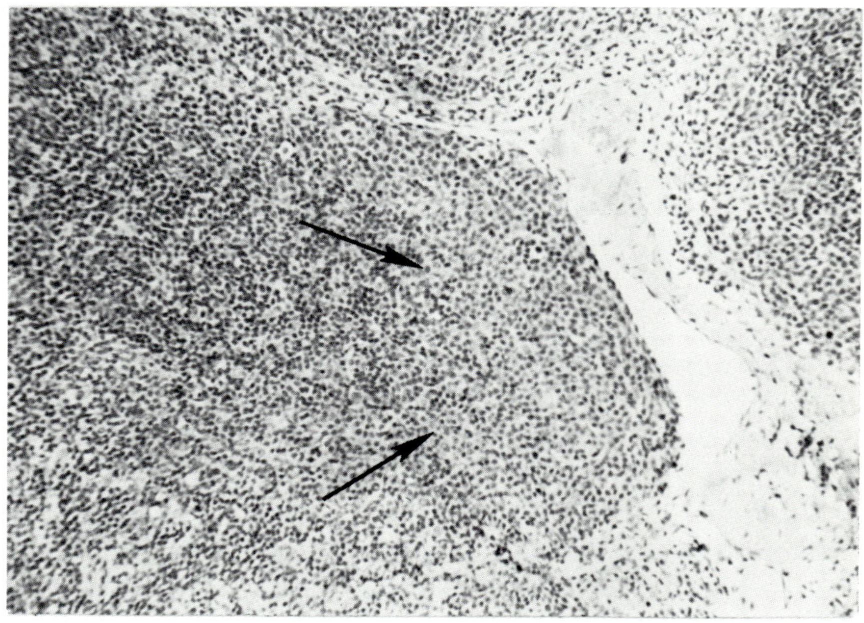

FIG. 10. Lymph node of a dog draining the site of a lung allotransplant. Status 10 years after transplantation and treatment with cyclophosphamide. Note aggregate of immature lymphoid cells (arrows). H&E; magnification ×150.

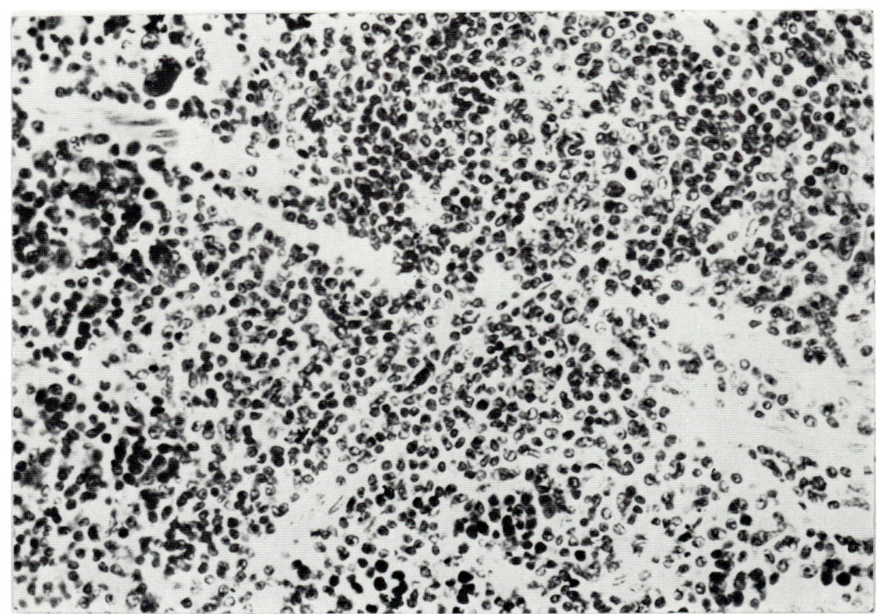

FIG. 11. Spleen of a mouse treated with triethylenemelamine (TEM) for 2 months. Note focal increase of hemopoietic precursor cells in the red pulp. H&E; magnification ×375.

same time (for instance by repeated bovine serum albumin injections). Thymuses were moderately to markedly atrophic as demonstrated by a narrowing of the cortex and loss of small lymphocytes. The medulla contained many histiocytes and reticulum cells diffusely dispersed or arranged in small clusters (Fig. 12).

Proceeding one step further from these observations, one comes to reports about an increased incidence of lymphomas after treatment with alkylating agents (Cardell, 1961; Karnofsky, 1967). Karnofsky (1967) classifies these as thymic lymphomas, which correlates well with the proliferates of immature reticulum cells in the thymus and paracortical regions of lymph nodes. It is my impression that it is a combination of antigenic stimulation and administration of alkylating agents rather than alkylating agents alone that initiates the hyperplastic or eventually neoplastic reticulum cell response. Reticulum cell saroma has also been described after longstanding treatment with another alkylating compound, namely busulfan (Sykes, 1958). As pointed out earlier in this chapter, the number and variety of compounds in the group of alkylating agents is large, and their function is not uniform. Anatomic records especially with regard to late effects are incomplete. It must be stressed at this point that investigation of immunosuppressive drugs for only their depressive effect on the production of circulating antibodies is inadequate, since no conclusions can be drawn as to their effect on cell proliferation in immunocompetent tissues. These, however, are of great significance in estimating the capacity to recover of chemotherapeutically treated tissues and in estimating the risk of tumor induction by the drugs used for immunosuppression. The hyperplastic response is somewhat surprising, since rapidly dividing cells appear most sensitive to the effect of alkylating agents; this obvious contradiction needs further investigation in the future. It may be regulated by quantitative influences relating to drug dosage and extent of antigenic stimulation, i.e., intense antigenic stimulation may decrease the cell-killing effect of alkylating agents at a given dose. A certain number of dead cells then stimulate cell proliferation for repair (Wassermann, 1929; Wrba, 1962; Altmann, 1966; Pardee, 1964). Therefore, from the point of view of an anatomic pathologist, a reconsideration and probably a limitation is needed of Berenbaum's (1967) statement that "probably the most important

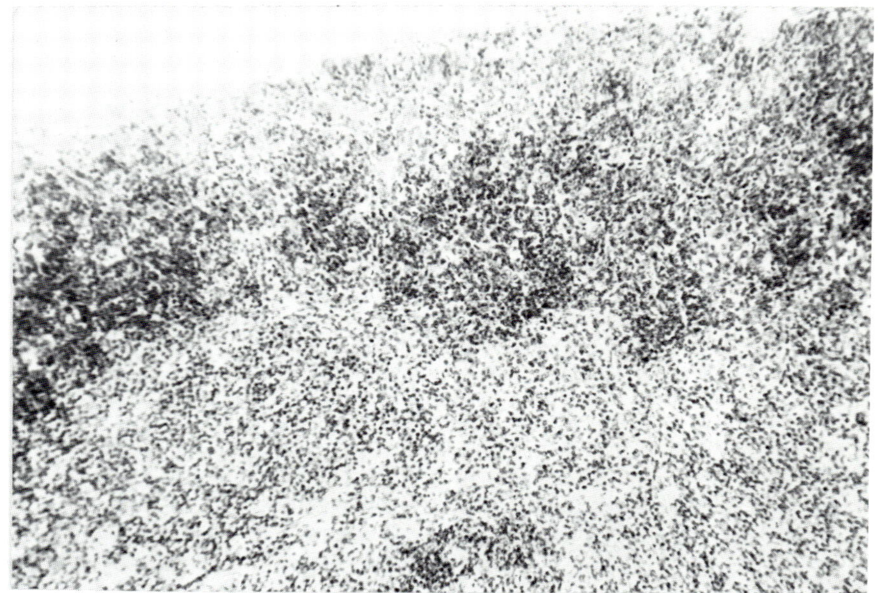

FIG. 12. Thymus of a mouse treated with triethylenemelamine (TEM) for 2 months. Note marked cortical atrophy. H&E; magnification ×150.

features of immunosuppressive agents (are), to prevent cells from proliferating and to kill them."

3. *Antimetabolites*

As indicated before, among antagonists of nucleic acid bases, purine antagonists show marked immunosuppressive effects. Since pyrimidine antagonists are of rather limited practical use as immunosuppressants, we shall focus in this paragraph on the morphological effects of purine antagonists. Among these, 6-mercaptopurine (6-MP) and azathioprine (AZA-T) are of great interest. Treatment with 6-MP of antigenically stimulated animals does not prevent the usual morphological changes in lymphoreticular tissues related to antibody formation. Development of secondary follicles is observed and basophilic reticulum cells appear in the paracortex and plasma cells in the medullary cords (Sahiar and Schwartz, 1966; Miller and Cole, 1967). There are, however, quantitative variations in different animals. Dogs, for instance, appear quite susceptible (Zukosky, 1964). In mice the follicular activation appears less prominent than in man. This effect becomes even more marked when AZA-T instead of 6-MP is used. The acute response of lymphoreticular tissues, especially of the thymus, is characterized by a decrease in the number of small lymphocytes which, however, is much less than after the use of alkylating agents. However, apart from our own experience, other investigations described a severe depletion of lymphocytes and a marked atrophy of lymph nodes draining a renal allograft in AZA-T-treated dogs (Good and Kelly, 1970). Regional and distant lymph nodes from AZA-T-treated, human, renal allotransplant recipients who died within 1 week after transplantation showed only a moderate atrophy and a prominent sinus histiocytosis. The findings are of interest since 6-MP apparently has quite a narrow effectiveness: the suppression of natural antibody production equals zero, the suppression of IgM production remains nearly normal, and the induction of immunological memory is blocked only with large doses of 6-MP (Sahiar and Schwartz, 1966; Schwartz, 1968). Again, as with alkylating agents, it is our impression, that the effectiveness of these drugs on the morphology of lymphoreticular tissues is influenced by the intensity of simultaneous antigenic "background stimulation." Although it was our impression, that chronic antigenic stimulation had a protective effect on AZA-T-treated mice in terms of survival time, Zschiesche (1968) reported earlier deaths and a higher incidence in amyloidosis in mice treated with 6-MP and receiving casein injections; however, this author used 10–20 times larger amounts of antigen than we used in our experiments as well as a different strain of mice. The protective effect of antigens observed by us may be similar to the protective effect of phytohemagglutinin on hemopoiesis in chemotherapeutically treated patients (Israel *et al.*, 1965). Discontinuation of short-term therapy with 6-MP of skin allograft recipients was followed by a rapid activation of lymphoreticular tissues (Laurentaci and Berardi, 1970): a marked proliferation of pyroninophilic reticulum cells was observed in the paracortex of lymph nodes as is usually seen in the development of cellular immunity. Also, secondary follicles increased in number, and many macrophages laden with nuclear debris (germinal center macrophages or tingible body macrophages) indicated a rapid lymphocyte turnover. A similar proliferative response of activated reticulum cells was noted in the peripheral zone of splenic follicles.

Chronic AZA-T administration in long-term experiments and in patients with autoimmune disorders or allotransplants was accompanied by diffuse or focal reticulum cell proliferation in the paracortical region of lymph nodes and in the peripheral zone of splenic follicles. The lymph node cortex in experimental mice appeared narrow and inactive but contained many small lymphocytes; the diameter of the intermediate zone of the splenic

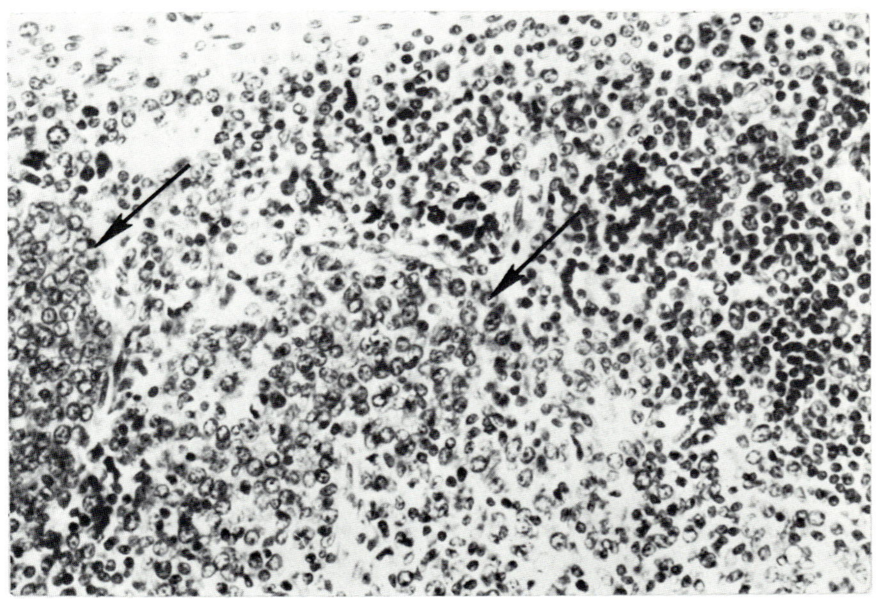

FIG. 13. Thymus of a mouse treated with azathioprine and stimulated with bovine serum albumin for 3 months. Note cortical atrophy and focal aggregates of activated reticulum cells, probably representing early lymphomatous change (arrows). H&E; magnification ×375.

follicle was reduced but also contained small lymphocytes. The thymus was homogeneously atrophic, showing occasional focal reticulum cells in the medulla. These changes became more severe when AZA-T-treated mice were antigenically stimulated at the same time (Krüger, 1970a; Krüger *et al.*, 1971b): paracortical reticulum cell hyperplasia was marked, and 20–60% thymic lymphomas developed in BALB/c and DBA mice. These lymphomas became generalized and finally killed the animal (Figs. 13–16) (Krüger *et al.*, 1971b; Krüger, 1971b). Casey reported a similar high lymphoma incidence in mice with autoimmune disorders and AZA-T treatment (Casey, 1968).

We observed in human kidney and bone marrow allograft recipients that received AZA-T and survived several months, occasional focal reticulum cell proliferates in lymph nodes. These lesions, however, were inconspicious and might easily be overlooked by investigators who are not sensitized by the above-mentioned experimental data. Nevertheless, the incidence of malignant lymphomas in human allograft recipients is 200 times higher than the expected incidence in the average population (McKhann, 1969; Penn and Starzl, 1970). In retrospect, this high incidence may render the focal reticulum cell proliferates highly significant.

Previously it has been demonstrated that, in acute experiments with the pyrimidine antagonists, 5-fluoro-2-deoxyuridine and 5-bis(2-chloroethyl)-aminouracil, the development of pyroninophilic reticulum cells reactive to

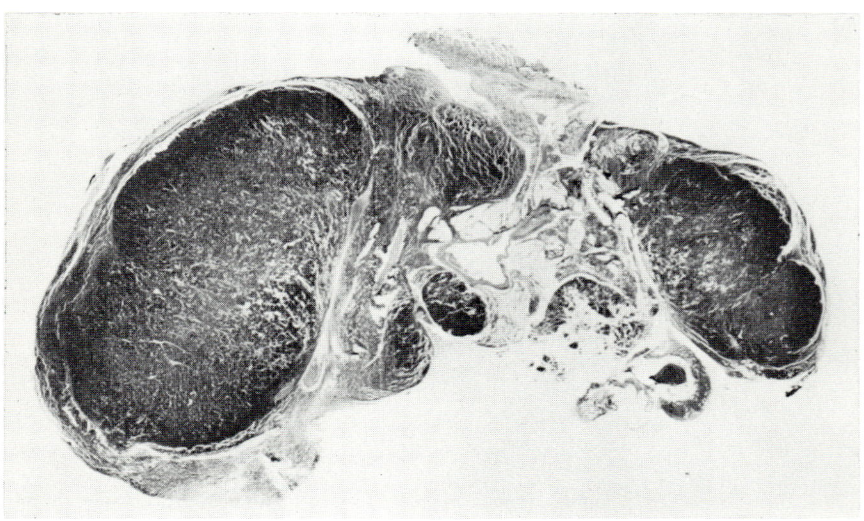

FIG. 14. Thymus of a mouse treated with azathioprine and stimulated with bovine serum albumin for 5 months. Note complete replacement of thymic tissue by lymphoma with extensive invasion of cervical tissues. H&E; magnification ×3.

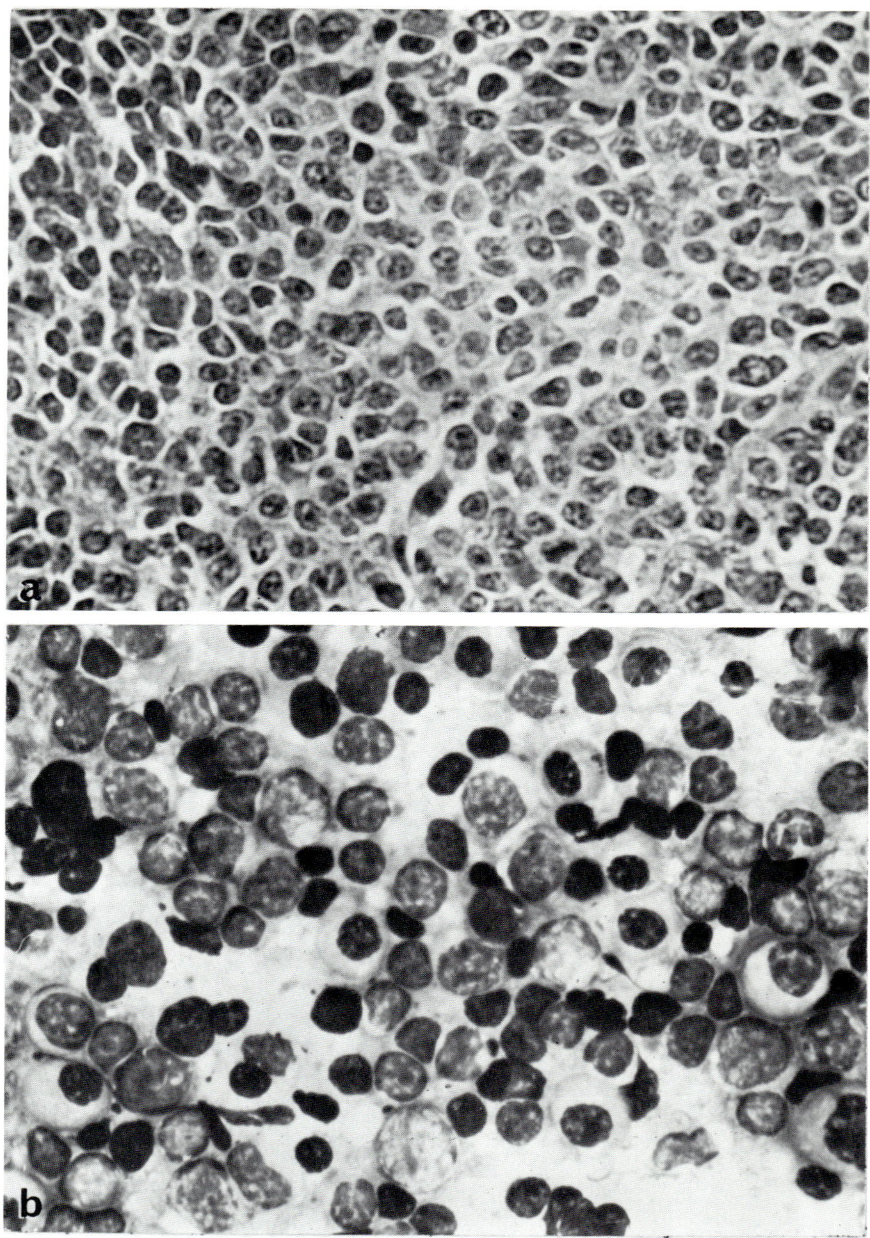

FIG. 15. (a) Cytological detail of the lymphoma shown in Fig. 14. Note dense population of atypical lymphoid cells and reticulum cells. H&E; magnification ×675. (b) Imprint from the lymphoma shown in Fig. 14. Note mixture of lymphoid cells, reticulum cells, and a few plasmacytoid cells. May-Grünwald-Giemsa; magnification ×1500.

antigenic stimulation is not inhibited by these drugs (Johnson *et al.*, 1966). 9-β-D-Arabinofuranosylcytosine apparently acts on proliferating pyroninophilic reticulum cells and leads to a marked depression in antibody formation in terms of decrease in plaque-forming cells and to a depression of the graft-vs.-host reaction (Gray *et al.*, 1968a,b). Another group of antimetabolites, the folic acid antagonists, aminopterin (methotrexate, MTX) and amethopterin, induce morphological changes in lymphoreticular tissues that are quite similar to the ones described following the use of purine antagonists (Krüger, 1970c; Laurentaci and Berardi, 1970). In experimental mice, the atrophy of lymphoreticular tissues is only moderate after MTX treatment (3 mg/kg/day). With increasing length of the experiment, the number of small lymphocytes is slightly reduced in lymph node cortices and splenic follicles. The thymus, however, shows a moderate to marked homogeneous atrophy. Different from the usual effect of alkylating agents is a marked stimulation of hemopoiesis in the red pulp of the spleen with prevalence of immature stem cells and many megakaryocytes (Fig. 17).

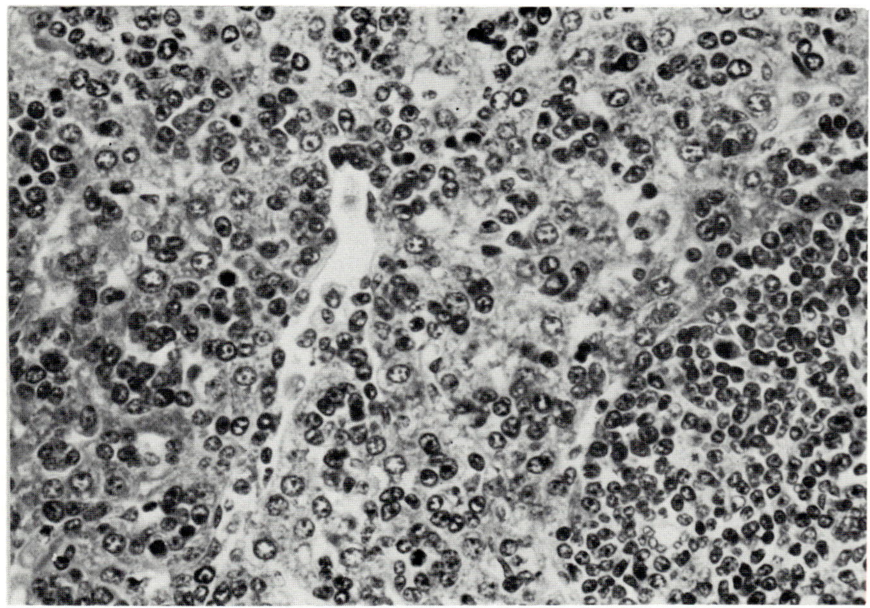

FIG. 16. Liver of a mouse treated with azathioprine and stimulated with bovine serum albumin for 5 months. Note dense nodular and sinusoidal infiltration by lymphoma cells. H&E; magnification ×375.

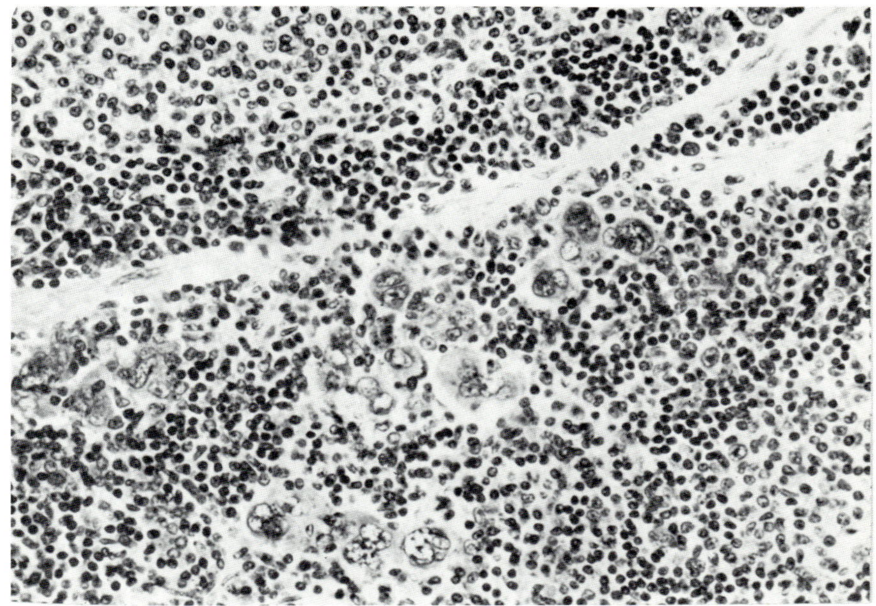

FIG. 17. Spleen of a mouse treated with methotrexate for 3 months. Note increase in hemopoiesis and in megakaryocytes in red pulp. H&E; magnification ×275.

This effect corresponds to findings in mice on a folic acid-free diet (Dunn, 1969), and probably also to the enhancing effect of MTX on the vaccine-induced leukemoid reaction in mice (Cooney *et al.*, 1965). Also, there is a marked hypertrophy of the paracortical zone of lymph nodes in chronically MTX-treated mice, yet cellular atypia in this region is less prominent than in mice receiving alkylating agents. No lymphoma development has yet been reported in experimental animals on MTX treatment, and our own experiments that were undertaken with the intention of inducing lymphomas have been negative so far.

4. *Antibiotics*

Many antibiotics including streptomycin, chloramphenicol, neomycin, and the tetracyclines act on a subcellular level by blocking the synthesis of rRNA and tRNA (Siebert, 1968), and this may interfere nonspecificly with the synthesis of antibody protein. No overt changes in lymphoreticular tissues of unstimulated animals which correlate with clinical symptoms of immune deficiency are known after use of these drugs. However, a marked

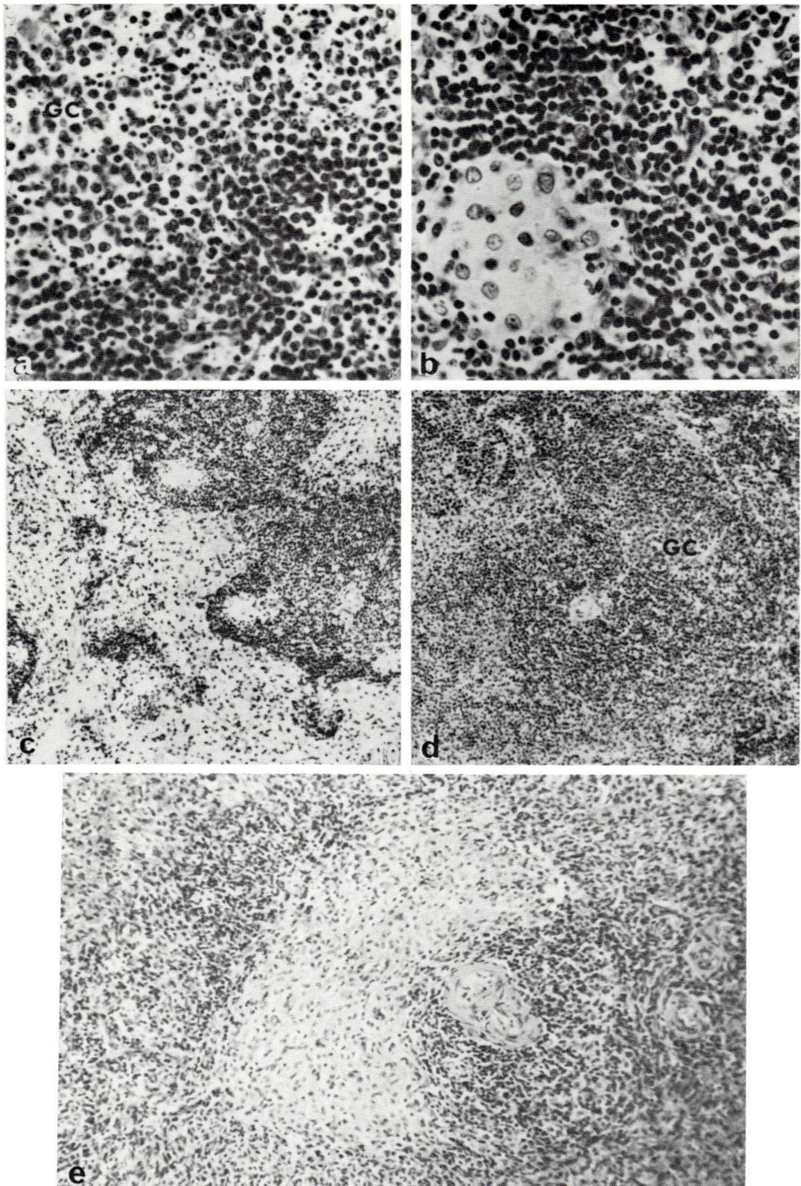

FIG. 18. (a–d) Lymphatic nodules of mice treated with actinomycin D (12 mg/mouse) and stimulated with sheep erythrocytes. (a) Note karyopyknosis of lymphoid cells and phagocytosis of nuclear debris in secondary follicle (GC) 6 hours after antigen

reactive formation of secondary follicles in antigenically stimulated animals, following the discontinuation of chloramphenicol treatment, suggests that this reaction had been inhibited during treatment. This assumption has been further substantiated by Hurlimann and co-workers (Hurlimann *et al.*, 1966) who found the number of secondary follicles decreased and their development delayed when antigenically stimulated animals were treated with chloramphenicol.

Actinomycin D depresses the activity of macrophages as evidenced by a decrease in pinocytosis, i.e., uptake of fluid droplets and materials in suspension (Roos, 1970); this may be recognized by phase-contrast microscopy. The number of phagocytes itself is not decreased. Cells in culture when treated with actinomycin D become swollen and contain increased numbers of mitochondria (Deitch and Goodman, 1967). Actinomycin also inhibits the increase in weight of lymphoreticular tissues after antigenic stimulation (Geller and Speirs, 1968; Hackmann, 1954). Secondary follicles in actinomycin-treated and antigenically stimulated mice are decreased in number and size, but the size of inactive primary follicles is not affected (Hanna and Wust, 1965). It has been suggested that actinomycin has a direct cytotoxic effect on pyroninophilic reticulum cells in the secondary follicle (Hanna and Wust, 1964) and, consequently, increased numbers of phagocytes containing nuclear debris, indicative of rapid lymphoid cell turnover, become visible. Secondary follicles which have already developed in the spleen became depleted of pyroninophilic cells and finally consisted entirely of a residual reticular stroma surrounded by small lymphocytes (Fig. 18a–e). From day 3 on, after actinomycin has been discontinued, recovery of lymphoreticular tissues takes place following a somewhat biphasic pattern: an increase in lymphocytes of the primary follicle accompanied by marked mitotic activity is followed by reconstruction of the secondary follicle caused by aggregation of large pyroninophilic reticulum cells (Hanna and Wust, 1964, 1965). The reappearance of secondary follicles is succeeded in a 5–7 day interval by a myeloid and erythroid hyperplasia in the splenic red pulp and by plasmacytosis of medullary cords of lymph nodes.

---

administration. H&E; magnification ×320. (b) Note reticular remnant of secondary follicle 2 days after antigen administration. H&E; magnification ×320. (c) Note homogeneous atrophy and reticular remnants of secondary follicles. H&E; magnification ×80. (d) Note reactive secondary follicles (GC) 14 days after antigen administration. H&E; magnification ×80. (e) Spleen of a mouse treated with actinomycin D (10 mg/day) for 1 month. Note atrophy of lymphatic nodule and reticular remnant of secondary follicle. H&E; magnification ×120. (Micrographs a–d were kindly supplied by Dr. M. G. Hanna, Biology Division, Oak Ridge National Laboratory, Tennessee.)

The acute response to actinomycin treatment of the thymus consists in a marked karyorhexis of lymphocytes and atrophy of the organ.

Electron microscopically, the cells of the reticular remnant of secondary follicles in actinomycin-treated animals show large nuclei with loosely organized or peripherally clumped chromatin; the cytoplasm contains large swollen mitochondria and numerous smooth-surfaced vesicles. A marked infolding of the plasma membrane of these reticulum cells is noted with extensive interdigitations of elongated cytoplasmic protrusions (Schwartzendruber, 1966). In addition, there is vacuolization of atypical lymphocytes.

Mitomycin C, another known immunosuppressant, has no uniform effect on lymphoreticular tissues. Although lymph nodes and spleen of dogs and rhesus monkeys show karyorhexis and depletion of small lymphocytes in the cortex and follicles in acute experiments, lymphoreticular tissues in rats are not overtly affected except for the thymus (Philips *et al.*, 1960). It has been suggested that the RNA synthesis of cells can be inhibited by mitomycin without interfering with their viability (Bloom *et al.*, 1964). This may account for the unimpressive morphological effect on lymphoid tissues in rats. Hemopoietic cells, however, which also rapidly synthesize nucleic acids, have been markedly reduced in number in all animals investigated (rats, cats, dogs, and monkeys). Since the mechanism of action of mitomycin C is similar to that of alkylating agents and since a variety of late effects after long-term treatment with alkylating agents has been described, it may be worthwhile to search in the future also for morphological late effects after mitomycin therapy. This is reasonable, especially since atrophy of the thymus is uniformly observed after mitomycin administration; this organ has a limited ability to recover even in animals with lifelong thymic persistency (Borum, 1969), yet its function apparently is necessary for the control of cellular immunity. This mechanism may be different in species without a persistent thymus, as for instance, man. Here it is reasonable to assume that the thymic-dependent part of lymphoreticular tissues, once completely destroyed, is unable to recover.

Long-term administration of mitomycin C to rats has led to the induction of malignant neoplasms in 34% of the animals (Schmähl, 1970). Puromycin markedly diminished splenic plaque-forming cells (Thiel *et al.*, 1967), an effect that apparently is secondary to polyribosomal disaggregation, as shown by electron microscopy of liver cells (Reid *et al.*, 1970).

The administration of daunomycin is limited by undesirable toxic side effects (see below); therefore, no information about morphological lesions after long-term treatment with this drug is available. Short-term administration, even with low doses of daunomycin, is followed by degeneration of lymphocytes and basophilic reticulum cells and by an inhibition of lymphocyte transformation in culture (Fig. 19) (Massimo, 1970; Costa and Astaldi, 1964). The cytoplasm of these cells becomes less basophilic and vacuolated, and the nuclei undergo chromatinolysis and rhexis. Small fluorescent endoplasmatic granules in these cells may represent the accumulation of daunomycin that is readily picked up by lymphoreticular tissues (Massimo, 1970; Rusconi *et al.*, 1968).

Bleomycin, despite its interference with cell division (Fujita and Kimura, 1970) and its DNA-binding activity (Ichikawa *et al.*, 1967), has no obvious effects on the immune response (Yamaki *et al.*, 1969). With high-dose levels, especially when given intravenously, bleomycin was found in splenic tissue, and this organ showed variable degenerative and hypertrophic regenerative changes (Ichikawa *et al.*, 1967; Ishizuka *et al.*, 1967). Lymphoreticular tissues from our human case material with combined chemotherapeutic regimens including bleomycin did not reveal any lesions specifically attributable to this drug. In general, an advanced homogeneous atrophy of lymph nodes and spleen was noted. In experimental dogs, low and intermediate doses of bleomycin (0.625–1.25 mg/kg/day) led to a

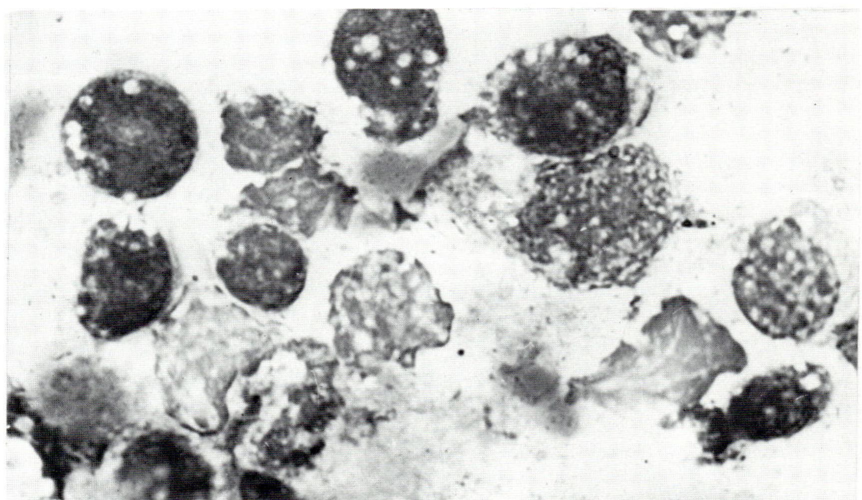

FIG. 19. Lymphocyte culture from a patient treated with daunomycin. Note numerous enlarged and degenerating cells. May-Grünwald-Giemsa; magnification about ×1700. (Micograph kindly supplied by Professor L. Massimo, Clin. Pediat. G. Gaslini, Genoa, Italy.)

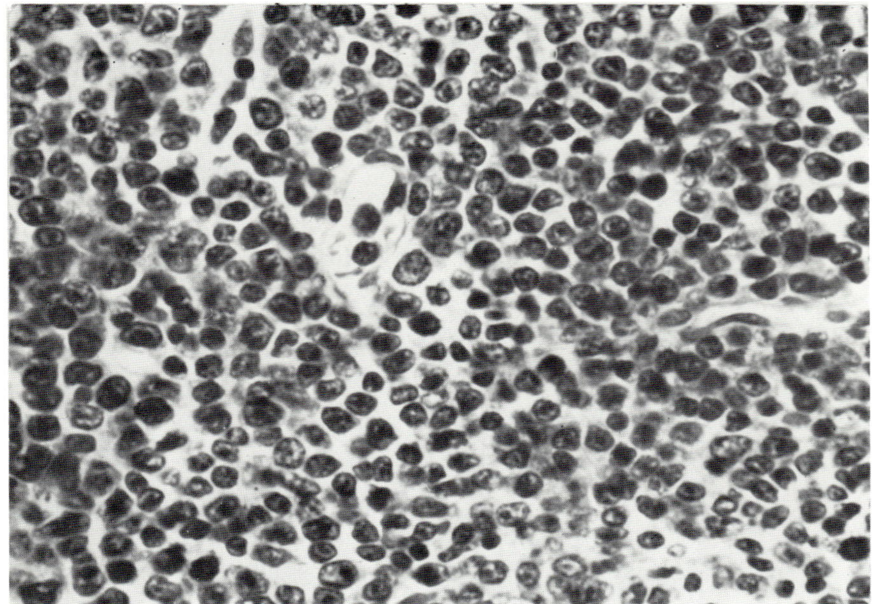

FIG. 20. Lymph node of a dog treated with intermediate doses of bleomycin. Note marked increase in immature lymphocytes in paracortex. H&E; magnification ×675.

marked stimulation of the paracortical region of lymph nodes (Fig. 20); larger doses (5 mg/kg/day) but produced a complete acute atrophy of this area.

Neocarzinostatin, when administered to mice in a short-term experiment, produces marked atrophy of lymph nodes, thymus, and spleen. Histologically, cortex and paracortex of lymph nodes as well as splenic follicles are depleted of small lymphocytes. The reticular stroma of lymph nodes and red pulp of the spleen appears "condensed" (Bradner and Hutchison, 1966). Concomitant with these lesions is a pronounced blood lymphocytopenia.

5. *Enzymes*

Besides its effectiveness on malignant lymphoma, L-asparaginase also interferes with the metabolism of normal lymphoreticular tissues (Grundmann, 1970a,b). This may arise from the fact that these tissues are sensitive to deprivation of L-asparagine. Injection of rabbits with L-asparaginase, interestingly enough, did not influence the formation of secondary follicles nor the plasma cell response in the spleen during a short-term experiment (Astaldi *et al.*, 1970; Micu *et al.*, 1970); there was, however, a decrease in number in small lymphocytes which was interpreted as correlating with a depression in cellular immunity. Hobik, in fact, did show a depression by L-asparaginase of cellular immune responses in terms of an inhibition of graft-vs.-host reaction (Hobik, 1969a,b). *In vitro* tests for lymphocytotoxicity of L-asparaginase have further proved the toxic effect of this drug; however, malignant lymphocytes were obviously more sensitive to L-asparaginase than were normal lymphocytes (Dolowy and Ameraal, 1967). The inhibition of blastic transformation of lymphocytes by L-asparaginase was mentioned earlier (Eridani *et al.*, 1970; Astaldi *et al.*, 1969a); this may relate to interference by this compound on the preparatory phase of immunocompetent cells for antibody synthesis. In addition to using L-asparaginase for interference with the aspartic acid metabolism of lymphoid cells, it has also been suggested that L-aspartic acid analogs may be used (Hirano *et al.*, 1970). Some of the compounds tested have shown antitumor activity, and they may well be immunosuppressants also, since their morphological effects include thymic cortical atrophy and atrophy of the splenic white pulp, secondary to depletion of small lymphocytes.

The immunosuppressive action of RNase has been demonstrated by several investigators (Mowbray, 1967; Mowbray *et al.*, 1969; Davis *et al.*, 1969); both cellular and humoral immune responses were affected. Other investigators, however, even when they used quite sensitive methods were unable to demonstrate any immunosuppressive effects of this enzyme (Chakrabarty and Friedman, 1970; Pullar *et al.*, 1968). Blast formation of lymphocytes *in vitro* was inhibited by RNase (Mowbray *et al.*, 1969), and cells that were already transformed when the enzyme was added, died. This probably also applies to lymphoid cells *in vivo* which were activated (transformed) by antigenic stimulation. After removal of RNase, small lymphocytes retain their ability for transformation completely.

We tested the effect of RNase on the lymphoreticular tissue in mice (Krüger and Yun, unpublished data) and observed at dose levels of 5 mg/mouse/day (crude bovine pancreatic RNase) a moderate-to-marked diminution of small lymphocytes in the cortex and paracortex of lymph nodes; this was accompanied by a marked nuclear pyknosis of lymphocytes and medullary plasma cells. Occasional atypical enlarged lymphoid cells were noted as well as many large histiocytes with water-clear cytoplasm (Fig. 21). In mice that were stimulated with an antigenic while under RNase treatment, the lesions were essentially the same. Secondary follicles, however, were less prominent and contained multiple pyknotic cells and debris-laden macrophages.

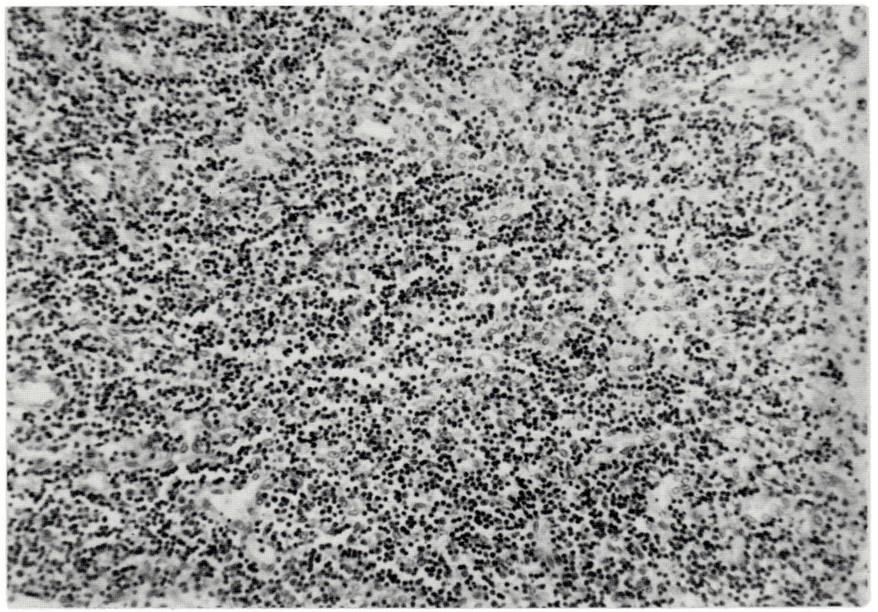

FIG. 21. Lymph node of a mouse treated for 1 month with ribonuclease. Note moderate homogeneous atrophy and sinus histiocytosis. H&E; magnification ×150.

6. *Mitosis Inhibitors*

In general, not much is known about morphological effects of mitotic inhibitors on lymphoreticular tissues. It appears that primarily cell proliferation is blocked. The transformation of small lymphocytes to blast cells, however, is not inhibited, as shown after treatment with colchicine (Astaldi *et al.*, 1967). When administered during the proliferative phase of immunoresponsive cells stimulated by an antigen, colchicine has an inhibitory effect on the formation of secondary follicles (Hurlimann *et al.*, 1967). Similar morphological lesions may also be expected after administration of colchicine derivatives, such as demecolcine, and of podophyllin derivatives. Trowell (1966) described the immediate toxic effect of mitotic poisons on lymphocytes as "radiomimetic" and compared these drugs with X-rays and corticosteroids. Lymphocytes showed early condensation of the cytoplasm with increase in ribosomes, membrane-associated cytoplasmic vacuoles, and disruption of the nuclear membrane. Subsequently, cellular disintegration occurred with the appearance of "naked" nuclei.

The group of mitotic poisons in most common use today is represented by *Vinca rosea* alkaloids. Like other mitotic inhibitors, these compounds (vinblastine and vincristine) act primarily on cells entering division and cause irreversible disruption of the spindle apparatus with consequent aberrant metaphases (Journey *et al.*, 1968). No lesions have been observed in interphase cells at the light microscopic level except for "ruffling" of cellular membranes.

7. *Polyanions*

Although a fair number of publications are available on the effects of polyanions, no detailed descriptions exist of their morphological effects on tissues. Several substances in this group of compounds have antimitotic activity (Regelson, 1968a,b) and, supposedly, may interfere with the germinal center formation and proliferation of basophilic reticulum cells (immunoblasts) in lymphoreticular tissues. Others stimulate the reticuloendothelial system or may block its function. Cytoplasmic granular inclusions were described in a variety of cells including hemo- and lympho-

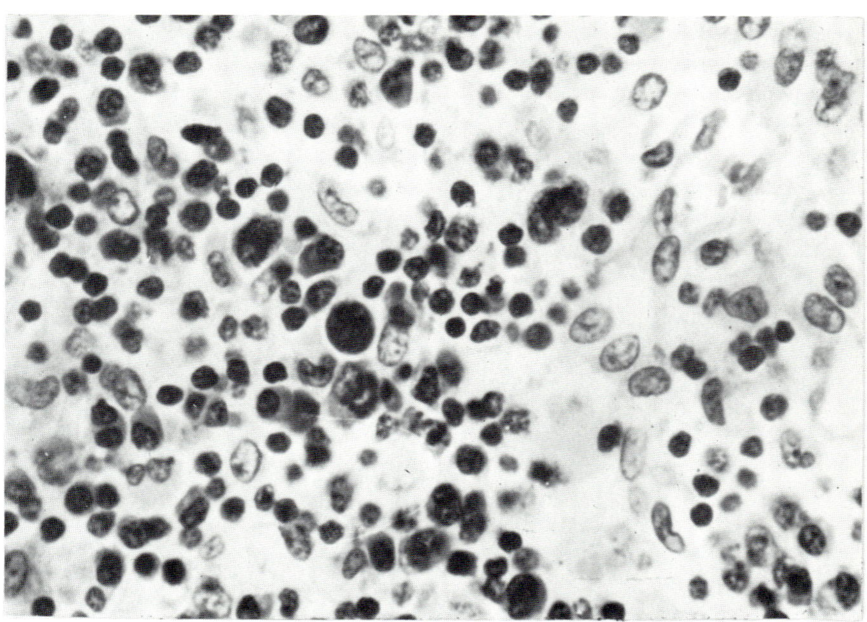

FIG. 22. Lymph node of a patient treated with poly I:C for systemic lupus erythematosus. Note atypical enlarged lymphoid cells with marked nuclear hyperchromasia. H&E; magnification ×675.

reticular cells when pyran copolymers were given (Regelson, 1968a,b). Despite the possible antimitotic activity and despite the effect on lymphoid cell lines, the polyanion, poly I:C, is not able to suppress cell proliferation in lymphoreticular tissues absolutely, as is clearly shown by its failure to inhibit "spontaneous" leukemia development in mice (Meier *et al.*, 1970a,b).

In reviewing our own case material of patients who came to autopsy after combination therapy including poly I:C for autoimmune diseases (lupus erythematosus) or cancer, the usual advanced depletion of lymphoid cells was noted in lymphoreticular tissues, but no changes were seen that may have been specific for the action of poly I:C. There was, however, a regular occurrence of lymphoid cells with enlarged nuclei (Fig. 22).

8. *Miscellaneous Substances*

Methylhydrazine derivatives as, for instance, procarbazine are immunosuppressive (Bollag, 1963; Amiel *et al.*, 1964a) and have a lymphocytopenic effect in certain experimental animals. This was interpreted as secondary to an inhibition of lymphopoiesis (Schmähl, 1970). Histologically a mild-to-moderate depletion from small lymphocytes of lymphoreticular tissues is noted accompanied by a sinus histiocytosis secondary to iron deposition from hemolysis.

Drugs BCNU and CCNU [1-(2-chloroethyl)-3-cyclohexyl-1-nitrosourea] cause a severe generalized atrophy of lymphoreticular tissues. The atrophy is initiated by a depletion from small lymphocytes of tissue affecting initially lymph node and splenic follicles. This extends to the entire lymphoreticular tissue components and is accompanied often by focal hemorrhages.

C. Tissue Site of Antigen–Antibody Reactions

1. *Normal Morphology*

In this section we describe the metamorphosis of the immune reaction which develops at the target site of antibodies or immune lymphocytes. This site usually is represented by the antigen itself and varies with the type of antigen. The following may serve as examples: the intracutaneous tubercle protein pool in a tuberculin test, the graft in a transplant rejection, the skin in a graft-vs.-host reaction, and the thyroid in Hashimoto's autoimmune thyroiditis. The general pathology of an immune reaction has been extensively described (Letterer, 1967; Wiener, 1970; Krüger *et al.*, 1971a; Feldman, 1964; Porter *et al.*, 1965; Grundmann, 1970a), and will not be repeated in detail here. In essence, immediate hypersensitivity reactions

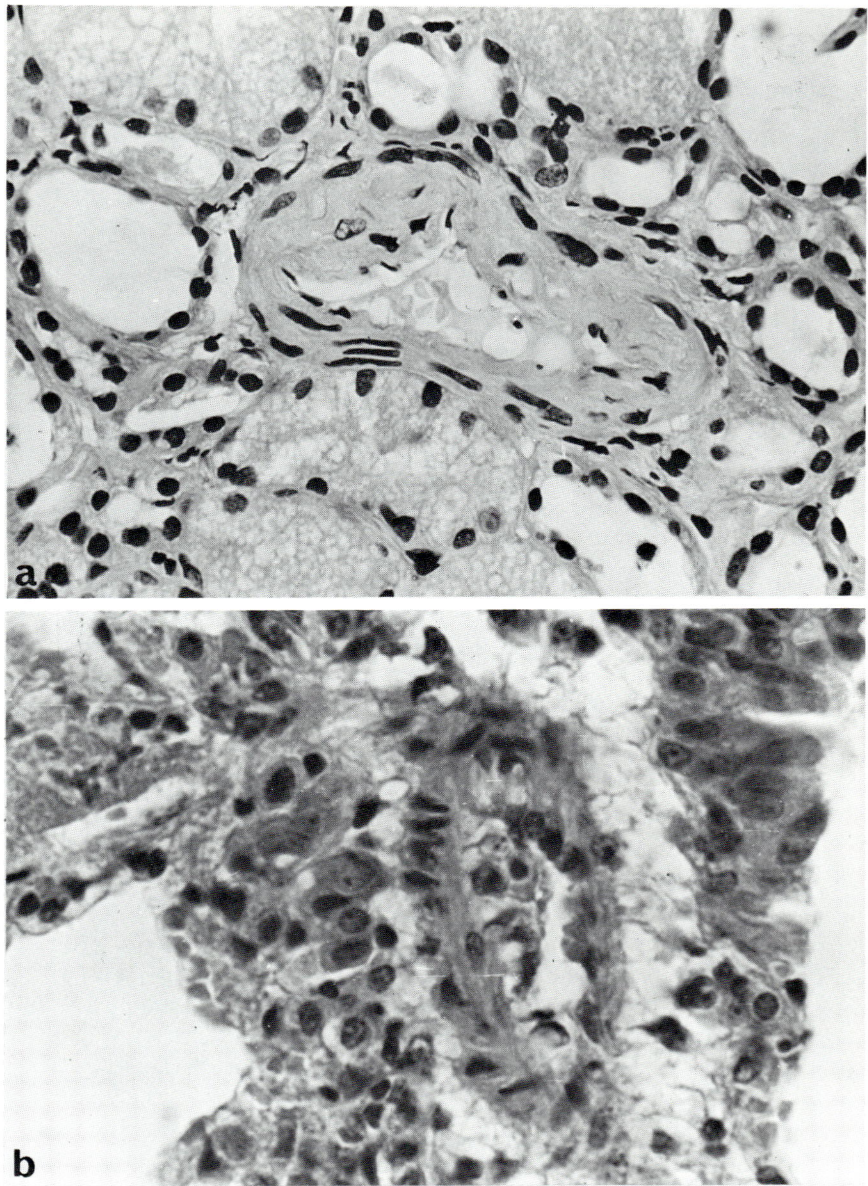

FIG. 23. (a) Human kidney allotransplant 6 days after transplantation. Note fibrinoid necrosis of a small artery. H&E; magnification ×680. (b) Lung of a mouse that died of shock after repeated administration of foreign serum. Note marked swelling of vascular endothelial cells, contraction of the vessel wall (lining-up of nuclei), and perivascular edema. H&E; magnification ×675.

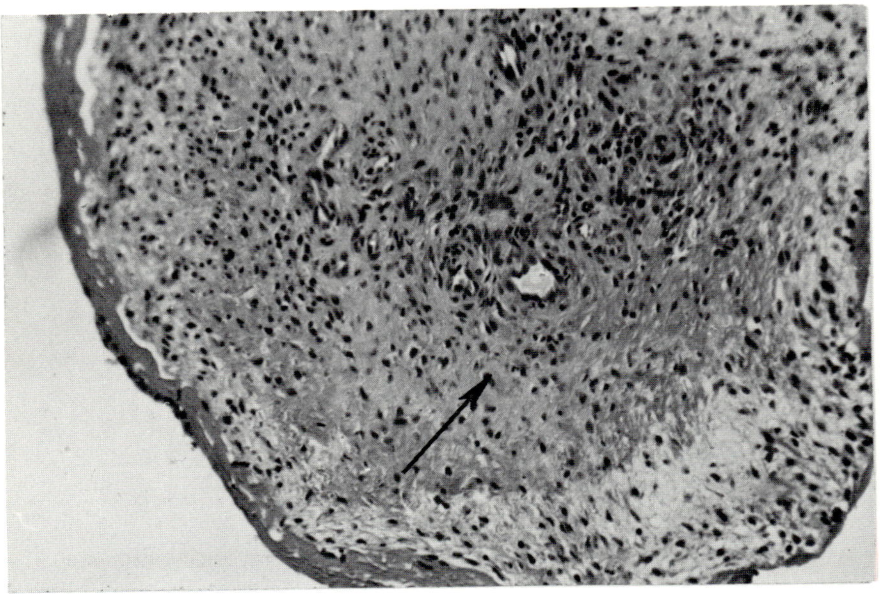

FIG. 24. Synovial villus of a patient with rheumatoid arthritis in acute exacerbation. Note perivascular insudation of the stroma (arrow) with focal fibrinoid necrosis and superficial fibrinoid necrosis. H&E; magnification ×150.

caused by circulating antibodies must be differentiated from delayed hypersensitivity reactions that are caused by immune lymphocytes. Under natural conditions, both reactions often occur more or less in combination, and suppression of one may enhance the other (Krüger and Harris, 1970; Parish, 1971). Both the immediate and the delayed hypersensitivity reaction *in vivo* are represented by a compound reaction of the *histion*, i.e., the unit of vessel and perivascular tissue. It includes nerves and, depending on its location, also parenchymal cells (liver, thyroid, pancreas, testes) and differentiated mesenchymal elements, such as muscle cells. The morphogenesis of the immediate hypersensitivity reaction of the histion is induced by immediate effects of antigen–antibody complexes themselves and in combination with complement and mediator substances such as histamine and serotonin. The morphological appearances in the vascular periphery during an immediate reaction, as in the Arthus phenomenon or the passive cutaneous anaphlyaxis, are composed of primary and secondary lesions. Primary lesions include swelling of vascular endothelial cells, thickening of the vascular basement membrane with deposition of immunoprecipitates between capillary endotheliai cells and basement membrane, contraction of smooth muscle causing narrowing of the vascular lumen, and folding of the basement membrane. In addition, hyaline (platelet) thrombi may be noted in the vessel lumen and eosinophilic homogenization of the vessel wall (Fig. 23a and b). Secondary lesions include perivascular edema, hemorrhage, fibrinous insudation, and necrosis (Fig. 24). Connective tissue elements show swelling and decollagenization of collagen fibers and swelling and rupture of reticulin fibers; cells show swelling and varying degrees of degeneration. In the further course of the reaction, leukocyte emigration, phagocytosis, and reparative fibroplasia occur, as in every other lesion. The extent of the entire reaction is influenced by the amount and "strength" of antigen and antibody as well as by nonspecific neural and hormonal influences. Variations may be caused by the route of entrance of the antigen. For instance, in bronchial asthma the antigen enters through the airways and in contact dermatitis it gains access through the skin.

The delayed hypersensitivity reaction of the histion is characterized by emigration of cells from capillaries without gross lesions of the vessel itself.

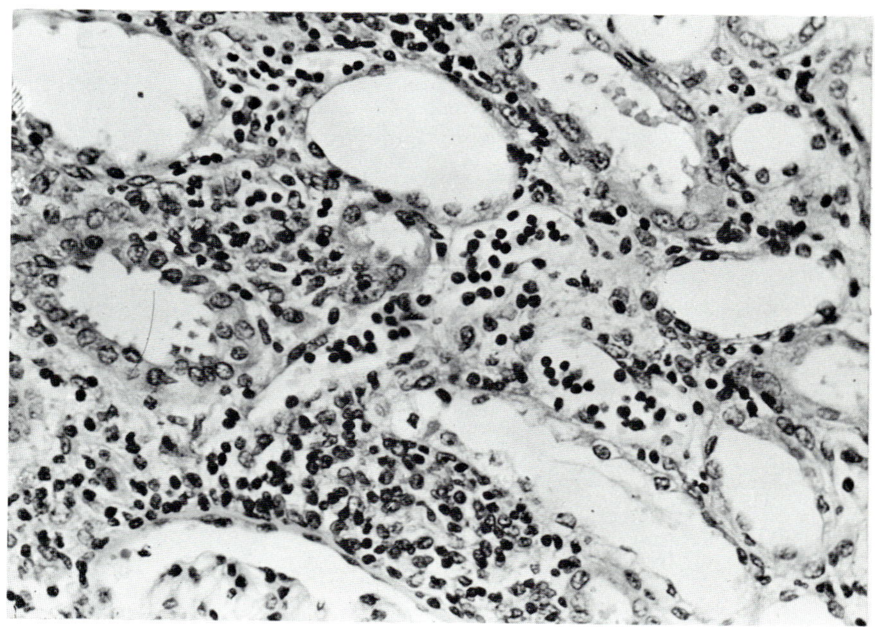

FIG. 25. Human kidney allotransplant 6 days after transplantation. Note the infiltration of the interstitial tissue by lymphocytes derived from peritubular capillaries. H&E; magnification ×275.

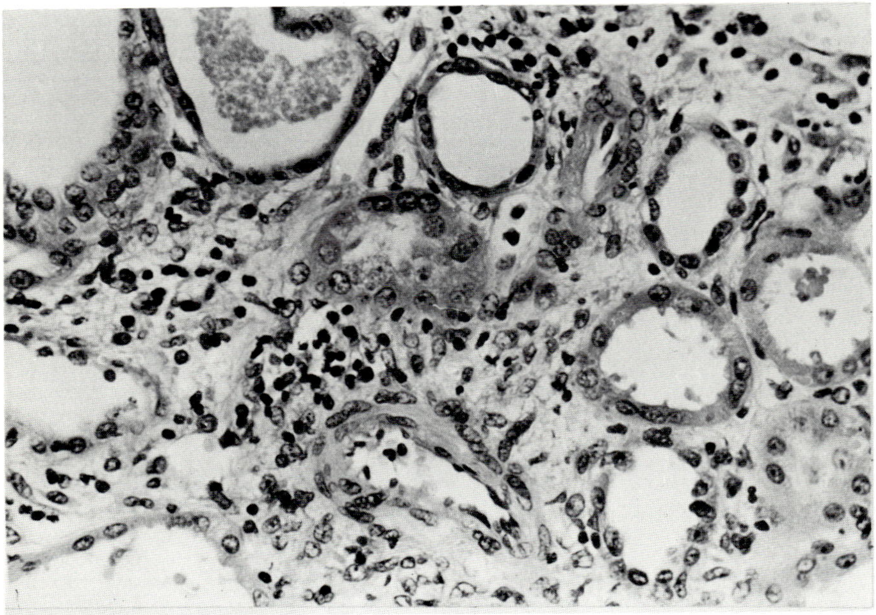

FIG. 26. Human kidney allograft 3 weeks after transplantation and treatment with azathioprine. Note reduction in small lymphocytes in interstitial tissue and increase in local mesenchymal cells. H&E; magnification ×275.

Within the first 3 hours after repeated antigenic stimulation, granulocytes outnumber mononuclear cells in the local perivascular infiltrate. The number of lymphocytes increases progressively after about 6 hours (Fig. 25). The extent of the early granulocytic infiltrate depends upon the mass and the strength of the antigen administered at the test site. Cell identification studies by use of cell markers suggest a progressive participation of local mesenchymal cells with increasing chronicity of the reaction. Morphologically, the mononuclear cells of the early phase resemble those of the chronic phase; however, histiocytic cell types dominate the late phase and the number of lymphocytes decreases (Fig. 26). This late phase in delayed hypersensitivity reactions, as in the immediate reaction, represents probably a nonspecific secondary phase of resorption and repair. Repair finally is characterized by fibrosis.

2. *Morphology under Immunosuppression*

Information about the metamorphosis by immunosuppression of the peripheral immune reaction is available from experimental and clinical studies of infections, transplantation, and autoimmune disease. Despite the large number and variety of drugs with immunosuppressive potentials as described, only a few of these are in practical use as immunosuppressants. All other compounds serve largely as cancer chemotherapeutic agents, and the morphological evaluation of the peripheral immune response in cancer patients as effected by these drugs is difficult, since the neoplastic process itself usually changes the immunological reactivity of the patient. This group of patients, therefore, will not be included in the present discussion.

Among hormones used for immunosuppression, glucocorticosteroids have been used for years as anti-inflammatory drugs. Despite their lymphocytotoxic effect as described, the anti-inflammatory potential of corticosteroids probably represents the main immunosuppressive mechanism. Cortisone inhibits the increase in vascular permeability following an antigen–antibody reaction. Therefore, edema, hemorrhage, and cell emigration is decreased in acute hypersensitivity reactions (Scheiffarth and Zicha, 1967; Derbes *et al.*, 1950; Gell and Hinde, 1951; Vollmer, 1951; Harris and Harris, 1950). Also, the secondary lesion initiating repair in immediate and delayed reactions is inhibited by cortisone and derivatives so that proliferation of capillaries and fibroblasts is reduced. Besides, corticosteroids probably interfere with the mobility of histiocytes, decrease phagocytosis (Spain *et al.*, 1950; Heller, 1955; Furness, 1959; Meier and Ecklin, 1960), and diminish the digestive efficiency of phagocytes (Forshter, 1951).

Similar to glucocorticosteroids, estrogens inhibit the acute immunologically induced inflammation (Müller-Beissenhirtz *et al.*, 1971). Also these compounds apparently decrease the vascular permeability so that edema and cell emigration are diminished.

In contrast, when synthetic progesterone derivatives are administered to kidney allograft recipients, these compounds do not inhibit the morphological development of a graft rejection—the graft is grossly swollen secondary to edema and hemorrhage, and mononuclear and polymorphonuclear cell infiltrates are seen as in untreated control animals (Turcotte *et al.*, 1968), but the survival time of the graft was significantly prolonged. When the progesterone derivative is administered, however, in combination with azathioprine, the graft rejection signs are markedly diminished, and the survival time of the graft on the average is 3 times as long as the survival time in animals treated with azathioprine only. It is suggested that progesterone acts on lymphoreticular tissues directly, leading to a decrease in circulating lymphocytes (Turcotte *et al.*, 1968).

Of all members in this group of compounds, cyclophosphamide is the alkylating agent probably in most common use for immunosuppression.

Consequently, it may serve as an indicator for possible effects of alkylating agents on the peripheral immune response.

In animal experiments using guinea pigs and rats infected with *Mycobacterium tuberculosis* or *Brucella abortus* or *Brucella melitensis* (Ullmann, 1969; Stender *et al.*, 1963; Potel and Brock, 1965; Potel, 1965) and treated with cyclophosphamide, a marked depression of the specific antibody to these organisms has been demonstrated. This immunosuppression was paralleled by a leukopenia and decrease of the usual plasma cell response during antibody formation, and cell proliferation was significantly decreased. The size of the tuberculous granuloma at the initial injection site was decreased and did not show the central granulocytic infiltrate with liquefaction as noted in guinea pigs not treated with cyclophosphamide. Accordingly, the number of acid-fast organisms counted in these lesions was initially larger in treated animals than in untreated ones, suggesting that the phagocytosis and digestion of these organisms was delayed. Dissemination of mycobacteria consequently occurred earlier and more

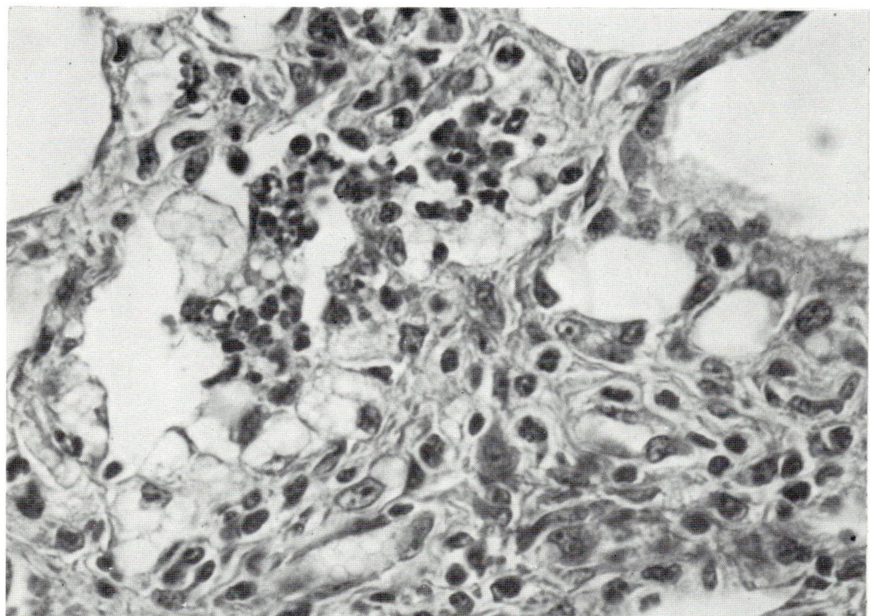

FIG. 27. Site of injection with tubercle bacteria in adjuvant of a mouse sensitized by tubercle bacteria and treated with azathioprine. Note absence of the usual lymphocyte response of chemically untreated animals, and replacement by granulocytes and atypical large mesenchymal cells. H&E; magnification ×675.

extensively in cyclophosphamide-treated animals than in untreated controls (Ullmann, 1969). Related to these findings is the assumption of Folb and Trounce (1970) that cellular immunity is primarily impaired in cyclophosphamide-treated patients. This is further supported by the suppression of the morphogenesis of tuberculin tests and contact hypersensitivity reactions by cyclophosphamide in guinea pigs (Maguire and Maibach, 1961; Turk, 1964b). However, cyclophosphamide must be given simultaneously with the sensitizing antigen in order to suppress the immune reaction; an already established hypersensitivity is not adequately suppressed.

Azathioprine and methotrexate are members of the group of antimetabolites which are the most widely used immunosuppressive agents for the treatment of allograft rejection and graft-vs.-host reaction. We studied the influence of both drugs in experimental animals and in human patients with antigenic stimulation, using several different antigens (Krüger, 1971b; Krüger *et al.*, 1971b; Krüger, 1970a), and in kidney and bone marrow allotransplantation (Krüger *et al.*, 1971a; Masshoff and Krüger, 1968). Administration of azathioprine markedly decreased the number of small lymphocytes in the delayed hypersensitivity reaction, as noted from the tuberculin footpad test of sensitized mice. Granulocytes usually replaced lymphocytes in the test injection site of azathioprine-treated mice (Fig. 27). A nonspecific local reaction consisting of swelling of mesenchymal cells, edema, and focal necroses was observed, in addition. This morphological pattern is not indicative of delayed hypersensitivity. It correlates well with the reduction in small lymphocytes at the site of the sensitizing antigen injection.

In kidney allotransplant recipients treated with azathioprine the early lymphohistiocytic response was not markedly diminished. The effect of azathioprine treatment, therefore, was augmented by adding prednisone and actinomycin C. During later stages, however, lymphocytes were markedly reduced in number in the graft; instead, a stationary reticulohistiocytic interstitial infiltrate was noted together with marked inflammatory and degenerative lesions of medium-sized and larger vessels. Bone marrow allograft recipients on methotrexate treatment showed less frequently the morphological changes of acute lethal graft-vs.-host reaction (Krüger *et al.*, 1971a,d) instead, the numbers of lymphocytes and immunoblasts invading epidermis, liver parenchyma, and intestinal mucosa were often decreased to an extent that the diagnosis of graft-vs.-host reaction was rendered quite difficult (Figs. 28 and 29).

These observations are in keeping with findings of other investigations in human and dog kidney allografts and azathioprine treatment (Porter, 1967; Porter *et al.*, 1965; Dammin, 1966). Also in these cases, despite the

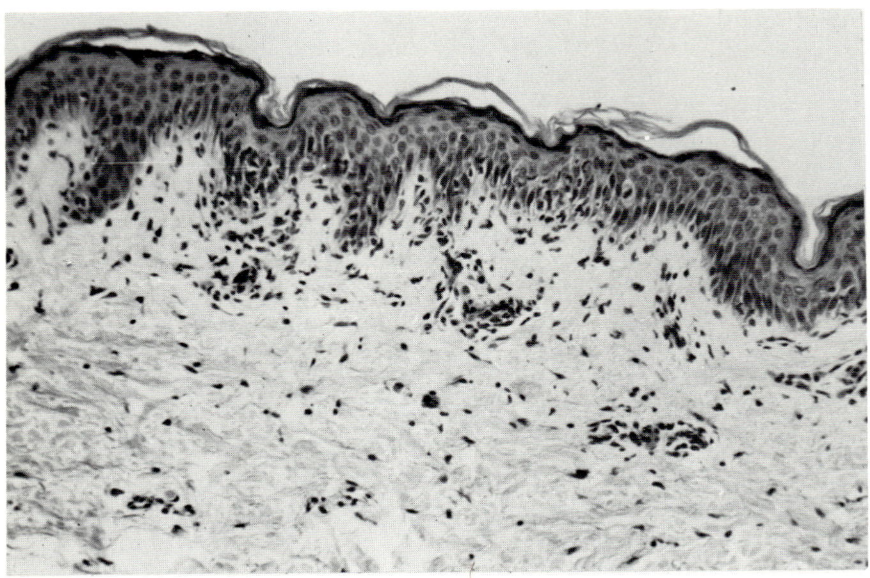

FIG. 28. Skin biopsy of a patient with graft-vs.-host disease after bone marrow allotransplantation. Note lymphocytes coating dermal vessels and invading epidermis. H&E; magnification ×150.

prolonged graft survival, the cellular equivalent of graft rejection often was present; in other patients, where cellular responses were suppressed, acute vascular lesions were observed quite frequently, which suggested the effect of circulating antibodies. Both were probably the result of a quantitative imbalance between antigenic stimulation by the graft and therapeutic immunosuppression.

6-Mercaptopurine is similar to azathioprine in that it inhibits the infiltration of allografts by lymphocytes (Schwartz and Damashek, 1962); the accumulation of mononuclear cells at the site of the inflammatory response is also suppressed by this drug (Page *et al.*, 1963). This observation corresponds well with the suppression of the tuberculin skin test that has been reported in 6-mercaptopurine-treated guinea pigs (Zweiman and Phillips, 1970), although the response to antigens of lymphocytes themselves was not inhibited.

Methotrexate markedly supported the generalization of experimental histoplasmosis infections but did not inhibit the local granulomatous response (Berry, 1969).

The antibiotic, chloramphenicol, prolongs allograft survival in experimental animals (Weisberger *et al.*, 1964a), indicating its interference with the cellular hypersensitivity reaction. Significant morphological lesions that could be correlated with this immune suppression have not yet been observed.

Actinomycin D shows a peripheral effect on the inflammatory exudate (Geller and Speirs, 1968), which is marked during the secondary response to antigenic stimulation. The significant decrease of the total cell count in inflammatory exudates was due to diminution of granulocytes, eosinophiles, and mononuclear cells. Similar to actinomycin are the anti-inflammatory effects of puromycin (Page, 1965).

Almost no information is available about the effect on the peripheral immune response of the remaining compounds (enzymes, mitotic inhibitors, polyanions, and miscellaneous agents), so that one has to refer to the

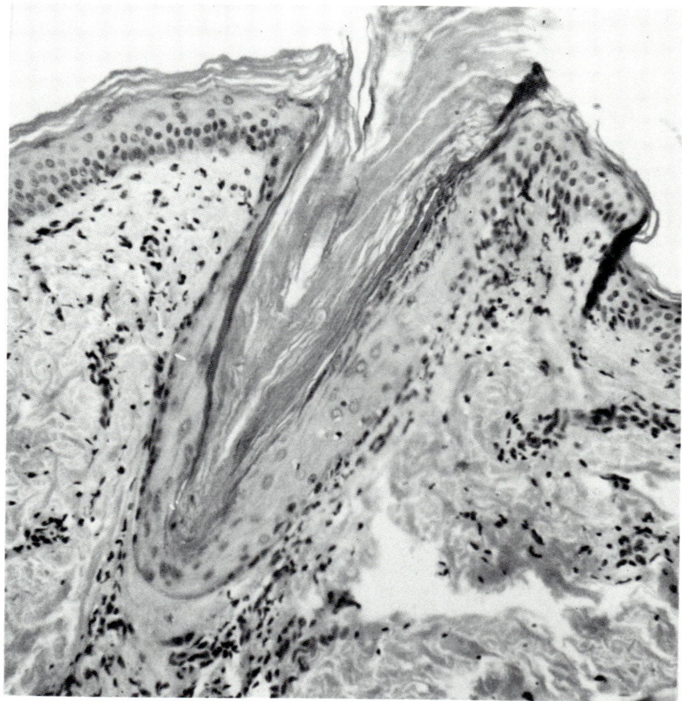

FIG. 29. Skin biopsy of a patient with chronic graft-vs.-host disease after bone marrow allotransplantation and treatment with methotrexate. Note occasional dermal lymphoid cells (not obviously increased in number), hyperkeratosis, and follicular plugging. H&E; magnification × 150.

lesions produced in the antibody-forming tissues themselves and then deduce the possible effect of antigen–antibody on the periphery. Compounds that damage the follicle–plasma cell system of lymph nodes, as for instance, mitosis inhibitors, would be expected also to interfere with the immediate hypersensitivity reaction. Compounds that reduce the number of small lymphocytes in the paracortex of lymph nodes, as does L-asparaginase, should be able to depress delayed hypersensitivity reactions. These correlations between morphology and function, however, cannot be taken absolutely, but rather serve as indicators of dysfunctions that may be expected. Also, most chemotherapeutic agents do not show specific effects on either cellular or humoral immunity, but act nonspecificly. For instance, BCNU depresses hemopoiesis and causes lymphocytopenia (Preisler and Henderson, 1969; Rall *et al.*, 1963) and, therefore, must depress peripheral inflammatory responses as well (an effect which certainly is dose-dependent). This compound also decreases the morphogenic effect of lymphocytic choriomeningitis virus and, therefore, depresses delayed hypersensitivity reactions (Sidwell *et al.*, 1965).

Our own studies with RNase (Krüger and Yun, unpublished data), as well as the studies of others with L-asparaginase (Hobik, 1969a,b), have shown a depression of cellular immune response, although the extent of atrophy of the paracortical zone of lymph nodes is not impressive. Thus, even a moderate reduction of small lymphocytes in this area may suffice readily to interfere with a cellular immune response. Nevertheless, some of these compounds may alter the function of these lymphocytes without causing lesions recognizable with the light microscope. In all these instances the stimulation test of lymphocytes by phytohemagglutinin may be helpful in estimating functional abnormalities.

D. Lesions Unrelated to Immune Reactions

These lesions represent the so-called side effects. It is impossible to review within this paragraph the complete spectrum of side effects that can be caused by immunosuppressive chemicals, since this would occupy the space of at least another chapter if not a complete book. In addition, the pathological anatomy of these untoward effects has not been completely described.

At the present time, however, the reader may refer for detailed listings of the clinical symptomatology of side effects to Meyler (1958–1966). The pathological anatomy, unfortunately, has not yet passed the period of occasional reports of side effects, and rather incomplete reviews are available (Karnofsky, 1967; Thurner, 1970; Albahary, 1953; Lampert, 1964; Spitz, 1948; Goldeck, 1950; Karrer and Wurnig, 1958; Letterer, 1948;

TABLE III
SIDE EFFECTS OF CHEMOTHERAPY[a]

Compound	Clinicopathological side effects
A. Hormones and antihormones	
Glucocorticosteroids	Cushingoid facies, fluid retention, osteoporosis, hypertension, peptic ulcers, pancreatitis, infections, leukocytosis, vasculitis, mental changes (euphoria, insomnia), endocrine dysfunctions (diabetes, growth delay, adrenal function suppression)
Estrogens and androgens	Fluid retention, mild gastrointestinal disturbances, gynecomastia, hypercalcemia and calcifications
Mitotane (o,p_1-DDD)	Anorexia, nausea, somnolence, lethargy, dermatitis
B. Alkylating agents	
Nitrogen mustard	Bone marrow depression, dermatitis (maculopapular eruptions), vomiting, nausea, anorexia, teratogenesis, local thrombophlebitis
Cyclophosphamide	Nausea, vomiting, dizziness, alopecia, skin pigmentation, ulcerative stomatitis, hepatotoxicity, hemorrhagic urocystitis, teratogenesis, widespread cellular atypia
Chlorambucil	Gastrointestinal disturbances, nausea, anorexia, hepatotoxicity, dermatitis, bone marrow depression
Uracil mustard	Nausea, vomiting, diarrhea, bone marrow depression, dermatitis
Phenylalanine mustard	Ulcerative stomatitis, hemorrhagic urocystitis, skin pigmentation, teratogenesis, dizziness, nausea vomiting
Myleran	Bone marrow depression, skin pigmentation, nausea, vomiting, diarrhea, anorexia, hyperuricemia, glossitis, gynecomastia, anhidrosis, teratogenesis, alopecia, interstitial pulmonary fibrosis, gastrointestinal dysfunction, fatigue, muscular weakness, cheilosis, amenorrhea
C. Antimetabolites	
6-Mercaptopurine	Bone marrow depression, anorexia, nausea, vomiting, hepatic necroses, cholestasis, renal tubular necroses, hyperuricemia, dermatitis
Azathioprine	Nausea, vomiting, diarrhea, bone marrow depression, allergy, radiculitis, infections
5-Fluorouracil	Anorexia, nausea, ulcerative stomatitis, bone marrow depression, dermatitis, alopecia, skin pigmentation and atrophy, myelopathy
Cytosine arabinoside	Bone marrow depression, gastrointestinal dysfunctions (mucosal lesions), stomatitis, hepatotoxicity, dermatitis, fever, local thrombophlebitis

(*continued*)

TABLE III (*continued*)

Compound	Clinicopathological side effects
Methotrexate	Bone marrow depression, ulcerative stomatitis, hemorrhagic enteritis, diarrhea, intestinal perforation, hepatotoxicity (fibrosis), dermatitis, alopecia
D. Antibiotics	
Actinomycin D	Anorexia, nausea, vomiting, bone marrow depression, glossitis, cheilitis, ulcerative stomatitis, proctitis, diarrhea, alopecia, skin erythema and pigmentation, desquamative dermatitis, diarrhea, teratogenesis
Mitomycin C	Nephrotoxicity (hyalinization of glomerular capillaries, tubular necrosis), hepatotoxicity, intestinal toxicity (necrosis of crypt epithelium), hemorrhages, granulocytopenia, skin pigmentation
Daunomycin	Myocardial toxicity, hepatotoxicity, nephrotoxicity (tubular necrosis), bone marrow depression with megaloblastic changes, gastrointestinal toxicity, ulcerative stomatitis, allergy, alopecia
Mithramycin	Bone marrow depression, hepatotoxicity, nephrotoxicity, calcium metabolism disturbances, blood coagulation disturbances
Bleomycin	Anorexia, alopecia, edema, phlebitis, chronic pneumonitis and fibrosis, sclerodermoid
E. Enzymes	
L-Asparaginase	Nausea, vomiting, headache, chills, fever, allergy, bone marrow depression (leukopenia, anemia), ulcerative stomatitis, hemorrhagic diathesis, hepatotoxicity (fatty metamorphosis), central nervous system toxicity (depression, personality changes, delirium), nephrotoxicity, pancreatitis, hyperglycemia, cardiovascular disorders, alopecia, blood coagulation defects
Ribonuclease	Hypersensitivity reactions (shock)
F. Mitotic inhibitors	
Colchicine derivatives	Gastrointestinal toxicity, central nervous system toxicity, bone marrow depression
Vinca rosea alkaloids	Bone marrow depression, neurotoxicity (depression, paresthesias, convulsions, headache, psychoses, reflex abnormalities, paralytic ileus, sinus tachycardia), gastrointestinal toxicity (diarrhea), nausea, vomiting, dermatitis, stomatitis, alopecia, local phlebitis, polyuria, fever, teratogenesis

TABLE III (*continued*)

Compound	Clinicopathological side effects
G. Polyanions	
Poly I:C	Anemia, hepatotoxicity, teratogenesis
H. Miscellaneous substances	
Hydrazine derivatives (including procarbazine)	Bone marrow depression, nausea, vomiting, dermatitis, pruritus, gastrointestinal toxicity, psychic abnormalities (depression), paresthesia
BCNU [1,3-bis(2-chloro-ethyl)-1-nitrosourea]	Bone marrow depression, anorexia, diarrhea, dysphagia, esophagitis

[a] Data collected in cooperation with Dr. David M. Young, Laboratory of Toxicology, National Cancer Institute.

Masshoff *et al.*, 1948). Until more information is at hand about the morphology of drug-induced diseases, it may suffice at this point to list the major clinical and morphological side effects so far known (Table III).

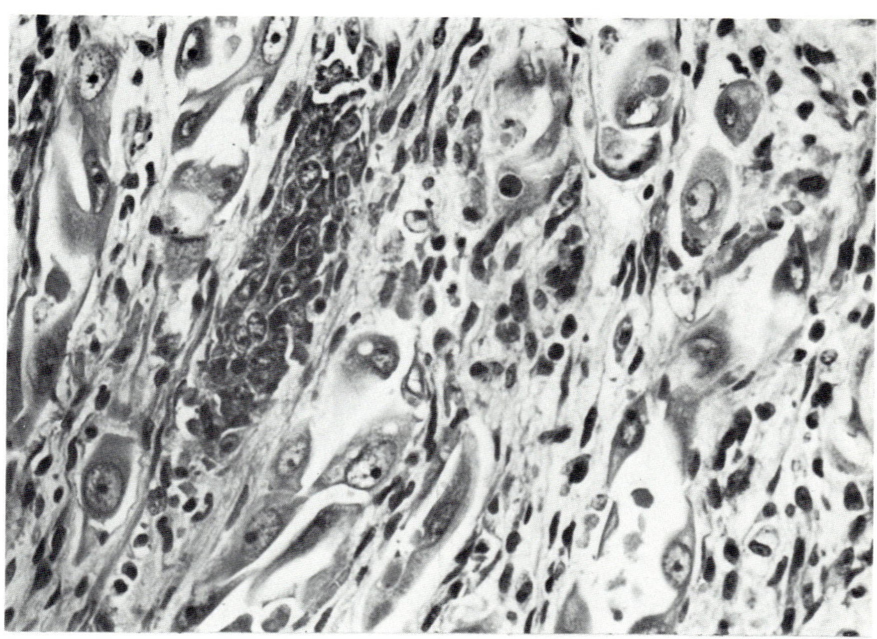

FIG. 30. Stomach of a dog treated with cyclophosphamide in preparation for bone marrow transplantation (100 mg/kg). Note marked cellular atypia and degeneration. H&E; magnification × 675.

VI. Pathological and Pathophysiological Synthesis

The ultimate task of pathological, pathophysiological, and biochemical correlations is to become able in future drug developments to deduce from chemical formulas the potential function and morphological lesions, as well as to deduce from morphological lesions the functional disturbances, of drugs of which the chemical structure is known. Pathological investigations in this schedule, although often neglected, are of major importance because (*1*) they are cheap and relatively easy to perform; (*2*) they are widespread in use in human disease and, therefore, constitute a unique source of information, if adequately evaluated by comparison with results from experimental pathology; (*3*) they may present immediate insight into functional disturbances by applying histochemical and ultrastructural methods; (*4*) they allow calculations about a chance of recovery by immediate observations of the damaged tissue; and (*5*) they may allow, ultimately, calculations about the risk of neoplastic transformation.

An example is given here of correlating chemical structure with function

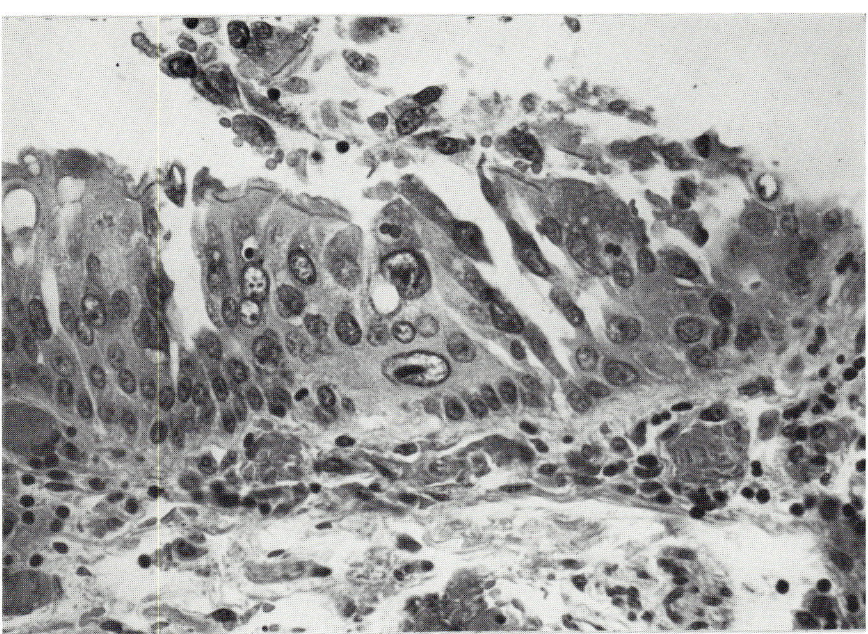

FIG. 31. Trachea of a dog treated with cyclophosphamide in preparation for bone marrow transplantation (100 mg/kg). Note anaplastic changes in columnar cells. H&E; magnification × 675.

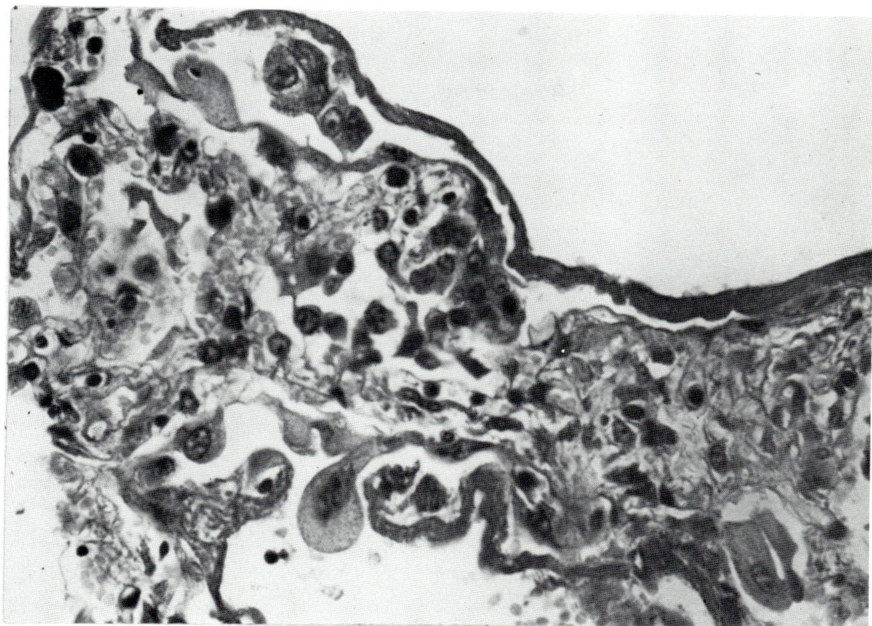

FIG. 32. Lung of a girl with bone marrow transplantation; cyclophosphamide was given in the pretransplant phase. Note atypia of alveolar lining cells and early hyaline membrane formation. H&E; magnification × 675.

and pathological findings. Following certain chemical criteria, alkylating groups are identified on a variety of biologically active substances (Baker, 1960); these alkylating groups are able to replace active hydrogens in functional groups such as amino, carboxyl, carboxamide, hydroxyl, and mercapto groups. Among the alkylating groups are carboxazides, epoxides, ethyleneimines, mono(β-chloroethyl)amines, bis(β-chloroethyl)amines, and others including diazonium salts, diazoketones, and halomethylketones. As discussed in Section IV,B, compounds containing these chemical groups may interfere with such important biological functions as nucleic acid replication and synthesis of proteins and enzymes; physiologically, this effect means disturbance of antibody synthesis, stop in production of specifically immunoreactive lymphocytes, and, dependent upon dosage, also inhibition of cell division or cell death. The expected morphological reaction to these functional disturbances are slow depopulation and atrophy of nonpostmitotic tissues, such as skin, bone marrow, lymphoreticular tissues, and intestinal mucosa. Antigenic stimulation does not respond as usual by germinal center formation, plasmacytosis, and activation of the

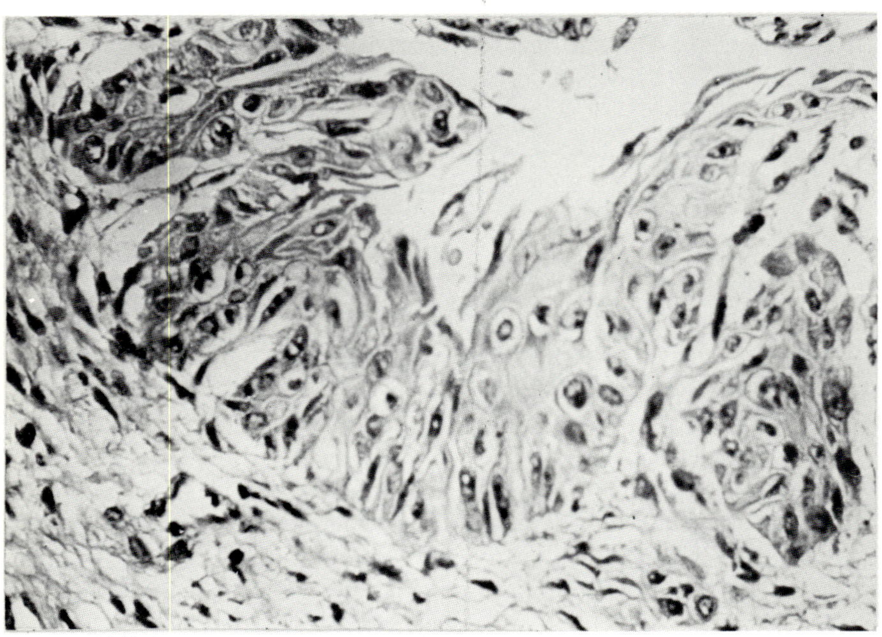

FIG. 33. Cervix uteri of a girl with bone marrow transplantation who received cyclophosphamide in the pretransplant phase. (same patient as in Fig. 32). Note derangement and atypia of epithelium. H&E; magnification × 675.

paracortex, but, instead, lymphoreticular tissues remain inactive, and already developing germinal centers become necrotic (Fig. 11). All these expected lesions, indeed, can be observed after administration of alkylating agents. High-dose treatment and treatment over a protracted period of time also produce complete atrophy of lymphoreticular tissues, necrosis, and hemorrhage, supporting the concept of a cytocidal effect of alkylating agents. From these descriptions it may seem that morphological lesions are predictable and, therefore, do not need to be further investigated. However, the extent of these anatomical findings varies in almost every individual case, and limited to this extent, certain predictions about the further course of the disease are possible. For instance, complete atrophy and necrosis of lymphoreticular tissues in athymic individuals renders recovery of lymphoid organs improbable, and the further course of the disease is complicated by an acquired immune deficiency syndrome. Most of these syndromes per se have an unfavorable prognosis. Also, when recovery of lymphoreticular tissues appears satisfactory, the therapeutically induced intestinal atrophy (Fig. 30) may cause a symptomatic malabsorption syndrome which complicates recovery.

Aside from these expected morphological changes, unexpected ones occur that are of immediate diagnostic value and these also make possible certain predictions for future developments. For instance, marked cellular enlargement and atypia were observed in patients and experimental animals treated with alkylating agents. We may mention here only cellular atypia in the gastrointestinal tract (Fig. 30), the tracheobronchial tree (Fig. 31), the alveolar lining cells (Fig. 32), the cervix uteri (Fig. 33), the prostate gland (Fig. 34), and the lymphoreticular tissue (Figs. 9a and b). The extent of alveolar lining cell atypia may permit predictions about susceptibility to toxic effects of oxygen and the development of hyaline membrane disease when the patient is treated with a respirator. Cellular atypia of the cervix uteri and the prostate gland must be differentiated from early malignancies. Also, there may exist an actual pathogenetic relationship between the development of these atypical cells and the development of a neoplasm in these tissues when the patient survives for longer periods of

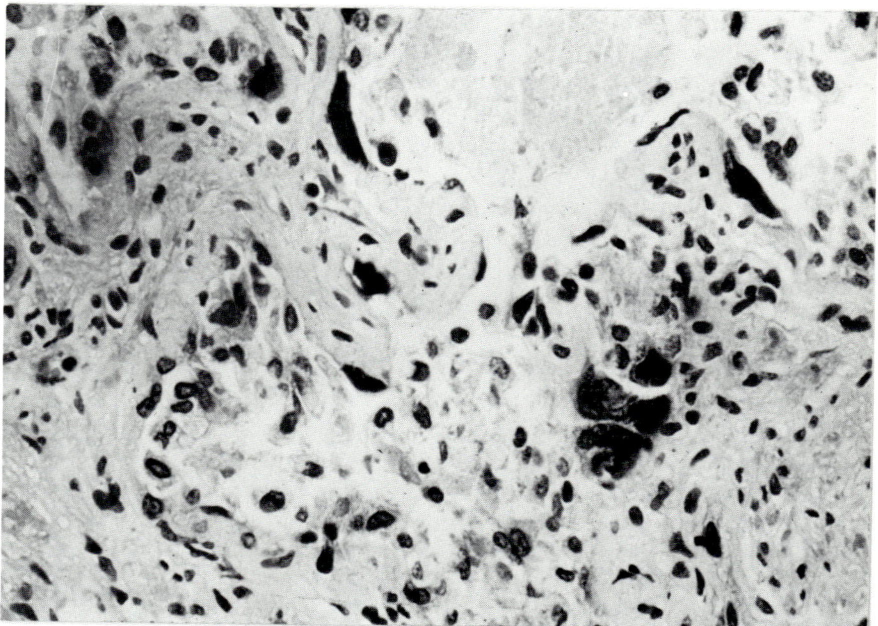

FIG. 34. Prostate of a dog treated with cyclophosphamide in for bone marrow transplantation. Note foci of atypical cells with hyperchromatic nuclei. H&E; magnification × 675.

time. Indeed, malignant neoplasms were described in 11 to 30% in experimental animals treated with various kinds of alkylating agents (Schmähl, 1970). It is well known that malignancies may develop after use of radioactive regimens that cause cell changes similar to those produced by alkylating agents. In consequence, exact pathological investigations may add to the evaluation of the effectiveness of chemotherapy, and may also permit the prediction of lesions that may be expected in drugs with comparable biological activity, as for instance, by comparison of mitomycin C or porfiromycin with the usual alkylating agents.

Besides the example given above, this type of investigation applies also to the evaluation of other substances as was stressed for the antimetabolites earlier in this chapter. However, much needs to be done in the future for biochemical, physiological, and anatomical correlations of the effects of the remaining drugs.

VII. Clinical Implications

A. Transplantation

Immunosuppressive therapy finds its major application today in transplantation biology. Substances that are in practical use include 6-mercaptopurine, azathioprine, methotrexate, cyclophosphamide, actinomycins, and glucocorticosteroids. Cyclophosphamide and corticosteroids are effective when administered before antigenic stimulation, i.e., before transplantation, and thus render the host unresponsive during the first few days after transplantation.

6-Mercaptopurine, azathioprine, and methotrexate are effective when administered after antigenic stimulation. The compounds of the first group appear to interact with antigen-sensitive cells and to interfere with cell proliferation, whereas the compounds of the second group interfere with cell transformation, cell differentiation, and initiation of antibody formation. Besides these, there are anti-inflammatory effects of compounds in both groups that inhibit the nonspecific secondary inflammation following an antigen–antibody interaction. Details have been discussed repeatedly elsewhere and need no further repetition here (Schwartz, 1968; Aisenberg, 1971; Good and Kelly, 1970; Parker and Vavra, 1969).

Histopathological studies in immunosuppressed transplant recipients represent an effectful tool to evaluate the possible extent of immunosuppression and the recovery potential of immunocompetent tissues. Such studies also provide information about the risk of graft rejection and graft-vs.-host reaction, and, finally, may provide a means for gaining insight into the mechanism of tumor formation in long-term survivors. Demonstration in our own studies of graft-vs.-host reaction in a bone marrow allograft recipient without proven engraftment (Krüger *et al.*, 1971a) and in patients transfused with cells from a donor with chronic myelogenous leukemia (Graw *et al.*, 1970) may be recalled here as examples.

In addition, morphological investigations can support the selection for practical use of newly developed drugs and also facilitate the selection of commonly known compounds for any specific case.

B. Autoimmune Diseases

Autoimmune diseases constitute probably the second largest group in which treatment with immunosuppressive agents has been tried. These diseases include idiopathic thrombocytopenic purpura (Schwarz and André, 1962), lupus erythematosus (Lee *et al.*, 1961), autoimmune hemolytic anemia (Schwartz and Damashek, 1962), autoimmune thyroiditis in animals (Spielberg and Miescher, 1963), chronic liver diseases or chronic renal diseases (Page *et al.*, 1963; Merrill, 1962), psoriasis and psoriatic arthritis (Van Scott, 1963; O'Brien *et al.*, 1962), autoimmune encephalomyelitis as well as lymphocytic choriomeningitis in animals (Paterson, 1968; Sidwell *et al.*, 1965), periarteritis nodosa (Merrill, 1962), scleroderma (Demis *et al.*, 1964), dermatomyositis (Eisen *et al.*, 1962), and ulcerative colitis (Bean, 1962). Among immunosuppressive compounds used to treat these diseases are cyclophosphamide, methotrexate, 6-mercaptopurine, 6-thioguanine, azathioprine, chlorambucil, BCNU, corticosteroids, and poly I:C. The effect of these agents on autoimmune diseases is quite variable and this may relate to the fact that an autoimmune pathogenesis is not unequivocally evident in all of these cases. Amelioration of the course of disease in which an autoimmune etiology appears controversial can be secondary to the nonspecific anti-inflammatory effect of immunosuppressive agents. Also, it must be borne in mind that certain immunosuppressive agents may act as chemical sensitizers and further complicate the disease. Among such compounds are L-asparaginase, poly I:C, RNase, and daunomycin. We observed a case of disseminated lupus erythematosus which, after treatment with poly I:C, changed to a rapidly progressive course with lethal outcome. Others have reported also the enhancement by poly I:C of autoimmune disease in New Zealand mice (Carpenter *et al.*, 1970). As in the homograft situation, careful morphological investigations of biopsy materials in autoimmune disorders may add to the pathogenetic clarification of the disease itself, allow predictions of its further course, and help to evaluate the effect of treatment.

C. Infectious Diseases

The influence of immunosuppressive drugs on various infections was mentioned in Section V,C,2. Best known of all is the exacerbation and generalization of tuberculous foci during corticosteroid treatment (Hart and Rees, 1950; Traut and Ellman, 1952; Werner and Prechtel, 1968). The present author autopsied a 67-year-old white woman whom corticosteroid therapy had rendered areactive and, thereby, caused exacerbation of an old fibrocaseous lung focus to an acute tuberculous sepsis (typhobacillosis LANDOUZY) accompanied by hematological changes resembling acute leukemia. In animal experiments, immunosuppression with cyclophosphamide enhances the spread of tuberculous and *Brucella* infections (Ullmann, 1969; Stender *et al.*, 1963; Potel and Brock, 1965; Potel, 1965). Commonly known are also systemic mycoses in patients undergoing cancer chemotherapy (Craig and Farber, 1953; Gruhn and Sanson, 1963; Sabesin *et al.*, 1963). Septic infections caused by *Pseudomonas*, *Pneumocystis*, *Candida*, *Aspergillus*, and *Cryptococcus* organisms in patients under extensive combination chemotherapy are observed so frequently at autopsy today that the question arises in several cases whether the patient actually died of his primary disease or rather of therapy-induced unresponsiveness that permitted these infections to develop and progress.

D. Neoplastic Diseases

Compounds used for the chemotherapy of neoplastic diseases are essentially the same as the ones for immunosuppressive use discussed in this chapter with the exception perhaps of chloramphenicol and cetophenicol. The selection of a certain drug or drug combination depends on the type and stage of the neoplasm to be treated, and for this histopathological methods are essential. Extensive cancer chemotherapy, as discussed above, interferes with the immune response and, therefore, is able to abolish the biological host response to the neoplasm. The morphological evaluation of this immunosuppression as exerted by chemotherapy often is impossible, since the tumor itself may cause immunological unresponsiveness. It has been claimed, however, that certain immunosuppressive drugs may also enhance antibody formation (Merritt and Johnson, 1963; Frisch and Davies, 1962a,b). This enhancement usually is accompanied also by hyperplastic changes in the immunocompetent tissues (Sahiar and Schwartz, 1966), but this effect on antibody formation applies only to a few quite specific models.

VIII. Comparative Pathology of Other Immunosuppressive Patterns

A. General Considerations

It is of considerable value for the morphologist to compare the lesions in states of immunological unresponsiveness caused by other mechanisms than chemical immunosuppression with those described so far in this chapter. Such comparative study permits insight into quantitative relationships between treatment and morphogenesis as, for instance, in immunosuppression by X-irradiation; or it allows a better correlation of morphological lesions with defects in certain immunological systems as in inherited immune deficiency diseases. Beside these, comparative investigations of lymphoreticular tissues in immunological tolerance or in biological immunosuppressive measures such as the administration of antilymphocytic serum (ALS) may be informative. These studies have also a certain value since chemical immunosuppressive treatment may be given in combination with ALS and since the patient may be in a state of immunological tolerance when immunosuppressive treatment is initiated. The latter applies especially to cancer chemotherapy.

B. Irradiation

Immunosuppression after irradiation is effective only when total-body X-irradiation is performed shortly before antigen administration, and the effect on the humoral immune response is more prominent than on the cellular response (Dixon *et al.*, 1952; Parker and Vavra, 1969). Histologically, all lymphoreticular tissues appear equally sensitive to the effect of irradiation, and these tissues probably are most sensitive of all (Zollinger, 1960). About 30 minutes after lethal irradiation (mice 800 R, guinea pigs 800 R, dogs 1000 R and 1100 R), lymphocytes and lymphoblasts become necrotic; this phase is followed by degeneration of secondary follicles in lymph nodes and spleen and by invasion of the damaged tissues by granulocytes. The next phase, about 24 hours after irradiation, is characterized by phagocytosis of cellular debris, and diffusely scattered macrophages are prominent in lymphoreticular tissues; macrophages also tend to accumulate in secondary follicles and in sinuses. Regeneration, dependent upon the extent of radiological damage, starts after a few days to 1 week, and is initiated by increased mitotic activity of remnants of cortical lymphoid cells in lymph nodes or by remnants of follicular lymphoid cells in the spleen. Complete morphological regeneration may take about 1 month, although often a moderate interstitial fibrosis and sinus fibrosis remain. The most sensitive constituent of lymphoreticular tissues to irradiation effects are small lymphocytes, which show pyknosis and rhexis after only 20–50 R (DeBruyn, 1948; Pizon, 1955). Therefore, morphological lesions induced by irradiation or by action of radioactive substances, such as Thorotrast, in general, are quite comparable to those induced by corticosteroids or alkylating agents.

C. Antilymphocytic Sera

Treatment of experimental animals with ALS causes a depression of cellular and humoral immune reactions (Waksman *et al.*, 1961; Lance and Medawar, 1970; Levey, 1970; Monaco *et al.*, 1966) and inhibits the transformation of lymphocytes by phytohemagglutinin (Mosedale *et al.*, 1968). The morphological effects on lymphoreticular tissues of ALS have been described by several investigators (Turk, 1970; Krüger *et al.*, 1971b; Turk and Willoughby, 1967). The paracortical region of lymph nodes becomes depleted of small lymphocytes, which correlates well with the decrease in circulating lymphocytes. Primary and secondary follicles as well as the plasma cell reaction in medullary cords are not obviously affected. This immediate effect of ALS on lymph nodes is similar to the effect of thymectomy on these organs. Prolonged administration of ALS, besides causing a marked depletion of the lymph node paracortex and a loss of small lymphocytes from splenic follicles, also enhances the formation of secondary follicles in lymph nodes and spleen and leads to an extensive plasmacytosis in lymphoreticular tissues. It may well be that the antigenicity of the ALS itself accounts for these lesions. When footpad tests were done for evaluation of delayed hypersensitivity in ALS-treated mice with antigenic stimulation, no perivascular lymphohistiocytic infiltrates indicative of a cellular immune response were noted. Instead, swelling of local mesenchymal cells and granulocytic infiltrates were observed at the site of the test injection (Krüger, 1971c).

In conclusion, ALS causes morphological lesions that differ from almost all lesions caused by chemical immunosuppressants. From both morphology and immunological tests, it appears that ALS affects primarily the cellular immune response. It should be, therefore, a valuable supplement to chemical immunosuppressants that affect germinal center formation and the production of circulating antibodies.

D. Immunological Tolerance

The problem of immunological tolerance is much too complicated to be discussed even in slight detail here. The proceedings of a recent international conference may serve as further reference (Landy and Braun, 1970). In the context of this chapter it it of interest to mention, however, that chemical immunosuppressants, under certain circumstances, can induce tolerance against antigens administered at a given time and dose. Schwartz (1967) demonstrated this by the use of sheep red blood corpuscles and cyclophosphamide. Also chloramphenicol and 6-mercaptopurine administration led to the induction of immunological tolerance (Cruchaud, 1965). Histologically, even though the usual picture associated with antibody production is not seen, a profuse activation of lymphoid cells to pyroninophilic blast cells is noted (Cerney and Viklicky, 1957) during tolerance. This phenomenon is interpreted as proliferation of stem cells, but differentiation of these cells to antibody-producing cells is blocked. This lesion, however, produced by the mechanism of high zone tolerance, is highly artificial. Under physiological conditions of a specific tolerance toward a certain antigen, no histological findings that differ from the normal appearance of lymphoreticular tissues are visible.

E. Immune Deficiency Syndromes

A short comparative note about the human defect immunopathies in chemically immunosuppressed patients may assist the clinicopathological correlation. Extensive testing for humoral and cellular reactivity has led to the characterization of certain syndromes with quite specific defects in immunological reactivity, and in many of these syndromes coincident anatomic lesions have been described (Hess, 1970; Engle and Wallis, 1969; Bergsma, 1968). Comparison of these lesions with the ones described in chemical immunosuppression may make it possible for conclusions to be drawn as to the immunological defect in immunosuppressed patients. For instance, the sex-linked (male) recessively inherited agammaglobulinemia of Bruton (1952) is characterized morphologically by absence of secondary follicles and plasma cells in lymphoreticular tissues, whereas the thymus and thymic-dependent paracortex of lymph nodes are less obviously changed. This anatomical defect is accompanied by a hypogammaglobulinemia and an inability to form sufficient circulating antibodies. Transformation by phytohemagglutinin and antigenic substances of lymphocytes, as well as cellular immune reactions, are inconsistently impaired (Hess, 1970). This syndrome is comparable to some extent with an immune deficiency caused by immunosuppressants of the radiomimetic type (alkylating agents, colchicine derivatives), actinomycins, and mitomycin C. These agents also affect primarily proliferating cells in the secondary follicle of lymphoreticular tissues and, therefore, interfere with the humoral immune response. The immediate effect of these compounds on lymphocytes, however, differs from findings in Bruton's syndrome.

Similar histologically and functionally to Bruton's agammaglobulinemia is the Swiss-type agammaglobulinemia which is not sex-linked (Hitzig *et al.*, 1968).

In contrast, patients with lymphopenic thymic dysplasia with dysgammaglobulinemia (Hoyer *et al.*, 1968b) show a depletion of lymphocytes in the thymus-dependent lymph node paracortex, but secondary follicles and plasmacytosis are present after antigenic stimulation. Serum γ-globulin levels are variable but usually IgG and IgA are deficient. This syndrome compares morphologically to lesions in lymphoreticular tissues caused by L-asparaginase treatment—despite an obvious decrease in small lymphocytes, the formation of secondary follicles and plasma cells is not obviously suppressed.

The remaining types of immune deficiency syndromes are morphologically more complex, as are the lesions caused by the remaining immunosuppressive chemicals. High-dose treatment with cyclophosphamide or combination chemotherapy of cancer patients, however, may cause lymph node changes and functional insufficiencies that compare superficially to the most primitive type of defect immunopathies, i.e., the reticular dysgenesis (DeVaal and Seynhaeve, 1959; Hoyer *et al.*, 1968a). It is of interest, also, that in reticular dysgenesis part of the pathogenetic mechanism is felt to be a graft-vs.-host reaction of maternal immunocompetent cells in the newborn. There are also morphological lesions suggestive of chronic graft-vs.-host reaction in chemotherapeutically treated patients who received blood transfusions (Krüger, 1971a).

IX. Conclusions

Immunosuppressive agents and cancer chemotherapeutic agents, in general, are synonymous; that is, the therapist must expect immunosuppressive effects when cancer chemotherapeutic drugs are used. This does not imply, however, that all compounds effective for the treatment of neoplastic disease may be also useful to treat disease caused by immune reactions. Screening of newly developed compounds for immunosuppressive effects is possible in part by comparison of the chemical structure of these agents with others that are known immunosuppressants [see, for instance, newly developed alkylating agents (Hirano *et al.*, 1970)]. Further selection can be made according to known biochemical and pathophysiological activities. For instance, substances that interfere with nucleic acid metabolism or with protein synthesis may also interfere with the immune response;

substances that inhibit cell proliferation in general are able to inhibit the immune response; and, finally, substances that possess nonspecific anti-inflammatory activity also suppress the inflammatory reaction following an antigen-antibody reaction.

The actual extent of immunosuppression caused by drugs preselected in such a way must then be tested in short-term and long-term experiments, and effects on both cellular and humoral immunity must be considered, since these are not necessarily suppressed in a parallel fashion. Last but not least, no tests for immunosuppressive activity of yet unknown compounds are complete without careful histological investigation.

Anatomical studies of immunocompetent tissues provide information about the potential interference of drugs with humoral or cellular immune responses, about the ability of these tissues to recover, and probably also about the risk of tumor development in these tissues; the last two subjects pertain mainly to long-term investigations. In this chapter attention was drawn to morphological lesions caused by immunosuppressive chemicals in order to familiarize the nonpathologist investigator of cancer and immunosuppressive therapy with this valuable tool of research. It was chosen to concentrate only on light-microscopic findings so that the matter would not become complicated. In fact, the light microscope can provide all information about investigations that are suggested in this chapter. Additional information pertaining to a specific drug and its action on a subcellular level may be obtained from individual publications.

Acknowledgments

I am gratefully indebted for active help and advice during the preparation of this paper to Professor L. Massimo, Dr. K. Snell, Dr. R. G. Graw, Dr. D. M. Young, Dr. M. G. Hanna, and Dr. R. J. Schnitzer. I also have to mention the careful assistance in the literature search by Mrs. Eileen Sussman and Miss Duran Harris, as well as in photographic documentation by Mr. R. Isenburg, and secretarial assistance by Mrs. Becky Coughlin.

References

Abe, T. and Nomura, M. (1970). *J. Nat. Cancer Inst.* **45,** 597.

Abe, T., Shimada, S., and Osaka, R. (1969). *J. Nat. Cancer Inst* **43,** 459.

Abell, C. W., Rosini, L. A., and Ramseur, L. A. (1965). *Proc. Nat. Acad. Sci. U.S.* **54,** 608.

Abramoff, P., and LaVia, M. (1970). "Biology of the Immune Response." McGraw-Hill New York.

Ada, G. L., Parish, C. R., Nossal, G. J. V., and Abbot, A. (1967). *Cold Spring Harbor Symp. Quant. Biol.* **32,** 381.

Adamson, R. H., Fabro, S., Homan, E. R., O'Gara, R. W., and Zendzian, R. P. (1969). *Antimicrob. Ag. Chemother.* p. 148.

Aisenberg, A. C. (1971). *Advan. Pharmacol. Chemother.* **8,** 31.
Aisenberg, A. C., and Davis, C. (1968). *J. Exp. Med.* **128,** 35.
Aisenberg, A. C., and Wilkes, B. (1964). *J. Clin. Invest.* **43,** 2394.
Akiyama, T. (1965). *Proc. Jap. Soc. Reticuloendothel. Syst.* **5,** 140.
Albahary, C. (1953). "Maladies Médicamenteuses d'Ordre Thérapeutique et Accidentel." Masson, Paris.
Altmann, H. W. (1966). *Verh. Deut. Ges. Pathol.* **50,** 15.
Amiel, J. L., Brezin, C., Sekiguchi, M., Mery, A. M., Hoerni, B., Garattini, S., Daguet, G., and Mathé, G. (1964). *Rev. Fr. Etud. Clin. Biol.* **9,** 636.
Armborst, V., and Maass, H. (1964). *Naturwissenschaften* **51,** 271.
Askonas, B. A., and Rhodes, J. M. (1965). *Nature (London)* **205,** 470.
Aso, Y., Asano, M., Hirose, K., and Takayasu, H. (1970). *Progr. Antimicrob. Anticancer Chemother.* **2,** 295.
Aspinall, R. L., Meyer, R. K., and Rao, M. A. (1961). *Endocrinology* **68,** 944.
Astaldi, G., Gociu, M., and Airó, R. (1967). *Exp. Cell Res.* **46,** 22.
Astaldi, G., Burgio, G. R., Krc, J., Genova, R., and Astaldi, A. A. (1969a). *Lancet* **i,** 423.
Astaldi, G., Eridani, S., Ponti, G. B., Valentini, R., and Giangrande, A. (1969b). *Blut* **19,** 8.
Astaldi, G., Bruckner, I., Micu, D., Maximilian, G., Leahu, S., and Burgio, G. (1970). *Proc. 6th Int. Meet. Reticuloendothel. Soc., Freiburg* Abstr., p. 4.
Avrameas, S., and Lespinats, G. (1967). *C. R. Acad. Sci., Ser. D* **265,** 302
Baker, B R. (1960). *Nat. Cancer Inst. Monogr.* **3,** 9.
Baltch, A. L., Lepper, M. H., and Lolans, V. T. (1966). *J. Immunol.* **96,** 149.
Barranco, S. C., and Humphrey, R M. (1970). *Proc. 10th Int. Cancer Congr., Houston, Tex.* Abstr. 433, No. 702.
Bean, R. H. (1962). *Med. J. Aust.* **2,** 592.
Bellelli, L. (1961). *Oncologia (Basel)* **14,** 254.
Benvenisti, D. S., Burchenal, J. H., and Ochoa, M. (1970). *Proc. 10th Int. Cancer Congr., Houston, Tex.* Abstr. 440, No. 714.
Berenbaum, M. C. (1967). *J. Clin. Pathol.* **20,** Suppl., 471.
Berenbaum, M. C., and Brown, I. N. (1964). *Immunology* **7,** 65.
Bergenstal, B. M., Hertz, R., Lipsett, M. B., and Moy, R. H. (1960). *Ann. Intern. Med.* **53,** 672.
Bergsma, D., ed. (1968). *Birth Defects, Orig. Artic. Ser.* **4.**
Berry, C. L. (1969). *J. Pathol.* **97,** 653.
Bertino, J. R., Hillcoat, B. L., and Johns, D. G. (1967). *Fed. Proc. Fed. Amer. Soc. Exp. Biol.* **26,** 893.
Biesele, J. J. (1963). *Exp. Cell Res. Suppl.* **9,** 525.
Bloom, B. R., Hamilton, L. D., and Chase, M. W. (1964). *Nature (London)* **201,** 689.
Boll, I., Mersch, G., Schoen, S., Göttke, U., Boxheimer, D., and Lucke, G. (1968). *Klin. Wochenschr.* **46,** 608.
Bollag, W. (1963). *Experientia* **19,** 304.
Bonadonna, G., Monfordini, S., and DiPietro, S. (1970). *Proc. 10th Int. Cancer Congr., Houston, Tex.* Abstr. 478, No. 774.
Bonmassar, E., Vieira, W., Vadlamudi, S., and Goldin, A. (1962). *Arch. Ital. Patol. Clin. Tumori* **12,** 163.
Borel, Y., and Schwartz, R. S. (1964). *J. Immunol.* **92,** 754.
Borel, Y., Fauconnet, M., and Miescher, P. A. (1965). *J. Exp. Med.* **122,** 263.

Borum, K. (1969). *Acta Pathol. Microbiol. Scand.* **76,** 515.
Bradner, W. T., and Hutchison, D. J. (1966). *Cancer Chemother. Rep.* **50,** 79.
Braunstein, H., Freimann, D. G., and Gall, E. A. (1958). *Cancer* (*Philadelphia*) **11,** 829.
Breinl, F., and Haurowitz, F. (1930). *Hoppe-Seyler's Z. Physiol. Chem.* **192,** 45.
Bresnick, E. (1959). *Fed. Proc. Fed. Amer. Soc. Exp. Biol.* **18,** 371.
Brewer, H. B., Comstock, J. P., and Arnow, L. (1961). *Biochem. Pharmacol.* **8,** 281.
Brinck-Johnson, T., and Dougherty, T. F. (1965). *Acta Endocrinol.* (*Copenhagen*) **49,** 471.
Brodsky, I., and Kahn, S. B., eds. (1967). "Cancer Chemotherapy: Basic and Clinical Applications." Grune & Stratton, New York.
Brookes, P., and Lawley, P. D. (1961). *Biochem. J.* **80,** 496.
Brookes, P., and Lawley, P. D. (1964). *J. Cell. Comp. Physiol.* **64,** 111.
Brown, D. M., and Todd, A. R. (1952). *J. Chem. Soc., London* p. 52.
Brown, I. N., and Berenbaum, M. C. (1964). *Nature* (*London*) **201,** 1340.
Bruton, O. C. (1952). *Pediatrics* **9,** 722.
Buchanan, J. M., and Wilson, D. W. (1953). *Fed. Proc. Fed. Amer. Soc. Exp. Biol.* **12,** 646.
Bukantz, S. C., Dammin, D. S., Johnson, M. D., and Alexander, H. L. (1949). *Proc. Soc. Exp. Biol. Med.* **72,** 21.
Burchenal, J. (1963). *Cancer Res.* **23,** 1181.
Burnet, F. M. (1959). "The Clonal Selection Theory of Acquired Immunity." Cambridge Univ. Press, London and New York.
Busch, L. (1955). *Ther. Ber.* **8,** 227.
Calendi, E., DiMarco, A., Reggiani, M., Scarpinato, B., and Valentini, (1965). *Biochim. Biophys. Acta* **103,** 25.
Cameron, G. R., Cowitice, R. C., and Jones, R. P. (1947). *J. Pathol. Bacteriol.* **59,** 425.
Cardell, B. S. (1961). *Brit. Med. J.* **i,** 1145.
Cardinali, G., Cardinali, G., and Blair, J. (1961). *Cancer Res.* **21,** 1542.
Carpenter, D. F., Steinberg, A. D., Schur, P. H., and Talal, N. (1970). *Lab. Invest.* **23,** 628.
Carter, S. K. (1968a). *Cancer Chemother. Rep.* **1,** 81.
Carter, S. K. (1968b). *Cancer Chemother. Rep.* **1,** 99.
Carter, S. K. (1968c). *Cancer Chemother. Rep.* **3,** 207.
Casey, T. P. (1968). *Blood* **31,** 396.
Cerney, J., and Viklicky, V. (1957). *In* "Germinal Centers in Immune Responses" (H. Cottier, N. Odartchenko, R. Schindler, and C. C. Congdon, eds.), pp. 319–328. Springer-Verlag, Berlin and New York.
Chakrabarty, A. K., and Friedman, H. (1970). *Clin. Exp. Immunol.* **6,** 619.
Claesson, M. H., and Ropke, C. (1969). *Acta Pathol. Microbiol. Scand.* **76,** 37.
Clarke, D. A., Reilly, H. C., and Stock, C. C. (1957). *Antibiot Chemother.* (*Washington, D.C.*) **7,** 653.
Clifford, P., Singh, S., Stjernswärd, J., and Klein, G. (1967). *Cancer Res.* **27,** 2578.
Congdon, C. C. (1962). *J. Nat. Cancer Inst.* **28,** 305.
Congdon, C. C. (1964). *Arch. Pathol.* **78,** 83.
Congdon, C. C. (1969). *Progr. Biophys. Mol. Biol.* **19,** 309.
Congdon, C. C., and Makinodan, T. (1961). *Amer. J. Pathol.* **39,** 69.
Cooney, D., Eckhardt, S., and Goldin, A. (1965). *Antimicrob. Ag. Chemother.* p. 509.
Cooper, M. D., and Weller, E. M. (1969). *Advan. Exp. Med. Biol.* **5,** 277.

Costa, H., and Astaldi, H. (1964). *Tumori* **50,** 471.
Cottier, H., Hess, M. W., Roos, B., and Grétillat, P. A. (1969). *In* "Handbuch der Allgemeinen Pathologie" (H. W. Altmann, F. Büchner, H. Cottier, E. Grundmann, G. Holle, E. Letterer, W. Masshoff, H. Meessen, F. Roulet, G. Seifert, G. Siebert, and A. Studer, eds.), Vol. VI/2, pp. 496–766. Springer-Verlag, Berlin and New York.
Craig, J. M., and Farber, S. (1953). *Amer. J. Pathol.* **29,** 601.
Creasey, W. A. (1967). *Pharmacologist* **9,** 192.
Creasey, W. A. (1968). *Cancer Chemother. Rep.* **52,** 501.
Creasey, W. A., and Markin, M. E. (1964). *Biochem. Pharmacol.* **13,** 135.
Cronkite, E. P., and Chanana, A. D. (1968). *In* "Human Transplantation" (F. T. Rapaport and J. Dausset, eds.), pp. 423–439. Grune & Stratton, New York.
Cruchaud, A. (1965). *Int. Arch. Allergy Appl. Immunol.* **27,** 373.
Csaba, G., Kiss, J., and Dunay, C. (1967). *Experientia* **23,** 267.
Curreri, A. R., and Ansfield, F. J. (1960). *Cancer Chemother. Rep.* **8,** 18.
Cutts, J. H. (1961). *Cancer Res.* **21,** 168.
Dammin, G. J. (1966). *In* "The Kidney" (F. K. Mostofi and D. E. Smith, eds.), pp. 445–468. Williams & Wilkins, Baltimore, Maryland.
Darken, M. A. (1964). *Pharmacol. Rev.* **16,** 233.
Davis, R. C., Cooperband, S. R., and Mannick, J. A. (1969). *J. Immunol.* **103,** 1029.
DeBruyn, P. P. (1948). *In* "Histopathology of Irradiation From External and Internal Sources" (W. Bloom, ed.), p. 348. McGraw-Hill, New York.
Deitch, A. D., and Goodman, G. C. (1967). *Proc. Nat. Acad. Sci. U.S.* **5,** 1607.
Delmonte, L., and Jukes, T. H. (1962). *Pharmacol. Rev.* **14,** 91.
Demis, D. J., Brown, C. S., and Crosby, W. H. (1964). *Amer. J. Med.* **37,** 195.
DePetris, S., and Karlsbad, G. (1965). *J. Cell Biol.* **26,** 759.
DePetris, S., Karlsbad, G., and Pernis, B. (1963). *J. Exp. Med.* **117,** 849.
Derbes, V. J., Dent, J. H., Weaver, N. K., and Vaughan, D. D. (1950). *Proc. Soc. Exp. Biol. Med.* **75,** 423.
DeVaal, O. M., and Seynhaeve, V. (1959). *Lancet* **ii,** 1123.
Diener, E. (1970). *In* "Handbuch der Allgemeinen Pathologie" (H. W. Altmann F. Büchner, H. Cottier, E. Grundmann, G. Holle, E. Letterer, W. Masshoff, H. Meessen, F. Roulet, G. Seifert, G. Siebert, and A. Studer, eds), Vol. VII/3, pp. 250–325. Springer-Verlag, Berlin and New York.
Diener, E., and Nossal, G. J. V. (1966). *Immunology* **10,** 535.
DiMarco, A. (1967). *In* "Antibiotics. I: Mechanism of Action" (D. Gottlieb and P. D. Shaw, eds.), pp. 190–210. Springer-Verlag, Berlin and New York.
DiMarco, A., Gaetani, M., Orezzi, P., Scarpinato, B. M., Silvestrini, R., Soldati, M., Dastia, T., and Valentini, L. (1964). *Nature (London)* **201,** 706.
DiMarco, A., Gaetani, M., and Scarpinato, B. (1969). *Cancer Chemother. Rep.* **53,** 33.
Dixon, F. J., Talmage, W., and Maurer, P. H. (1952). *J. Immunol.* **68,** 693.
Dold, V. M., Mielsch, M., and Holzer, H. (1962). *Z. Krebsforsch.* **65,** 13.
Dolowy, W. C., and Ameraal, A. N. (1967). *Science* **155,** 329.
Dougherty, T. F. (1952). *Pharmacol. Rev.* **32,** 379.
Dougherty, T. F., Berliner, M. L., Schneebeli, G. L., and Berliner, D. L. (1964). *Ann. N.Y. Acad. Sci.* **113,** 825.
Dougherty, T. F. (1951). *Amer. J. Pathol.* **27,** 714.
Dumonde, D. C. (1967). *Brit. Med. Bull.* **23,** 9.
Dunn, T. B. (1969). Personal communication.
Dustmann, H. O., and Stolpmann, H. J. (1968). *Virchows Arch., A* **345,** 121.

Eckhardt, S., Humphreys, S. R., and Goldin, A. (1965). *Antimicrob. Ag. Chemother.* p. 503.

Eisen, B., Demis, D. J., and Crosby, W. H. (1962). *J. Amer. Med. Ass.* **179,** 789.

Elion, G. B. (1967). *Fed. Proc. Fed. Amer. Soc. Exp. Biol.* **26,** 898.

Elion, G. B., Callahan, S. W., Hitchings, G. H., Rundles, R. W., and Laszlo, J. (1962). *Cancer Chemother. Rep.* **16,** 197.

Engle, R. L., and Wallis, L. A. (1969). "Immunoglobulinopathies." Thomas, Springfield, Illinois.

Epstein, W. L., and Maibach, H. I. (1965). *Arch. Dermatol.* **91,** 599.

Eridani, S., Esposito, R., Ponti, G. B., and Uderzo, C. (1970). *Proc. 6th Int. Meet. Reticuloendothel. Soc., Freiburg* Abstr. p. 42.

Ernström, U., and Larsson, B. (1967). *Acta Pathol. Microbiol. Scand.* **70,** 371.

Feigelson, P., and Feigelson, M. (1968). *In* "Actions of Hormones and Molecular Processes" (G. Litwack and D. Kritchewsky, eds.), pp. 218–233. Wiley, New York.

Feldman, J. D. (1964). *Advan. Immunol.* **4,** 175.

Feldman, M., and Gallily, R. (1967). *Cold Spring Harbor Symp. Quant. Biol.* **32,** 415.

Fischel, E. E., Stoerk, H. C., and Bjorneboe, M. (1951). *Proc. Soc. Exp. Biol. Med.* **77,** 111.

Fishman, M., and Adler, F. L. (1963a). *Immunopathology* **3,** 79.

Fishman, M., and Adler, F. L. (1963b). *J. Exp. Med.* **117,** 595.

Folb, P. I., and Trounce, J. R. (1970). *Lancet* **ii,** 1112.

Forshter, K. K. (1951). *J. Microbiol. Epidemiol. Immunbiol.* **28,** 603.

Freedman, H. H., Fox, A. E., and Willis, R. S. (1968). *Proc. Soc. Exp. Biol. Med.* **129,** 796.

Frei, P. C., Benacerraf, B., and Thorbecke, G. J. (1965). *Proc. Nat. Acad. Sci. U.S.* **53,** 20.

Friedman, H. (1964). *Science* **156,** 934.

Friedman, H. P., Stavitzky, A. B., and Solomon, J. M. (1965). *Science* **149,** 1106.

Friedman, R. M. (1964a). *Nature (London)* **201,** 848.

Friedman, R. M. (1964b). *Proc. Soc. Exp. Biol. Med.* **116,** 471.

Friedman, R. M., and Baron, S. (1961). *J. Immunol.* **87,** 379.

Friedman, R. M., and Buckler, C. E. (1963). *J. Immunol.* **91,** 846.

Frisch, A. W., and Davies, G. H. (1962a). *Proc. Soc. Exp. Med.* **110,** 444.

Frisch, A. W., and Davies, G. H. (1962b). *J. Immunol.* **88,** 269.

Frisch, A. W., Davies, G. H., and Milstein, V. (1962). *J. Immunol.* **89,** 300.

Fujikami, S., Kajikawa, K., and Ozaki, T. (1962). *Cancer Chemother. Rep.* **3,** 1584.

Fujita, H., and Kimura, K. (1970). *Progr. Antimicrob. Anticancer Chemother.* **2,** 309.

Furness, G. (1959). *J. Bacteriol.* **77,** 461.

Gabourel, J. D., and Arnow, L. (1962). *J. Pharmacol. Exp. Ther.* **136,** 213.

Gabrielsen, A. E., and Good, R. A. (1967). *Advan. Immunol.* **6,** 91.

Galton, D. A. (1956). *Advan. Cancer Res.* **4,** 73.

Gardner, W. U. (1950). *Proc. Soc. Exp. Biol. Med.* **75,** 434.

Gardner, W. U., Kirschbaum, A., and Strong, L. C. (1940). *Arch. Pathol.* **29,** 1.

Garvey, J. S., and Campbell, D. H. (1957). *J. Exp. Med.* **105,** 361.

Gell, P. G. H., and Coombs, R. R. A. (1968). "Clinical Aspects of Immunology." Davis, Philadelphia, Pennsylvania.

Gell, P. G. H., and Hinde, I. T. (1951). *Brit. J. Exp. Pathol.* **32,** 516.

Geller, B. D., and Speirs, R. S. (1968). *Immunology* **15,** 707.

Gentry, G. A., Dorsett, M. T., and Morse, P. A. (1970). *Proc. 10th Int. Cancer Congr., Houston, Tex.* Abstr. 397, No. 643.

Gieldanowski, J., Pelczarska, A., Patkowski, J., Michalski, Z., and Szaga, B. (1969). *Arch. Immunol. Ther. Exp.* **17,** 380.
Gill, F. A., and Cole, R. M. (1965). *J. Immunol.* **94,** 898.
Göing, H., Günther, G., Gujarathi, S., and Kaiser, P. (1970). *Int. Arch. Allergy Appl. Immunol.* **38,** 420.
Goldberg, I. H. (1965). *Amer. J. Med.* **39,** 732.
Goldeck, H. (1950). *Sang* **21,** 390.
Goldin, A., Kaziwara, K., Kinosita, R., and Yamamura, Y., eds. (1970). *Gann Monogr.* **2.**
Good, R. A., and Kelly, W. D. (1970). *In* "Organ Transplantation" (F. Largiader, ed.), pp. 31–49. Thieme, Stuttgart.
Gordon, A. S. (1955). *Ann. N.Y. Acad. Sci.* **59,** 907.
Gottlieb, A. A., Glisin, V. R., and Doty, P. (1967). *Proc. Nat. Acad. Sci. U.S.* **57,** 1849.
Graw, R. G., Buckner, C. D., Whang-Peng, J., Leventhal, B. G., Krüger, G., Berard, C., and Henderson, E. S. (1970). *Lancet* **ii,** 338.
Gray, G. D., Crim. J. A., and Mickelson, M. M. (1968a). *Transplantation* **6,** 818.
Gray, G. D., Mickelson, M. M., and Crim, J. A. (1968b). *Transplantation* **6,** 805.
Gregoire, C. (1946). *J. Endocrinol.* **5,** 68.
Gross, U. M. (1964). *Verh. Deut. Ges. Pathol.* **48,** 135.
Gruhn, J. G., and Sanson, J. (1963). *Cancer (Philadelphia)* **16,** 61.
Grundmann, E. (1970a). *Verh. Deut. Ges. Pathol.* **54,** 65.
Grundmann, E. (1970b). *Progr. Antimicrob. Anticancer Chemother.* **2,** 273.
Hackmann, C. (1952). *Z. Krebsforsch.* **58,** 607.
Hackmann, C. (1954). *Z. Krebsforsch.* **60,** 250.
Hakim, A. A. (1957). *J. Biol. Chem.* **228,** 459.
Hakim, A. A. (1960). *Enzymologia* **22,** 73.
Halkerston, I. D. K., Scully, E., Feinstein, M., and Hechter, O. (1965). *Life Sci.* **4, 1473.**
Hamilton, L., Philips, F. S., Sternberg, S. S., Clarke, D. A., and Hitchins, G. H. (1954). *Blood* **9,** 1062.
Hanna, M. G., and Wust, C. J. (1964). *Exp. Hematol.* **7,** 63.
Hanna, M. G., and Wust, C. J. (1965). *Lab. Invest.* **14,** 272.
Hansen, H. G. (1957). *Proc. 6th Eur. Haematol. Congr., Copenhagen* **2,** 59.
Hansen, M. M., Hertz, H., and Videback, A. A. (1966). *Acta Med. Scand.* **180,** 211.
Harris, S., and Harris, T. N. (1950). *Proc. Soc. Exp. Biol. Med.* **74,** 186.
Harris, T. N., and Harris, S. (1956). *Amer. J. Med.* **20,** 114.
Hart, P., and Rees, R. J. W. (1950). *Lancet* **ii,** 391.
Hartman, S. C., Levenberg, B., and Buchanan, J. M. (1956). *J. Biol. Chem.* **221,** 1057
Hashimoto, T., Miura, K., and Nagai, R. (1965). *Proc. Jap. Soc. Reticuloendothel. Syst.* **5,** 116
Hata, Z., Sano, Y., Sugawara, R., Kanamori, K., Shima, T., and Hoshi, T. (1956). *J. Antibiot.* **9,** 141.
Haurowitz, F. (1965). *Physiol. Rev.* **45,** 1.
Hayashi, S., Ueki, H., and Komija, J. (1964a). *Gann* **55,** 289.
Hayashi, S., Ueki, H., and Ueki, Y. (1964b). *Gann* **55,** 1.
Heller, J. H. (1955). *Endocrinology* **56,** 80.
Henderson, J. F., LePage, G. A., and McIver, F. (1957). *Cancer Res.* **17,** 609.
Heppel, L. A., Whitfield, P. A., and Markham, R. (1955). *Biochem. J.* **60,** 8.
Herrmann, R. L., Day, R. A., and Buchanan, J. M. (1959). *Amer. Chem. Soc., 135th Meet.* Abstr., p. 45C.
Hess, M. W. (1970). *In* "Handbuch der Allgemeinen Pathologie" (H. W. Altmann, F. Büchner, H. Cottier, E. Grundmann, G. Holle, E. Letterer, W. Masshoff, H.

Messen, F. Roulet, G. Seifert, G. Siebert, and A. Studer, eds.), pp. 183–236. Springer-Verlag, Berlin and New York.

Hilz, H., Hubmann, B., Oldekop, M., Scholz, M., and von Gossle, M. (1962). *Biochem. Z.* **336**, 62.

Hirano, M., Miura, M., Kakizowo, H., Morita, A., Uetani, T., Ohno, R., and Yamada, K. (1970). *Progr. Antimicrob. Anticancer Chemother.* **2**, 200.

Hitzig, W. H., Barandun, S., and Cottier, H. (1968). *Ergeb. Inn. Med. Kinderheil.* **27**, 79.

Hobik, H. P. (1969a). *Naturwissenschaften* **56**, 217.

Hobik, H. P. (1969b). *Verh. Deut. Ges. Pathol.* **53**, 525.

Hoehn, R. J. (1965). *Transplantation* **3**, 131.

Hölzel, F., Maass, H., and Kübjekm, G. A. (1961). *Naturwissenschaften* **48**, 627.

Hölzel, F., Pflüger, P., Barth, O., and Maass, H. (1965). *Z. Krebsforsch.* **66**, 559.

Hoyer, J. R., Cooper, M. D., Gabrielsen, A. E., and Good, R. A. (1968a). *Medicine (Baltimore)* **47**, 201.

Hoyer, J. R., Cooper, M. D., Gabrielsen, A. E., and Good, R. A. (1968b). *Birth Defects, Orig. Artic. Ser.* **4**, 91.

Huennekens, F. M. (1963). *Biochemistry* **2**, 151.

Hume, D. M. (1966). *In* "The Kidney" (F. K. Mostofi and D. E. Smith, eds.), pp. 409–432. Williams & Wilkins, Baltimore, Maryland.

Hurlimann, J., Wakefield, J. D., and Thorbecke, G. J. (1966). *Exp. Hematol.* **11**, 19.

Hurlimann, J., Wakefield, J. D., and Thorbecke, G. J. (1967). *In* "Germinal Centers in Immune Responses" (H. Cottier, N. Odartchenko, R. Schnidler, and C. C. Congdon, eds.), pp. 225–233. Springer-Verlag, Berlin and New York.

Hutter, A. M., and Kayhoe, D. E. (1966). *Amer. J. Med.* **41**, 572.

Ichikawa, T., Matsuda, A., Miyamoto, K., Isubosaki, M., Kaihara, T., Sakamoto, K., and Umezawa, H. (1967). *J. Antibiot.* **20**, 149.

Isaacs, A. (1963). *Sci. Amer.* **209**, 46.

Ishizuka, M., Takayama, H., Takeuchi, T., and Umezawa, H. (1967). *J. Antibiot.* **20**, 15.

Israel, L., Delobel, J., and Bernard, E. (1965). *Pathol. Biol.* **13**, 887.

Jerne, N. K. (1955). *Proc. Nat. Acad. Sci. U.S.* **41**, 849.

Johnson, A. G., Jacobs, A., Abrams, G., and Merritt, K. (1966). *Exp. Hematol.* **11**, 20.

Johnson, B. T., Goodman, R. N., and Goldberg, H. S. (1967). *Science* **157**, 560.

Johnson, I. (1968). *Cancer Chemother. Rep.* **52**, 455.

Johnson, I. S., Armstrong, J. G., Gorman, M., and Burnett, J. P. (1963). *Cancer Res.* **23**, 1390.

Jolly, J., and Lieure, C. (1930). *C. R. Soc. Biol.* **104**, 451.

Journey, L. J., Burdman, J., and George, P. (1968). *Cancer Chemother. Rep.* **52**, 509.

Kabat, E. (1968). "Structural Concepts in Immunology and Immunochemistry." Holt, New York.

Kabat, E. A. (1966). *J. Immunol.* **97**, 1.

Karnofsky, D. A. (1967). *Fed. Proc. Fed. Amer. Soc. Exp. Biol.* **26**, 925.

Karrer, K., and Wurnig, P. (1958). *Klin. Med. (Vienna)* **13**, 196.

Kass, E. H., and Kendrick, M. (1952). *Fed. Proc. Fed. Amer. Soc. Exp. Biol.* **11**, 472.

Kidson, C. (1967). *Nature (London)* **213**, 779.

Kirschbaum, A., Liebelt, A. G., and Falls, N. G. (1955). *Cancer Res.* **15**, 685.

Kofman, S., and Ream, N. (1963). *Presbyterian St. Lukes Hosp. Med. Bull.* **2**, 16.

Kremer, W. B., and Laszlo, J. (1967). *Cancer Chemother. Rep.* **51**, 19.

Krüger, G. (1967a). *Exp. Hematol.* **14**, 12.

Krüger, G. (1967b). *J. Nat. Cancer Inst.* **39**, 1.

Krüger, G. (1968). *J. Nat. Cancer Inst.* **41,** 287.
Krüger, G. (1970a). *Verh. Deut. Ges. Pathol.* **54,** 175.
Krüger, G. (1970c). Unpublished observations.
Krüger, G. (1971a). Unpublished observations.
Krüger, G. (1971b). *Verh. Deut. Ges. Pathol.* **55,** 200.
Krüger, G. (1971c). *Pathol. Microbiol.* **37,** 436.
Krüger, G., and Harris, D. (1970). *J. Nat. Cancer Inst.* **45,** 801.
Krüger, G., and Stolpmann, H. J. (1971). *Z. Immunitaetsforsch. Allerg. Klin. Immunol.* **142,** 115.
Krüger, G., Berard, C. W., DeLellis, R. A., Graw, R. G., Yankee, R. A., Leventhal, B. G., Rogentine, G. N., Herzig, G. P., Halterman, R. H., and Henderson, E. S. (1971a). *Amer. J. Pathol.* **63,** 179.
Krüger, G., Malmgren, R. A., and Berard, C. W. (1971b). *Transplantation* **11,** 138.
Krüger, G., Berard, C. W., Elias, P., Graw, R. G., Rogentine, G. N., Leventhal, B. G., Yankee, R. A., Herzig, G. P., Halterman, R. H., and Henderson, E. S. (1971d). *Exp. Hematol* **21,** 4.
Kuchler, R. J. N., Arnold, N. J., and Grauer, R. G. (1962). *Proc. Soc. Exp. Biol. Med.* **111,** 798.
Kuff, E. L., and Roberts, N. E. (1967). *J. Mol. Biol.* **26,** 211.
Kumagai, K., Koide, T., Kikuchi, M., and Ishida, M. (1970). *Proc. 10th Int. Cancer Congr., Houston, Tex.* Abstr. 401, No. 649.
Lampert, F. (1964). *Med. Klin. (Munich)* **59,** 1001.
Lance, E. M., and Medawar, P. B. (1970). *Fed. Proc. Fed. Amer. Soc. Exp. Biol.* **29,** 151.
Landy, M., and Braun, W., eds. (1970). "Immunologic Tolerance." Academic Press, New York.
Lane, M. (1967). *Fed. Proc. Fed. Amer. Soc. Exp. Biol.* **26,** 890.
Lang, P. G., and Ada, G. L. (1967). *Immunology* **13,** 523.
LaPlante, E. S., Condie, R. M., and Good, R. A. (1962). *J. Lab. Clin. Med.* **59,** 542.
Laurentaci, G., and Berardi, T. (1970). *Proc. 6th Int. Meet. Reticuloendothel. Soc., Freiburg* Abstr., p. 80.
LaVia, M. F., Vatter, A. E., and Northrup, P. V. (1968). *Fed. Proc. Fed. Amer. Soc. Exp. Biol.* **27,** 318.
Leduc, E. H., Avrameas, S., and Bouteille, M. (1968). *J. Exp. Med.* **127,** 109.
Lee, S. L., Meiselas, L. E., Zingale, S. B., and Richman, S. M. (1961). *Arthritis Rheum.* **4,** 56.
Lennert, K. (1961). *In* "Handbuch der Speziellen Pathologischen Anatomie und Histologie" (O. Lubarsch, F. Henke, R. Rössle, and E. Uehlinger, eds.), Vol. I/3. Springer-Verlag, Berlin and New York.
Lennert, K., and Rinneberg, H. (1961). *Klin. Wochenschr.* **39,** 923.
Letterer, E. (1948). *Klin. Wochenschr.* **26,** 385.
Letterer, E. (1967). *In* "Handbuch der Allgemeinen Pathologie" (F. Büchner, E. Letterer, and F. Roulet, eds.), Vol VII/2, pp. 1–253. Springer-Verlag, Berlin and New York.
Lettré, H. (1943). *Hoppe-Seyler's Z. Physiol. Chem.* **278,** 201.
Lettré, H., and Lettré, R. (1946). *Naturwissenschaften* **33,** 283.
Levenberg, B., Hartman, S. C., and Buchanan, J. M. (1956). *J. Biol. Chem.* **220,** 379.
Levenberg, B., Melnick, I., and Buchanan, J. M. (1957). *J. Biol. Chem.* **225,** 163.
Levey, R. H. (1970). *Fed. Proc. Fed. Amer. Soc. Exp. Biol.* **29,** 156.

Levey, R. H., and Medawar, P. B. (1966). *Proc. Nat. Acad. Sci. U.S.* **56,** 1130.
Levis, A. G., Danieli, G. A., and Piccini, E. (1965). *Nature* (*London*) **207,** 608.
Levy, H. B., Law, L. W., and Rabson, A. S. (1969). *Proc. Nat. Acad. Sci. U.S.* **62,** 357.
Limburg, H., and Krahe, M. (1961). *In* "Krebsforschung und Krebsbekämptung" (H. A. Gottron, E. Ühlinger, T. Antoine, and W. Nikolowski, eds.), Vol. 4, p. 94. Urban & Schwarzenberg, Munich.
Liss, E., and Palme, G. (1964). *Z. Krebsforsch.* **66,** 196.
Lits, F. J. (1934). *C. R. Soc. Biol.* **115,** 1421.
Lührs, W. (1961). *In* "Krebsforschung und Krebsbekämpfung" (H. A. Gottron, E. Ühlinger, T. Antoine, and W. Nikolowski, eds.), Vol. 4, p. 111. Urban & Schwarzenberg, Munich.
Lundin, M., and Schelin, U. (1966). *Pathol. Eur.* **1,** 15.
McDevitt, H. O. (1968). *J. Reticuloendothel. Soc.* **5,** 256.
McKhann, C. F. (1969). *Transplantation* **8,** 209.
Maeda, H., and Meienhofer, J. (1970). *Proc. 10th Int. Cancer Congr., Houston, Tex.* Abstr. 400, No. 648.
Maguire, H. C., and Maibach, H. I. (1961). *J. Invest. Dermatol.* **37,** 427.
Maguire, H. C., and Stiers, E. (1963). *Experientia* **19,** 591.
Mahler, H. R., and Cordes, E. H. (1968). "Basic Biological Chemistry." Harper, New York.
Malmgren, R. A., Bennison, B. E., and McKinley, T. W. (1952a). *Proc. Soc. Exp. Biol. Med.* **79,** 484.
Malmgren, R. A., Bennison, B. E., and McKinely, T. W. (1952b). *J. Nat. Cancer Inst.* **12,** 807.
Mandel, H. G. (1959). *Pharmacol. Rev.* **11,** 743.
Mandel, H. G., and Carló, P. E. (1953). *J. Biol. Chem.* **201,** 335.
Mariani, T., Linna, T. J., and Good, R. A. (1971). *Exp. Hematol.* **21,** 26.
Masshoff, W., and Gross, U. (1962). *Virchows Arch. Pathol. Anat. Physiol.* **335,** 109.
Masshoff, W., and Krüger, G. (1968). Unpublished observations.
Masshoff, W., Heinzel, W., Von Rom, D., and Siess, M. (1948). *Klin. Wochenschr.* **26,** 397.
Massimo, L. (1970). *Blut* **20,** 44.
Mathé, G. (1966). "La Chimiotherapie des Cancers." Expansion Sci., Paris.
Mathé, G., Berumen, L., Schweisguth, O., Brule, G., Schneider, M., Cattan, A., Amiel, J. L., and Schwarzenberg, L. (1963). *Lancet* **ii,** 1077.
Matthews, R. E. F. (1958). *Pharmacol. Rev.* **10,** 359.
Meier, H., Hancock, R., and Huebner, R. J. (1970a). *Life Sci.* **9,** 641.
Meier, H., Myers, D. D., and Huebner, R. J. (1970b). *Life Sci.* **9,** 653.
Meier, R., and Ecklin, B. (1960). *Experientia* **16,** 204.
Melchers, F., and Knopf, P. M. (1969). *Cold Spring Harbor Symp. Quant. Biol.* **32,** 255.
Merrill, J. P. (1962). *Blood* **20,** 119.
Merritt, K., and Johnson, A. G. (1963). *J. Immunol.* **91,** 266.
Metschnikoff, E. (1892). "Lecons sur la Pathologie Comparée de l'Inflammation." Masson, Paris.
Meyler, L., ed. (1958–1966). "Side Effects of Drugs," Vols. I–VI. Exerpta Med. Found., Amsterdam.
Micu, D., Mihailescu, E., and Astaldi, A. (1970). *Proc. 6th Int. Meet. Reticuloendothel. Soc., Freiburg* Abstr., p. 98.

Mielsch, M., Grimberg, H., Dold, U., and Holzer, H. (1962). *Biochim. Biophys. Acta* **62,** 519.

Miescher, P. A., and Müller-Eberhard, H. J. (1968). "Textbook of Immunopathology." Grune & Stratton, New York.

Miller, J., and Cole, J. J. (1967). *J. Exp. Med.* **126,** 109.

Mitsui, A., Suzuki, S., Koyama, K., and Akiba, T. (1970). *Progr. Antimicrob. Anticancer Chemother.* **2,** 130.

Monaco, A. P., Wood, M. L., Gray, J. G., and Russell, P. S. (1966). *J. Immunol.* **96,** 229.

Mori, Y., and Lennert, K. (1969). "Electron Microscopic Atlas of Lymph Node Cytology and Pathology." Springer-Verlag, Berlin and New York.

Morrison, B. H., III, ed. (1960). *Nat. Cancer Inst. Monogr.* **3,**

Mosedale, B. K., Felstead, K. J., and Parke, J. A. C. (1968). *Nature (London)* **218,** 983.

Movat, H. Z., and Fernando, N. V. (1965). *Exp. Mol. Pathol.* **4,** 155.

Mowbray, J. F. (1967). *J. Clin. Pathol.* **20,** Suppl., 499.

Mowbray, J. F., Boylston, A. W., Milton, J. D., and Weksler, M. (1969). *Antibiot. Chemother. (Basel)* **15,** 384.

Müller-Beissenhirtz, P., Schmidt, J., Hilfrich, J., Althoff, J., and Mohr, U. (1971). *Transplantation* **11,** 102.

Müller-Bérat, C. N. (1969). *Acta Pathol. Microbiol. Scand.* **77,** 750.

Murphy, M. L., Ellison, R. R., Karnofsky, D. A., and Burchenal, J. H. (1954). *J. Clin. Invest.* **33,** 1388.

Nadler, S. H., and Moore, G. E. (1964). *Arch. Surg. (Chicago)* **89,** 592.

Neidhardt, M. (1969a). *Monatsschr. Kinderheilk.* **117,** 282.

Neidhardt, M. (1969b). *Z. Gesamte Exp. Med.* **150,** 161.

Neil, G. L., and Moxley, T. E. (1970). *Proc. 10th Int. Cancer Congr., Houston, Tex.* Abstr. 416, No. 674.

Nelson, A. A., and Woodard, G. (1949). *Arch. Pathol.* **48,** 387.

Nelson, J. H., and Hall, J. E. (1967). *In* "Germinal Centers in Immune Responses" (H. Cottier, N. Odartschenko, R. Schindler, and C. C. Congdon, eds.), pp. 432–437. Springer-Verlag, Berlin and New York.

Newton, B. A. (1965). *Annu. Rev. Microbiol.* **19,** 209.

Nicol, T., and Bilbey, D. L. J. (1960). *In* "Reticuloendothelial Structure and Function" (J. H. Heller, ed.), pp. 301–320. Ronald Press, New York.

Nossal, G. J. V., Ada, G. L., and Austin, C. M. (1964). *Aust. J. Exp. Biol. Med. Sci.* **42,** 311.

Obrecht, P., and Fusenig, N. (1965). *Z. Krebsforsch.* **66,** 496.

Obretenova, K. (1963). *Dokl. Bolg. Akad. Nauk* **16,** 677.

O'Brien, W. M., Van Scott, E. J., Black, R. L., Eisen, A. Z., and Bunim, J. J. (1962). *Arthritis Rheum.* **5,** 312.

Ochoa, M., Jr., and Hirschberg, E. (1967). *In* "Experimental Chemotherapy" (R. J. Schnitzer and F. Hawking, eds.), Vol. 5, pp. 1–132. Academic Press, New York.

Oerkermann, H., and Hirschmann, W. D. (1970). *Progr. Antimicrob. Anticancer Chemother.* **2,** 269.

Oleson, J. J., Bennett, P. L., Halliday, S. L., and Williams, J. H. (1955). *Acta Unio Int. Contra Cancrum* **11,** 161.

Ono, T., Terayama, H., Tokoku, F., and Nakao, N. (1968). *Biochim. Biophys. Acta* **161,** 361.

Oort, J., and Turk, J. L. (1965). *Brit. J. Exp. Pathol.* **46,** 147.

Page, A. R. (1965). *Ann. N.Y. Acad. Sci.* **116,** 950.

Page, A. R., Condie, R. M., and Good, R. A. (1962). *Amer. J. Pathol.* **40,** 519.
Page, A. R., Condie, R. M., and Good, R. A. (1963). *Blood* **20,** 118.
Palme, G., and Liss, E. (1964). *Proc. 6th Int. Congr. Biochem., New York* Abstr., p. 273.
Pardee, A. B. (1964). *Nat. Cancer Inst. Monogr.* **14,** 7.
Parish, C. R. (1971). *Ann. N.Y. Acad. Sci.* **181,** 108.
Parker, C. W., and Vavra, J. D. (1969). *Progr. Hematol.* **6,** 1.
Paterson, P. Y. (1968). *In* "Textbook of Immunopathology" (P. A. Miescher and H. J. Müller-Eberhard, eds.), Vol. I, pp. 132–149. Grune & Stratton, New York.
Peña, A., Dvorkin, B., and White, A. (1966). *J. Biol. Chem.* **241,** 2144.
Penn, E., and Starzl, T. E. (1970). *Int. Z. Klin. Pharmakol. Ther. Toxikol.* **3,** 49.
Pepper, F. (1961). *J. Endocrinol.* **22,** 335.
Pernis, B. (1967). *In* "Germinal Centers in Immune Responses" (H. Cottier, N. Odartschenko, R. Schindler, and C. C. Congdon, eds.), pp. 112–119. Springer-Verlag, Berlin and New York.
Petering, H. G. (1952). *Physiol. Rev.* **32,** 197.
Philips, F. S., Schwartz, H. S., and Sternberg, S. S. (1960). *Cancer Res.* **20,** 1354.
Pinchuck, P., Fishman, M., Adler, F. L., and Maurer, P. H. (1968). *Science* **160,** 194.
Pizon, P. (1955). *Presse Med.* **63,** 1158.
Porter, K. A. (1967). *J. Clin. Pathol.* **20,** Suppl., 518.
Porter, K. A., Marchioro, T. L., and Starzl, T. E. (1965). *Brit. J. Urol.* **37,** 250.
Potel, J. (1965). *Arzneim.-Forsch.* **15,** 527.
Potel, J. (1970). *Proc. 6th Int. Meet. Reticuloendothel. Soc., Freiburg* Abstr. p. 112.
Potel, J., and Brock, N. (1965). *Arzneim.-Forsch.* **15,** 659.
Preisler, H. D., and Henderson, *B.* S. (1969). *Proc. Amer. Ass. Cancer Res.* **10,** 70.
Press, E. M., and Butler, J. A. V. (1952). *J. Chem. Soc., London* p. 626.
Pribnow, J. F., and Silverman, M. S. (1967). *J. Immunol.* **98,** 225.
Pritchard, R. W., and Hayes, D. M. (1961). *Amer. J. Pathol.* **38,** 328.
Pütter, J. (1961). *Krebsarzt* **16,** 249.
Pullar, D. M., James, K., and Naysmith, S. D. (1968). *Clin. Exp. Immunol.* **3,** 457.
Rabson, A. S., Tyrrell, S. A., and Levy, H. (1969). *Proc. Soc. Exp. Biol. Med.* **131,** 495.
Rall, D. P., Ben, M., and McCarthy, D. M. (1963). *Proc. Amer. Ass. Cancer Res.* **4,** 55.
Ratner, S., and Petrack, B. (1953). *J. Biol. Chem.* **200,** 161.
Regelson, W. (1968a). *Advan. Cancer Res.* **11,** 123.
Regelson, W. (1968b). *Advan. Chemother.* **3,** 303.
Regelson, W., and Munson, A. (1970). *Proc. 10th Int. Cancer Congr., Houston, Tex.* Abstr. p. 403, No. 653.
Regelson, W., Munson, A. E., Munson, J. A., Mayer, G. D., and Krueger, R. F. (1970). *Proc. 6th Int. Meet. Reticuloendothel. Soc., Freiburg* Abstr., p. 116.
Reich, E. (1963). *Cancer Res.* **23,** 1428.
Reichard, P., and Lagerkvist, U. (1953). *Acta Chem. Scand.* **7,** 1207.
Reid, I. M., Shinozuka, H., and Sidransky, H. (1970). *Lab. Invest.* **23,** 119.
Reilly, H. C. (1958). *Amino Acids Peptides Antimetab. Activ., Ciba Found. Symp.* pp. 62–74.
Richards, J. F. (1968). *Cancer Chemother. Rep.* **52,** 463.
Richards, J. F., and Beer, C. T. (1964). *Lloydia* **27,** 346.
Ringertz, N., and Adamson, C. A. (1950). *Acta Pathol. Microbiol. Scand. Suppl.* **86,** 1.
Roberts, K. B., Florey, H. W., and Jorlik, W. K. (1952). *Quart. J. Exp. Physiol. Cog. Med. Sci.* **37,** 239.
Roos, B. (1970). *In* "Handbuch der Allgemeinen Pathologie" (H. W. Altmann, F. Büchner, H. Cottier, E. Grundmann, G. Holie, E. Letterer, W. Masshoff, H.

Meessen, F. Roulet, G. Seifert, G. Siebert, and A. Studer, eds.), pp. 1–128. Springer-Verlag, Berlin and New York.

Ross, W. C. J. (1958). *Ann. N.Y. Acad. Sci.* **68,** 669.

Ross, W. C. J. (1962). "Biological Alkylating Agents." Butterworth, London.

Rowland, G. F., and Edwards, A. J. (1969). *Eur. J. Cancer* **5,** 437.

Rusconi, A., DeFronzo, G., and DiMarco, A. (1968). *Cancer Chemother. Rep.* **52,** 331.

Rutman, R. J., Steele, W. J., Jones, J., and Price, C. C. (1961). *Cancer Chemother.* Abstr. **2,** 3261.

Sabesin, S. M., Fallon, H. J., and Andriole, V. T. (1963). *Arch. Intern. Med.* **111,** 661.

Sahiar, K., and Schwartz, R. S. (1966). *Int. Arch. Allergy Appl. Immunol.* **29,** 52.

Samaan, N. A. (1970). *Proc. 10th Int. Cancer Congr., Houston, Tex.* Abstr. 532, No. 860.

Santos, G., and Owens, A. H. (1964). *Bull. Johns Hopkins Hosp.* **114,** 384.

Santos, G., and Owens, A. H. (1966). *Nature* (*London*) **210,** 139.

Schabel, F. M., Johnston, T. P., McCaleb, G. S., Montgomery, M., Laster, W. R., and Skipper, H. E. (1963). *Cancer Res.* **23,** 725.

Scheiffarth, F., and Zicha, L. (1967). *In* "Handbuch der Allgemeinen Pathologie" (F. Büchner, E. Letterer, and F. Roulet, eds.), pp. 317–414. Springer-Verlag, Berlin and New York.

Schmähl, D. (1970). "Entstehung, Wachstum und Chemotherapie maligner Tumoren." Cantor, Aulendorf, Germany.

Schneiderman, M. A. (1962). *J. Chron. Dis.* **15,** 283.

Schnitzer, R. J., and Hawking, F., eds. (1966). "Experimental Chemotherapy," Vol. 4. Academic Press, New York.

Schoenberg, M. D., Muman, V. R., Moore, R. D., and Weisberger, R. S. (1964). *Science* **143,** 964.

Schwartz, R., ed. (1967). *Fed. Proc. Fed. Amer. Soc. Exp. Biol.* **26,** 880–960.

Schwartz, R., and Dameshek, W. (1962). *Blood* **19,** 483.

Schwartz, R., Stack, J., and Dameshek, W. (1958). *Proc. Soc. Exp. Biol. Med.* **99,** 164.

Schwartz, R. S. (1968). *In* "Human Transplantation" (F. T. Rapaport and J. Dausset, eds.), pp. 440–471. Grune & Stratton, New York.

Schwartzendruber, D. C. (1966). *Amer. J. Pathol.* **48,** 613.

Schwarz, R., and André, J. (1962). *In* "Mechanisms of Cell and Tissue Damage Produced by Immune Reactions" (P. Grabar and P. A. Miescher, eds.), p. 385. Schwabe, Basel.

Sellei, C., Eckhardt, S., and Németh, L. (1970). "Chemotherapy of Neoplastic Diseases." Akad. Kiadó, Budapest.

Shimoyama, M., and Hutchison, D. J. (1970). *Progr. Antimicrob. Anticancer Chemother.* **2,** 193.

Sidwell, R. W., Dixon, G. J., Sellers, S. M., and Schabel, F. M. (1965). *Appl. Microbiol.* **13,** 579.

Siebert, G. (1968). *In* "Handbuch der Allgemeinen Pathologie" (H. W. Altmann, F. Büchner, H. Cottier, E. Grundmann, G. Holle, E. Letterer, W. Masshoff, H. Meessen, F. Roulet, G. Seifert, G. Siebert, and A. Studer, eds.), pp. 1–237. Springer-Verlag, Berlin and New York.

Silberberg,M., and Silberberg,R. (1949). *Proc. Soc. Exp. Biol.Med.* **72,** 547.

Smiley, J. C., Heard, J. G., and Ziff, M. (1964). *J. Exp. Med.* **119,** 881.

Snell, J. F. (1960). *In* "Reticuloendothelial Structure and Function" (J. H. Heller, ed.), pp. 321–332. Ronald Press, New York.

Sonne, C. J., Lin, I., and Buchanan, J. M. (1956). *J. Biol. Chem.* **220,** 369.

Spain, D. M., Molomut, M. N., and Haber, A. (1950). *Science* **112,** 335.

Spielberg, H. L., and Miescher, P. A. (1963). *J. Exp. Med.* **118,** 869.

Spitler, L., and Fudenberg, H. H. (1970). *Vox Sang.* **18,** 450.

Spitz, S. (1948). *Cancer (Philadelphia)* **1,** 383.

Starzl, T. E., Marchioro, T. L., and Waddell, W. R. (1963). *Surg. Gynecol. Obstet.* **117,** 385.

Steele, W. J. (1962). *Proc. Amer. Ass. Cancer Res.* **3,** 364.

Stefani, S., and Oester, Y. T. (1967). *Transplantation* **5,** 317.

Stefani, S., and Schrek, R. (1964). *J. Lab. Clin. Med.* **63,** 1027.

Steffen, C. (1968). "Allgemeine und experimentelle Immunologie und Immunopathologie sowie ihre klinische Anwendung." Thieme, Stuttgart.

Steiner, L. A., and Porter, R. R. (1967). *Biochemistry* **6,** 3957.

Stender, H. S., Strauch, D., Winter, H., and Textor, W. (1963). *Arzneim.-Forsch.* **13,** 1031.

Swenson, R. M., and Kern, M. (1968). *Proc. Nat. Acad. Sci. U.S.* **59,** 546.

Sykes, M. P. (1958). *Ann. N.Y. Acad. Sci.* **68,** 1035.

Szakal, A. K., and Hanna, M. G. (1968). *Exp. Mol. Pathol.* **8,** 75.

Takabatake, T. (1961). *Osaka Shiritsu Daigaku Igaku Zasshi* **10,** 87.

Tan, C., Wollner, N., and Habhbin, M. (1970). *Proc. 10th Int. Cancer Congr., Houston, Tex.* Abstr. 479, No. 775.

Tasaka, S., Mashimo, K., Kuroda, Y., and Harada, T. (1965). Mitomycin C Fundamental and Clinical Reports. Kyowa, Hakko, Kogyo, Tokyo.

Thiel, N., L'Age-Stehr, J., and Wacher, A. (1967). *Hoppe-Seyler's Z. Physiol. Chem.* **348,** 1407.

Thurner, J. (1970). "Iatrogene Pathologie." Urban & Schwarzenberg, Munich.

Timmis, G. (1967). "Chemotherapy of Cancer." Butterworth, London.

Timmis, G. M., Lawley, P. D., Leese, C. L., Lister, J. H., and Hems, G. (1959). *Angew. Chem.* **71,** 44.

Traut, E. F., and Ellman, J. (1952). *J. Amer. Med. Ass.* **149,** 1214.

Travis, R. H., and Sayers, G. (1965). *In* "The Pharmaceutical Basis of Therapeutics" (L. S. Goodman and A. Gillman, eds.), pp. 1608–1648. Macmillan, New York.

Trowell, O. A. (1966). *Quart. J. Exp. Physiol. Cog. Med. Sci.* **51,** 207.

Troy, W., Smith, S., Personens, G., Moser, L., James, E., Sparks, S. J., Sevens, M., Halliday, S. L., McKenzie, D., and Oleson, J. J. (1954). *Antibiot. Annu.* 1953/1954, p. 186.

Turcotte, J. G., Haines, R. F., Brody, G. L., Meyer, T. J., and Schwartz, S. A. (1968). *Transplantation* **6,** 248.

Turk, J. L. (1964a). *Int. Arch. Allergy Appl. Immunol.* **24,** 191.

Turk, J. L. (1964b). *In* "Cyclophosphamide" (G. H. Fairley and J. M. Simister, eds.), p. 151. Wright, Bristol.

Turk, J. L. (1967). *Brit. Med. Bull.* **23,** 3.

Turk, J. L. (1970). *Fed. Proc. Fed. Amer. Soc. Exp. Biol.* **29,** 136.

Turk, J. L., and Oort, J. (1970). *In* "Handbuch der Allgemeinen Pathologie" (H. W. Altmann, F. Büchner, H. Cottier, E. Grundmann, G. Holle, E. Letterer, W. Masshoff, H. Meessen, F. Roulet, G. Seifert, G. Siebert, and A. Studer, eds.), Vol. VII/3, pp. 392–435. Springer-Verlag, Berlin and New York.

Turk, J. L., and Willoughby, D. A. (1967). *Lancet* **i,** 249.

Ullmann, U. (1969). *Zentralbl. Bakteriol. Parasitenk. Infektionskr. Hyg., Abt.* **1,** *Orig.* **209,** 377.

Umezawa, H. (1965). *Antimicrob. Ag. Chemother.* p. 1079.

Vadlamudi, S., Padarathsingh, M., Bonmassar, E., and Goldin, A. (1970). *Proc. Soc. Exp. Biol. Med.* **133,** 1232.
Van Scott, E. J. (1963). *Proc. 12th Int. Congr. Dermatol., Washington, D.C., 1962* Abstr., p. 9.
Venditti, J. M., Abbott, B. J., DiMarco, A., and Goldin, A. (1966). *Cancer Chemother. Rep.* **50,** 659.
Vogel, T. T., Mott, V., Minton, J. P., and Zollinger, R. M. (1970). *Proc. 10th Int. Cancer Congr., Houston, Tex.* Abstr. 533, No. 862.
Volkin, E., and Cohn, W. E. (1953). *J. Biol. Chem.* **205,** 767.
Vollmer, H. (1951). *J. Pediat.* **39,** 22.
von Möllendorff, W. (1939). *Klin. Wochenschr.* **18,** 1098.
Waksman, B. H., Arbouys, S., and Arnason, B. G. (1961). *J. Exp. Med.* **114,** 997.
Warner, N. L., and Burnet, F. M. (1961). *Aust. J. Exp. Biol. Med. Sci.* **14,** 58.
Wassermann, F. (1929). *In* "Handbuch der Mikroskopischen Anatomie des Menschen" (W. von Möllendorff, ed.), Vol. I, Part 2. Springer-Verlag, Berlin and New York.
Webster, G. C., and Johnson, M. P. (1955). *J. Biol. Chem.* **217,** 641.
Weisberger, A. S. (1967). *Annu. Rev. Med.* **18,** 483.
Weisberger, A. S., Daniel, T. M., and Hoffman, A. (1964a). *J. Exp. Med.* **120,** 183.
Weisberger, A. S., Wolfe, S., and Armentrout, S. (1964b). *J. Exp. Med.* **120,** 161.
Werkheiser, W. C. (1963). *Cancer Res.* **23,** 1277.
Werner, T., and Prechtel, K. (1968). *Muenchen. Med. Wochenschr.* **110,** 1118.
Werthamer, S., Hicks, C., and Amaral, L. (1969). *Blood* **34,** 348.
Wheeler, G. P. (1962). *Cancer Res.* **22,** 651.
Wheeler, G. P., and Alexander, J. A. (1964). *Cancer Res.* **24,** 1338.
Whitelock, O. von St., ed. (1958). *Ann. N.Y. Acad. Sci.* **68,** 661.
Wiener, J. (1970). *Curr. Top. Pathol.* **52,** 143.
Wiener, J., Cottrell, T. S., Margaretten, W., and Spiro, D. (1967). *Amer. J. Pathol.* **50,** 484.
Williamson, A. R., and Askonas, B. A. (1967). *J. Mol. Biol.* **23,** 201.
Wilmans, H. (1964). "Chemotherapie maligner Tumoren." Schattauer, Stuttgart.
Wrba, H. (1962). *Naturwissenschaften* **40,** 97.
Wust, C. J., Gall, C. L., and Novelli, D. G. (1964). *Science* **143,** 1041.
Yamaki, H., Tanaka, N., and Umezawa, H. (1969). *J. Antibiot.* **22,** 315.
Young, I., and Friedman, H. (1967). *In* "Germinal Centers in Immune Responses" (H. Cottier, N. Odartschenko, R. Schindler, and C. C. Congdon, eds.), pp. 102–111. Springer-Verlag, Berlin and New York.
Zollinger, H. U. (1960). *In* "Handbuch der Allgemeinen Pathologie" (F. Büchner, E. Letterer, and F. Roulet, eds.), pp. 127–28. Springer-Verlag, Berlin and New York.
Zschiesche, W. (1968). *In* "Proceedings of the Symposium on Amyloidosis" (E. Mandema, L. Ruinen, J. H. Scholten, and A. S. Cohen, eds.), pp. 327–334. Excerpta Med. Found., Amsterdam.
Zschiesche, W., and Augsten, K. (1970). *Proc. 6th Int. Meet. Reticuloendothel. Soc., Freiburg* Abstr. p. 162.
Zubrod, C. G. (1961). *J. Amer. Med. Ass.* **178,** 832.
Zukosky, C. F. (1964). *Exp. Hematol.* **7,** 66.
Zweiman, B., and Phillips, S. M. (1970). *Science* **169,** 284.

Latest Developments in the Treatment of Amebiasis

S. J. Powell

*Amoebiasis Research Unit**
Institute for Parasitology and Department of Medicine
University of Natal
Durban, South Africa

I. Introduction

Since effective drugs have been available for several decades it is paradoxical that amebiasis should still be widely regarded as a rather chronic condition of protean symptomatology which is frequently resistant to all forms of therapy. In view of the efficacy of amebicides it is more accurate to claim that amebiasis is nearly always readily curable, responding promptly and completely to correct management. Faulty diagnosis, together with erroneous assumptions regarding the pathogenicity of *Entamoeba histolytica* and of the symptoms and lesions for which it may reasonably be held responsible, are the commonest causes of apparent treatment failure. When diagnosis is correct inadequate response is most commonly due to neglect of the cardinal principle that therapy should be directed at

* The Amoebiasis Research Unit is sponsored by the following bodies: The South African Medical Research Council; The Natal Provincial Administration; The University of Natal; and The United States Public Health Service (Grant AI 09654–02).

the three possible sites where *E. histolytica* may be present. These sites are in the bowel lumen, in the gut wall, and systemically, particularly in the liver.

In the past changing concepts of the role of *E. histolytica* in producing disease have largely determined fashions in the choice of drugs. As was shown in a recent review of the therapy of amebiasis (Powell, 1971a), it is a story with relatively few landmarks.

II. Evolution of Chemotherapy in Amebiasis

A. Emetine Preparations

The foundations of our modern knowledge of clinical amebiasis date from the latter part of the last century and are based on a clearly described invasive disease, manifest as the often fatal conditions of amebic dysentery and liver abscess. Although ipecacuanha had long been used in treatment (Docker, 1858) the first landmark in therapy was the introduction of emetine hydrochloride by Rogers (1912). Its value rapidly became apparent and it has remained universally successful wherever severe invasive amebiasis is encountered. However, despite its efficacy as a tissue amebicide the drug frequently fails to eradicate amebas from the gut lumen, and, hence recurrence of symptoms is common.

In an attempt to achieve greater activity within the bowel lumen, oral emetine preparations were introduced (Du Mez, 1915). Emetine bismuth iodide (EBI) has yielded high cure rates in intestinal amebiasis and, preceded by a short course of emetine hydrochloride, is still widely used (Manson-Bahr, 1941; Woodruff, 1959). Gastrointestinal side effects are a major disadvantage.

B. Luminal Amebicides

Shortly after World War I, interest was aroused in the frequency of intestinal infections by *Entamoeba histolytica* in the temperate zones. The view became prevalent, particularly in the United States (Craig, 1926; Faust, 1941), that *E. histolytica* was an obligate pathogen which always invaded the tissues although many of those infected were symptomless and possibly even more had vague symptoms of extremely doubtful origin. It was implied that there were vast numbers of individuals with occult amebiasis in need of treatment and, hence, great impetus was given to the development of numerous luminal amebicides, chiefly arsenical and quinoline derivatives. In more recent years, diloxanide preparations have also become popular. Since all these drugs are capable to some degree of eradicating lumen-dwelling amebas, they have enjoyed a vogue for the treatment of symptomless and mildly symptomatic bowel infections, but wherever amebiasis is associated with a significant amount of tissue invasion they are inadequate.

C. Antibiotics

Soon after the advent of antibiotics, Hargreaves (1945) demonstrated the value of penicillin and sulfonamides in amebic dysentery. It was not long before this combination was replaced by the tetracyclines which have remained the antibiotics of choice, acting on *E. histolytica* apparently indirectly by modifying the bacterial flora of the bowel (McVay *et al.*, 1949; Armstrong *et al.*, 1950; Most and Van Assendelft, 1950). However, relapse may occur after apparent cure, and tetracyclines are not effective in treating hepatic amebiasis (Powell *et al.*, 1965).

D. Chloroquine

In contrast to the tetracyclines, chloroquine was found to be effective in amebic liver abscess (Conan, 1948) although it has little activity in the bowel. It has achieved wide usage as a less toxic alternative to emetine

TABLE I

Results of Treatment and Sites of Action of Amebicides on Amebic Dysentery

Therapy	Bowel lumen	Bowel wall	Liver	Percentage cure
Emetine HCl or dehydroemetine	−	+	+	30–50
Emetine HCl + EBI[a]	+	+	+	92
Luminal amebicides	+	−	−	20–50
Oral tetracycline	+	+	−	97
Chloroquine	−	−	+	10
Tetracycline + luminal amebicide + chloroquine	+	+	+	98
Tetracycline + luminal amebicide + emetine HCl or dehydroemetine	+	+	+	98

[a] Emetine bismuth iodide.

but it is less active (Harinasuta, 1951; Wilmot *et al.*, 1958). Nevertheless, it is still used as a supplementary medication.

E. Dehydroemetine

Dehydroemetine was introduced by Brossi *et al.* (1959) as an advance on natural emetine because of more rapid excretion and a more favorable liver–heart concentration ratio (Schwartz and Herrero, 1965). Although there is now doubt over claims of reduced toxicity (Johnson and Neal, 1968), in practice the synthetic preparation is a satisfactory alternative to emetine although it possesses precisely the same limitations (Powell, 1968a).

Until approximately 6 years ago, the above-described amebicides were the major drugs available for treatment. [See the reviews by Elsdon-Dew (1968), Woolfe (1963, 1966), and Wilmot (1961).] Our findings with them over 20 years of controlled trials in Durban are summarized in Tables I and II.

No single drug was effective at all the sites where *E. histolytica* might be present but when used in suitable combinations excellent cure rates could be obtained. It is by no means essential that these preparations should be entirely abandoned and under certain circumstances their use is still mandatory (see Section III, B, 4). However, in most instances they are now drugs of second choice, for, compared to the newest amebicides, such combinations are more complicated and tedious to use and some occasionally exhibit serious toxicity.

TABLE II

Results of Amebic Liver Abscess Treatment

Therapy[a]	Percentage cure
Emetine HCl (65 mg × 10 days)	88
Emetine HCl (65 mg × 2 courses)	100
Dehydroemetine (80 mg × 10 days)	88
Dehydroemetine (80 mg × 2 courses)	89
Chloroquine (× 28 days)	71
Emetine (65 mg) + chloroquine	98
Dehydroemetine (80 mg) + chloroquine	100

[a] In all instances a luminal amebicide was also given and when concomitant dysentery was present tetracycline was added.

III. More Recent Developments in Therapy

A. Niridazole

The introduction of a new series of compounds in therapy was heralded in 1964 by a preliminary report of the activity of a nitrothiazole derivative, niridazole, in amebic liver abscess (Kradolfer and Jarumilinta, 1966). It was soon demonstrated that this drug was capable of curing both intestinal and hepatic amebiasis, but more extensive trial showed it to possess undesirable toxicity (Powell *et al.*, 1969a). The significant fact remained that a compound had been discovered with a fairly high degree of activity against both intestinal and systemic infections.

B. Metronidazole

Cosar and Julou (1959) found 1-β-hydroxyethyl-2-methyl-5-nitroimidazole (metronidazole) to be systemically active against *Trichomonas vaginalis* infections when given by mouth. At a dosage of 200 mg 3 times per day for 7 days the drug rapidly came into wide usage for the treatment of urogenital trichomoniasis (Durel *et al.*, 1959, 1960). Soon after this it was also shown to possess useful activity against other infections, notably giardiasis and acute ulcerative gingivitis (Fowler, 1960; Shinn, 1962). However, its value in amebiasis was not realized until several years later (Powell *et al.*, 1966).

1. *Chemical, Physical, and Experimental Properties*

Metronidazole is a white crystalline powder which is only slightly soluble in water and ethanol, hence it must be administered orally. It has the following structural formula:

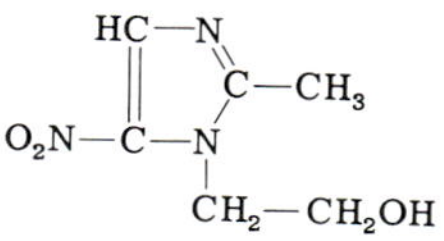

```
      HC—N
      ||  \\
      ||   C—CH3
      ||  /
O2N—C—N
       |
       CH2—CH2OH
```

A benzoyl ester suspension has been prepared for pediatric use.

The growth of intestinal protozoa *in vitro* is inhibited by metronidazole in the following minimum inhibitory concentrations: *Trichomonas vaginalis*, 0.25–1.0 μg/ml; *Trichomonas hominis*, 0.5 μg/ml; *Entamoeba histolytica*, 0.25–1.0 μg/ml; and *Balantidium coli*, 4.0–8.0 μg/ml (Powell, 1968b).

In experimental amebiasis, Cosar *et al.* (1961) found that a dosage of 100 mg/kg orally daily protected rats against intestinal infections, whereas 35 mg/kg orally daily sufficed against hepatic infections in hamsters. The precise mode of action of metronidazole against *Entamoeba histolytica* is not known although it is evident that it is a direct-acting amebicide. Since the drug is also active against some of the bacteria which inhabit the bowel, notably *Clostridium* and *Bacteroides*, it may also have some indirect activity against the parasite in the gut. It is noteworthy that other bacteria, for example, *Proteus*, *Pseudomonas*, and most strains of *Escherica coli*, are capable of inactivating metronidazole (McFadzean, 1969). This might explain failure of the drug to eradicate *Entamoeba histolytica* in some intestinal infections (see Section III, B, 3, *c*).

Absorption from the gut is rapid, peak levels in the serum being reached within 1 hour of a single dose. The bulk of the compound is excreted unchanged in the urine although two oxidation products, which are considerably less active than metronidazole against *E. histolytica*, have been isolated. Excretion is rapid and there is no evidence of a cumulative effect. Only small concentrations are found in the feces. High concentrations have been found in serum, cerebrospinal fluid (CSF), and pus aspirated from amebic liver abscess 48 hours after starting treatment (Kane *et al.*, 1961; Cosar *et al.*, 1962; Davies, 1967; McFadzean, 1969).

2. *Side Effects and Toxicity*

In animal studies metronidazole appears to be pharmacologically inert and nontoxic. The drug has a bitter taste and nausea, vomiting, drowsiness, headache, skin rashes, and pruritis have been noted. A moderate leukopenia has been observed, but there has always been a return to normal before or after completion of treatment. No effect on the cardiovascular system has been observed (Powell, 1967). Attempted suicide by the ingestion of 4.2 (Fluker, 1961), 3.6, and 12.0 gm (Lewis and Kenna, 1965) resulted in minimal disturbances.

In the dosage used for trichomoniasis and giardiasis, side effects are infrequent and rarely severe enough to stop treatment. Significant toxicity has not been observed in the high doses used in amebiasis but reports of intolerance, usually nausea and vomiting, vary. Such side effects appear to be most frequent when the disease is mild or the diagnosis of amebiasis is tenuous.

3. *Clinical Studies*

a. Amebic Dysentery. The results of our clinical trials are summarized in Table III.

In an initial trial of a dosage of 200 mg 3 times per day for 10 days, con-

TABLE III

RESULTS OF TREATMENT OF AMEBIC DYSENTERY WITH METRONIDAZOLE

Dosage[a]	No. of patients	Success (%)	Probable failure (%)	Parasitic failure (%)
200 mg t.d.s. × 10 days	11	45	0	55
400 mg t.d.s. × 10 days	20	55	30	15
800 mg t.d.s. × 10 days	50	92	4	4
800 mg t.d.s. × 5 days	30	93	7	0
800 mg t.d.s. × 2 days	10	40	0	60
2.4 gm × 1 dose	20	75	10	15
2.4 gm (single dose) daily × 2 days	30	87	0	13
2.4 gm b.d. × 1 day	20	85	0	15
2.4 gm (single dose) daily × 3 days	50	90	0	10
2.0 gm (single dose) daily × 2 days	20	95	0	5
2.0 gm (single dose) daily × 3 days	10	90	0	10

[a] Abbreviations: t.d.s., three times a day; b.d., twice a day.

ducted in 1960, the results were unsatisfactory. The potential value of the drug as an amebicide only became apparent in 1966 when a trial of 400 mg 3 times per day for 10 days was sufficiently promising to warrant testing an increased dosage of 800 mg 3 times per day for 10 days. This regimen yielded a cure rate of 90% which was almost equal in our experience to that obtained by any previous combination of amebicides (Powell *et al.*, 1966). Confirmation of these results was provided by André *et al.*, (1967).

A subsequent, more extensive trial of 800 mg 3 times per day for 10 days produced cure in 92% of patients, and it was shown that the duration of treatment could be halved to 5 days without effecting these results significantly (Powell *et al.*, 1967). Since better results were obtained by a total dose of 12.0 gm of metronidazole given over 5 days than by the same amount given as 400 mg 3 times per day for a 10-day period, it appeared that a high concentration of the drug might be more important than length of treatment. In a series of trials designed to test this possibility it was shown that a single dose of 2.4 gm was more effective than twice this amount of metronidazole given as 800 mg 3 times per day for 2 days (Powell *et al.*, 1969b). Single doses of 2.4 gm given on three successive days yielded results which were similar to our previous optimal regimen of 800 mg 3 times per day for 5 days (Powell, 1970). In our most recent studies, we have found single doses of 2.0 gm to be as effective as 2.4 gm (Powell and Elsdon-Dew, 1971). In infants and young children a regimen of 50 mg/kg/day for 7 days has been shown to equal the most satisfactory combinations of older amebicides (Rubidge *et al.*, 1970; Watson *et al.*, 1970).

Metronidazole has now been widely tested in amebic dysentery in many parts of the world, including West Africa, Pakistan, India, Malaysia, and the Americas, with almost uniformly satisfactory results although there has been a good deal of variation in dosage. In our experience a notable feature is the prompt relief of dysenteric symptoms, usually within 12 to 24 hours of beginning treatment.

b. Amebic Liver Abscess. The potential of metronidazole as a systemic amebicide became apparent during the early trials in amebic dysentery. If the latter condition is treated with a drug such as tetracycline, which has no activity against *Entamoeba histolytica* in the liver, up to 5% of patients will develop liver abscess despite cure of the intestinal infection. It is for this reason that a systemically active amebicide must be included in

TABLE IV

RESULTS OF TREATMENT OF AMEBIC LIVER ABSCESS WITH METRONIDAZOLE

Dosage[a]	No. of patients	No. cured
2.4 gm statim, 1.2 gm 6 hours later, then 800 mg t.d.s. × 9 days	20	20
800 mg t.d.s. × 10 days	20	20
2.4 gm statim, 1.2 gm 6 hours later, then 800 mg t.d.s. × 5 days	20	20
800 mg t.d.s. × 5 days	20	20
400 mg t.d.s. × 5 days	20	20
200 mg t.d.s. × 5 days + luminal amebicide (diloxanide furoate)	20	20
800 mg t.d.s. × 1 day + luminal amebicide (diloxanide furoate)	20	19 + 1 doubtful
2.0 gm (single dose)	100	96 + 2 doubtful
1.2 gm (single dose) + luminal amebicide (diloxanide furoate)	20	20
600 mg (single dose) + luminal amebicide (diloxanide furoate)	5	3
2.4 gm (single dose)	20	20

[a] Statim, at once; t.d.s., three times a day.

From Powell *et al.*, 1967, 1969b; Powell, 1970, by permission.

treatment regimens for amebic dysentery. Since none of the patients given metronidazole developed hepatic amebiasis, trials of the drug in amebic liver abscess were begun. The results of a series of trials in amebic liver abscess are summarized in Table IV.

Since small doses of metronidazole were known to be unreliable in eradicating concomitant bowel infection, an intestinal amebicide (diloxanide furoate) was added to the lowest dosage regimens. It was only at the lowest of these regimens, comprising a single dose of 600 mg that some patients with liver abscess failed to respond to treatment. It was evident that metronidazole was more potent as a tissue than intestinal amebicide and, although a choice of regimens is available, a dosage of 400 mg 3 times per day for 5 days has become widely used for the treatment of hepatic amebiasis (World Health Organization, 1969).

As in the case of amebic dysentery the drug has now been extensively tested in liver abscess in many parts of the world with excellent results. It should be stressed that the use of metronidazole has in no way altered the indications for closed aspiration in amebic liver abscess.

c. Chronic Intestinal Amebiasis. This condition includes both symptomless infections and patients with variable and often ill-defined symptoms who are found to be passing cysts of *E. histolytica*. The parasite may be scanty and inconstantly present in the feces, hence high standards of parasitological skill are required for both correct diagnosis and the assessment of cure. This may largely explain why conflicting results are often reported from different centers when evaluating amebicides in this condition.

Although a growing number of reports have appeared on the value of metronidazole in chronic intestinal amebiasis, it is prudent to view these with some caution. Success has been claimed for regimens that we find inadequate in amebic dysentery. One is reluctant to accept that there are significant regional variations in treatment response although this possibility cannot be entirely dismissed.

Although the precise place of metronidazole in the treatment of chronic intestinal amebiasis must await large-scale careful assessment, we have recently attempted to obtain a guide by studying the effect of the drug on the intestinal infection in patients with amebic liver abscess, about 50% of whom are found to be passing cysts of *E. histolytica* in the feces (Powell and Elsdon-Dew, 1971). The findings, which are summarized in Table V, indicate that, although all three regimens tested were capable of curing liver abscess, eradication of the intestinal infection was best achieved by a dosage of 800 mg 3 times per day for 5 days. Hence we now believe that this is the optimal regimen for the treatment of both liver abscess and

TABLE V

RESULTS OF TREATMENT OF AMEBIC LIVER ABSCESS WITH METRONIDAZOLE

Dosage[a]	No. of patients	No. cured	Cyst-passers after therapy
2.0 gm daily × 2 days	27	26	4/26
400 mg t.d.s. × 5 days	15	15	5/15
800 mg t.d.s. × 5 days	30	30	4/30

[a] t.d.s., three times a day.

amebic dysentery, and it is probable that not less than this dosage should be given for chronic intestinal amebiasis.

4. *Present Status of Metronidazole*

Of more than a hundred drugs and their combinations that have been evaluated by the Amoebiasis Research Unit during the past 25 years, metronidazole approximates most closely the ideal amebicide. It is easily administered, rapidly acting, well-tolerated in our experience, without significant toxicity, and effective in courses of short duration. Although the cure rates achieved are no better than those obtainable by combinations of other drugs, metronidazole is the nearest approach to an all-purpose amebicide. Nevertheless, its balance of activity at all sites is not perfect for it is more effective against *E. histolytica* in the tissues than in the intestine. Larger doses are needed to cure amebic dysentery than liver abscess.

Although the place of metronidazole in the therapy of invasive amebiasis is established, its status as a predominantly luminal amebicide for use against cyst-passers is less certain although it undoubtedly possesses significant activity. There are, however, many cheap alternative luminal amebicides.

Metronidazole can be given only by the oral route and, in the most severe cases of invasive amebiasis when peritonitis is threatened or already present, parenteral therapy is mandatory. In such instances the life-saving properties of emetine preparations in full dosage together with intravenous tetracycline should be borne in mind. Even under these circumstances it is advantageous to add metronidazole as soon as oral therapy is practicable. It is a drug which can safely be given with any other combination of amebicides.

C. New Nitroimidazole Preparations

The success of metronidazole has stimulated interest in the development of other nitroimidazole derivatives. Among these de Carneri (1969, 1970) has indicated that 1-(*N*, β-ethylmorpholine)-5-nitroimidazole (nitrimidazine, nimorazole) has been tested in intestinal and hepatic amebiasis although detailed results have not been published. The drug is well absorbed and reaches somewhat higher blood and urine levels than metronidazole. This would suggest that, although tissue activity may be enhanced, the drug is likely to be of less value against *E. histolytica* in the intestine.

Of several newer promising preparations with experimental activity against both *Trichomonas vaginalis* and *Entamoeba histolytica* only one, 1-methyl-2-(*p*-fluorophenyl)-5-nitroimidazole, has so far been subject to adequate clinical assessment. This compound was found to be seven to eightfold more potent than metronidazole in the laboratory (Cuckler *et al.*, 1970), and one favorable report of a clinical trial in amebiasis has appeared (Chari and Gadiyar, 1970). More extensive trials in both amebic dysentery and liver abscess at maximum dosages permitted by the toxicity data showed that, whereas tissue activity was comparable to that of metronidazole, the drug was less effective in eradicating *E. histolytica* from the bowel (Powell and Elsdon-Dew, 1971). Among compounds at present under clinical trial α-chloromethyl-2–methyl-5-nitro-1-imidazole ethanol is of promise (Brossi, 1969; Powell, 1971b).

IV. Conclusion

Metronidazole is an advance on older amebicides, but there remains room for improvement, and it is probable that in the near future other nitroimidazole derivatives as good, if not better, will appear. At present there is a tendency to work in the production of single new preparations superior to metronidazole against both *Trichomonas vaginalis* and *Entamoeba histolytica*. Nevertheless, this may not be the correct approach since the actions required against these two parasites are not identical. In trichomoniasis, high tissue levels are needed but in amebiasis there must also be activity within the large bowel. It must be borne in mind that laboratory evidence of increased potency is liable to be offset by increased absorption, and claims for enhanced activity in trichomoniasis are likely to be counterbalanced by reduced efficacy against intestinal amebas. Metronidazole would be an even better amebicide if it had greater activity within the bowel even at the expense of some systemic effect. All the same, among all the nitroimidazoles which have been evaluated up to the present time, it still strikes the best balance between systemic and intestinal efficacy.

References

André, L. J., Bon, J. F., Zerdani, S., and Bandelier, J. (1967). *Med. Trop. (Marseilles)* **27,** 245.
Armstrong, T. G., Wilmot, A. J., and Elsdon-Dew, R. (1950). *Lancet* **ii,** 10.
Brossi, A. (1969). *Pure Appl. Chem.* **19,** 171.
Brossi, A., Baumann, N., Chopard-dit-Jean, L. H., Würsch, J., Schneider, F., and Schnider, D. (1959). *Helv. Chim. Acta* **42,** 772.
Chari, M. V., and Gadiyar, B. N. (1970). *Amer. J. Trop. Med. Hyg.* **19,** 926.
Conan, N. J. (1948). *Amer. J. Trop. Med.* **28,** 107.
Cosar, C., and Julou, L. (1959). *Ann. Inst. Pasteur* **96,** 238.
Cosar, C., Ganter, P., and Julou, L. (1961). *Presse Med.* **69,** 1069.
Cosar, C., Dubost, M., Dubost, P., Devoize, P., and Palliere, M. (1962). *Ann. Pharm. Fr.* **20,** 872.
Craig, C. F. (1926). "Manual of Parasitic Protozoa of Man." Lippincott, Philadelphia, Pennsylvania.
Cuckler, A. C., Malanaga, C. M., and Conray, J. (1970). *Amer. J. Trop. Med. Hyg.* **19,** 916.
Davies, A. H. (1967). *Brit. J. Vener. Dis.* **43,** 197.
de Carneri, I. (1969). *Arzneim.-Forsch.* **19,** 382.
de Carneri, I. (1970). *J. Parasitol.* **56,** 69.
Docker, E. S. (1858). *Lancet* **ii,** 113.
Du Mez, A. G. (1915). *Philipp. J. Sci., Sect. B* **10,** 73.
Durel, P., Roiron, V., Siboulet, A., and Borel, L. J. (1959). *C. R. Soc. Fr. Gynecol.* **29,** 36.
Durel, P., Roiron, V., Siboulet A., and Borel, L. J. (1960). *Brit. J. Vener. Dis.* **36,** 21.
Elsdon-Dew, R. (1968). *Advan. Parasitol.* **6,** 1.
Faust, E. C. (1941). *Amer. J. Trop. Med.* **21,** 35.
Fluker, J. L. (1961). *Brit. J. Vener. Dis.* **37,** 280.
Fowler, W. (1960). *Brit. J. Vener. Dis.* **36,** 157.
Hargreaves, W. H. (1945). *Lancet* **ii,** 68.
Harinasuta, C. A. (1951). *Indian Med. Gaz.* **86,** 137.
Johnson, P., and Neal, R. A. (1968). *Ann. Trop. Med. Parasitol.* **62,** 455.
Kane, P. O., McFadzean, J., Squires, S., King, A. J., and Nichol, C. S. (1961). *Brit. J. Vener. Dis.* **37,** 273.
Kradolfer, F., and Jarumilinta, R. (1966). *Proc. 1st Int. Congr. Parasitol., Rome, 1964* p. 397.
Lewis, B. V., and Kenna, A. P. (1965). *J. Obstet. Gynaecol. Brit. Commonw.* **72,** 806.
McFadzean, J. A. (1969). *Med. Today* **3,** 10.
McVay, L. V., Laird, R. L., and Sprunt, D. H. (1949). *Science* **109,** 590.
Manson-Bahr, P. (1941). *Brit. Med. J.* **ii,** 255.
Most, H., and Van Assendelft, F. (1950). *Ann. N.Y. Acad. Sci.* **53,** 427.
Powell, S. J. (1967). *Amer. J. Trop. Med. Hyg.* **16,** 447.
Powell, S. J. (1968a). *Proc. 8th Int. Congr. Trop. Med. Malaria, Teheran* (Abstr.).
Powell, S. J. (1968b). *Med. Today* **2,** 44.
Powell, S. J. (1970). *Med. Today* **4,** 57.
Powell, S. J. (1971a). *Bull. N.Y. Acad. Med.* **47,** 469.
Powell, S. J. (1971b). Unpublished observations.
Powell, S. J., and Elsdon-Dew, R. (1971). *Amer. J. Trop. Med. Hyg.* **20,** 839.
Powell, S. J., MacLeod, I. N., Wilmot, A. J., and Elsdon-Dew, R. (1965). *Trans. Roy. Soc. Trop. Med. Hyg.* **59,** 709.

Powell, S. J., Wilmot, A. J., MacLeod, I. N., and Elsdon-Dew, R. (1966). *Lancet* **ii,** 1329.
Powell, S. J., Wilmot, A. J., and Elsdon-Dew, R. (1967). *Ann. Trop. Med. Parasitol.* **61,** 511.
Powell, S. J., Wilmot, A. J., and Elsdon-Dew, R. (1969a). *Ann. N.Y. Acad. Sci.* **160,** 749.
Powell, S. J., Wilmot, A. J., and Elsdon-Dew, R. (1969b). *Ann. Trop. Med. Parasitol.* **63,** 139.
Rogers, L. (1912). *Brit. Med. J.* **i,** 1424.
Rubidge, C. J., Scragg, J. N., and Powell, S. J. (1970). *Arch. Dis. Childhood* **45,** 196.
Schwartz, D. E., and Herrero, J. (1965). *Amer. J. Trop. Med. Hyg.* **14,** 78.
Shinn, D. L. S. (1962). *Lancet* **i,** 1191.
Watson, C. E., Leary, P. M., and Hartley, P. S. (1970). *S. Afr. Med. J.* **44,** 419.
Wilmot, A. J. (1961). "Clinical Amoebiasis." Blackwell, Oxford.
Wilmot, A. J., Powell, S. J., and Adams, E. B. (1958). *Amer. J. Trop. Med. Hyg.* **7,** 1958.
Woodruff, A. W. (1959). *Practitioner* **183,** 92.
Woolfe, G. (1963). *In* "Experimental Chemotherapy" (R. J. Schnitzer and F. Hawking, eds.), Vol. 1, pp. 355–443. Academic Press, New York.
Woolfe, G. (1966). *In* "Experimental Chemotherapy" (R. J. Schnitzer and F. Hawking, eds.), Vol. 4, pp. 432–439. Academic Press, New York.
World Health Organization (1969). *World Health Organ. Tech. Rep. Ser.* **421.**

Social Implications of Psychotropic Drugs*

F. M. Berger

Wallace Laboratories, Division of Carter-Wallace, Inc.
Cranbury, New Jersey

I. Introduction

Although the modern psychoactive drugs were introduced only within the past 15 years, they are today among the most often prescribed therapeutic agents. Since the use of these drugs has become so widespread, it seems appropriate to evaluate the social consequences resulting from their use.

Consideration will be given only to those psychotropic drugs that are used predominantly in the medical treatment of mental illness. These are the antipsychotic substances, such as phenothiazines and butyrophenones, the antidepressants, such as tricyclic dibenzocycloheptene derivatives and monoamine oxidase inhibitors, and the antianxiety tranquilizers, such as meprobamate and the benzodiazepines. Substances used primarily for psychological reasons, such as stimulants and hallucinogens, will not be discussed. The social implications of these have been reviewed by Cole and Wittenborn (1969), Kales *et al.* (1969), and Wittenborn *et al.* (1970).

The clinical effectiveness or pharmacological properties of individual drugs will not be considered. Instead, epidemiological data will be examined to see whether the introduction of these drugs was socially beneficial and

* Presented at the Menninger Foundation, Topeka, Kansas, February 8, 1971.

whether their use may have been reflected by changes in the population of mental hospitals or in the incidence of suicide. We shall also inquire whether the use of these substances, as many have feared, can cause damage to society by impairing initiative, performance, and creativity of the individual, whether these substances can be used to control the mind, whether they lead to habituation and dependence, and whether they are likely to induce asocial or dangerous behavior.

II. Decrease of Mental Hospital Population

Deaths from most infectious diseases have been steadily declining since the middle of the nineteenth century. This is illustrated in Fig. 1 showing the mean annual death rates from tuberculosis in England and Wales from 1850 to 1960. Similar declines in death rates have been reported for diphtheria, scarlet fever, rheumatic fever, pertussis, and many other infectious diseases. The mortality rates from these diseases have been declining in an almost linear fashion and do not seem to have been greatly influenced by the discoveries of the causative agents or the introduction of specific remedies. The decline in the overall rates of these diseases correlates much better with improving socioeconomic conditions than it does with advances in medicine (Kass, 1971). It is of interest to inquire whether there has been a similar decrease in the incidence of mental illness during

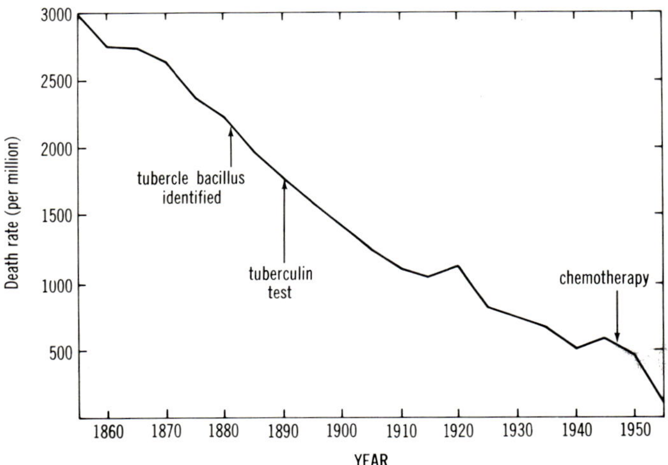

FIG. 1. Mean annual death rates from respiratory tuberculosis in England and Wales from 1860 to 1955.

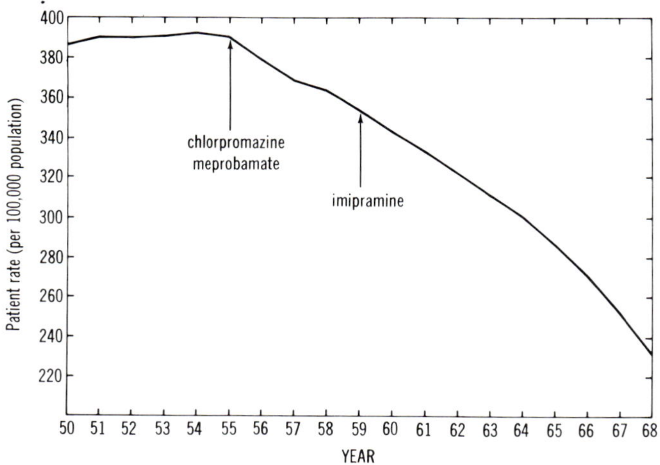

FIG. 2. Number of patients per 100,000 population in mental hospitals in the United States from 1950 to 1968.

the past 100 years and, if so, whether this has been due to an improvement of the social and economic environment, to the introduction of the psychotropic drugs, or to other factors.

Figure 2 shows the number of patients per 100,000 population resident in mental hospitals in the United States from 1950 to 1968 (Statistical Abstract, 1970). All mental hospitals have been counted including the federal, Veterans Administration, Public Health Service, state, county, and private hospitals and institutions. The patient rate was constant until 1955 when the first psychotropic drugs were introduced. Since then the patient rate has been steadily decreasing.

These trends are also apparent when the total number of patients resident in mental institutions is considered. These figures are given in Table I for the years 1935 to 1968, together with the number of patients treated in outpatient psychiatric clinics. The number of patients in mental hospitals increased from 422,000 in 1935 to 634,000 in 1955. It has been decreasing since, in spite of the continuing growth of the population, dropping to the figure of 457,000 in 1968. The number of patients treated in outpatient psychiatric clinics has been moving in the opposite direction. There were 181,000 outpatients treated in 1959, the first year for which data are available, and the number of outpatients increased to 711,000 in 1968.

Data obtained from state and county hospitals show similar but less marked trends. The number of resident patients in these hospitals has been

TABLE I

Number of Patients in Mental Hospitals and Outpatient Psychiatric Clinics in the United States (1935–1968)[a]

Year	Mental hospitals[b]	Outpatient clinics[b]
1935	422	NA
1940	479	NA
1945	522	NA
1950	580	NA
1955	634	NA
1960	611	211
1965	550	436
1968	457	711

[a] Data from Statistical Abstract (1970).

[b] Figures in thousands. Mental hospitals include federal, state, county, and private institutions. NA, not available.

gradually decreasing since 1956. Since that year there has been a greater increase in the rate of releases then in the rate of admissions year by year, although both have increased. These data are illustrated in Fig. 3 (Mental Health Statistics, 1968).

The duration of the stay has been drastically shortened. At the present

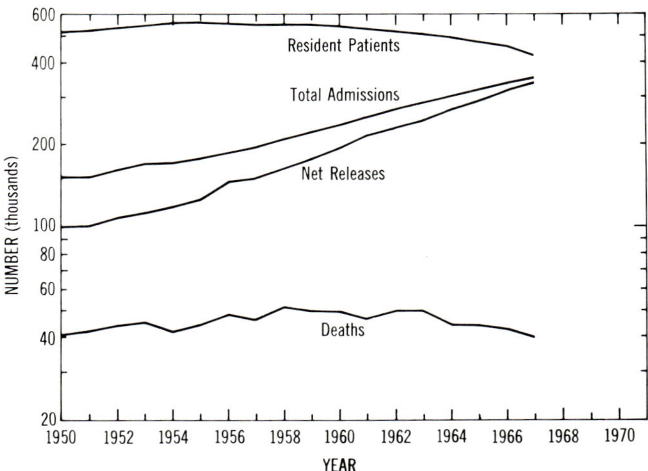

Fig. 3. Number of resident patients, total admissions, net releases, and deaths in state and county mental hospitals of the United States from 1950 to 1967.

time the vast majority of patients entering mental hospitals are released in less than a year. The readmission rate has also decreased. These trends become apparent from the data obtained from state and county mental hospitals for the year 1968 (Statistical Abstract, 1970). At the beginning of the year there were 426,364 resident patients in mental hospitals. During the year, 365,455 patients were admitted and 39,677 died. At the end of the year there were only 400,681 resident patients left in the hospitals, a decrease from the number of patients present at the beginning of the year. The net live releases, that is, the excess of patients released alive from hospitals over those remaining in or returning to hospitals, was 351,461.

III. Causes Responsible for the Decline in the Number of Mental Hospital Patients

There may be factors other than the introduction of the psychotropic drugs that could account for this reversal in the trend and the sustained decrease in the number of patients in mental hospitals since 1955. Such a decline in the number of patients in mental institutions could be due to a decrease in the spontaneous incidence of mental disease or the introduction of new administrative practices or to changes in social attitudes that were beneficial to mental patients.

There is no reason to believe that the smaller number of patients in mental hospitals is due to a spontaneous decrease in the incidence of mental disease. Indeed, the incidence of serious mental diseases, as judged by the admission rates to mental institutions, has not appreciably changed during the past 100 years. Goldhamer and Marshall (1949) compared the admission rates to mental hospitals in Massachusetts recorded from 1840 to 1885 with those recorded from 1917 to 1941. Only the first admission and not subsequent admissions of each patient were counted. These first admission rates for ages under 50 years were just as high during the last half of the nineteenth century as they were in the 1930s and early 1940s, suggesting that there has been little change in the incidence of psychosis during the past 100 years. There has, however, been a marked increase in the admission rates of the older age groups which is almost certainly to be due to a larger number of elderly people and to an increased tendency to hospitalize persons suffering from the mental diseases of the senium.

There is no question that continuous, devoted, and understanding care can greatly improve the condition and prognosis of many seriously disturbed mental patients. The outstanding humanitarian efforts of Samuel

Bayard Woodward, the Superintendent of the Worcester Hospital from 1833 to 1846, the only mental hospital in Massachusetts at that time, are of interest in this connection. He attempted to cure his mentally disturbed patients by "moral treatment," a therapeutic regimen which combined the judicious use of the then available drugs with something like contemporary milieu therapy. Among a selected sample of 1157 patients treated in this way, 58% were never readmitted to mental hospitals. Yet, moral treatment was gradually abandoned as the facilities became overcrowded. During the next decades, the number of recoveries steadily declined and during the 1870s and 1880s averaged about 23%. This trend persisted until the mid-1950s (Grob, 1966).

Studies of Pasamanick *et al.* (1964), carried out after the modern psychotropic drugs came into widespread use, indicate the joint beneficial influence of drugs and of the sejour of patients in their home environment. The authors evaluated, over a period of 18 months among 193 randomly assigned schizophrenic patients seeking hospitalization, the results obtained by subjecting some patients to community living where they received either placebo or drugs, with the results achieved in conventionally treated hospitalized patients. A surprisingly large number of outpatients were able to manage at home under placebo medication during the first few months. The superiority of the drug treatment became, however, clearly apparent after 6–18 months. In the community group, 82% of the drug-treated outpatients as compared with only 37% of the placebo subjects were successful in remaining continuously at home. In contrast, the hospital control patients spent 60% of the time in the community.

The decrease in the number of patients in mental institutions observed since 1955 cannot be due in its entirety to therapeutic practices, such as moral treatment, early discharge policy, therapeutic community concept, or the open door policy. Although envisaged and tried almost 200 years ago by Pinel (Selling, 1940), it was only after the introduction of the psychotropic drugs that these practices became acceptable and practical.

As a result of treatment with psychotropic drugs, many individuals who had to be hospitalized in the past can now be treated at home. This is apparent from the decline in the number of patients in mental hospitals since 1955, a decrease which was later accompanied by a proportionate increase in the number of patients treated in outpatient psychiatric clinics (Table I). If we assume, as we appear justified in doing, that the incidence of mental disease has not changed in the recent past, we must conclude that psychotropic drugs made it possible to treat seriously disturbed mental patients in outpatient clinics and in many cases made hospitalization unnecessary.

IV. Suicide and Antidepressants

An epidemiological evaluation of the effectiveness of antidepressants presents even greater difficulties than that of the antipsychotic drugs. Only relatively few depressed patients are admitted to mental hospitals. Suicide rates, however, may be a useful index of the prevalence of serious depressions. Barraclough *et al.* (1968) found a psychiatric diagnosis of depression in 80% of consummated suicides. If it is assumed that depression is the main cause of suicide, a decrease in suicides since the introduction of antidepressant drugs would be a measure of their effectiveness.

The number of suicides and self-inflicted injuries per million population in England and Wales from 1945 to 1967 is shown in Fig. 4 (Roth and Schapira, 1970). The rate of suicide in males has been steadily decreasing since the year 1963 and by 1967 attained a lower level than had ever been observed in the past. The suicide rates in females have also been falling significantly since 1964 but have not yet reached the low rates observed in the 1948 to 1953 period of time.

The suicide rate for the general population of the United States has been relatively constant and has fluctuated only between 9.8 and 11.1 per

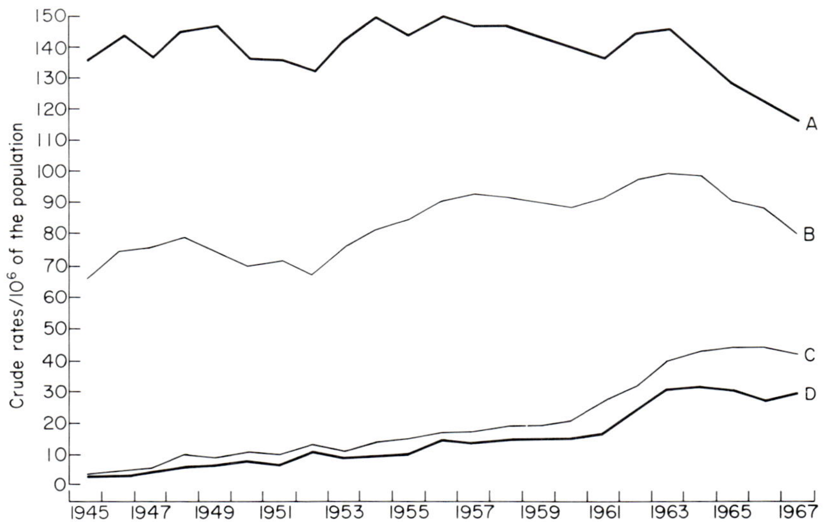

FIG. 4. Number of suicides and self-inflicted injuries per million population in England and Wales from 1945 to 1967. (A, B) Total number of suicides and self-inflicted injuries; (C, D) cases of suicide by poisoning with soporific and analgesic substances. — males; — females. (Reproduced, by permission, from Roth and Schapira, 1970.)

100,000 between 1951 and 1967. There are, however, great differences in suicide rates among various subgroups of the general population of the United States depending on race, sex, age, and social status (Berger, 1967a). Thus, the incidence of suicide among white males at all ages is appreciably higher than that of white females and that of nonwhite males or nonwhite females. In white males older than 44 years the suicide rate is more than two-thirds higher than in the other groups. Persons insured under standard policies in the Metropolitan Life Insurance Company (Statistical Bulletin, 1970) may represent a more homogeneous and suitable population sample than the general population. The policyholders are predominantly male whites, belonging to the middle class, and are presumably sufficiently intelligent and conscientious to seek medical advice when sick. In this group, suicide rates have been steadily declining since 1958. The 1969 suicide rate of 7.5 per 100,000 was the lowest ever recorded among the policyholders. The corresponding rate for the white males for the general population of the United States for the age group 25 or older fluctuated between 14.6 and 16.9 per 100,000 during this period (Table II). Since 1958, about a year after the antidepressants came into widespread use in the United States, suicide rates among policyholders have been less

TABLE II

Suicide Death Rates per 100,000 Population (1955–1969)

Year	White males U.S. over 25 years[a]	Metropolitan Life Insurance standard ord. policyholders[b]
1955	16.3	10.3
1956	16.0	9.6
1957	15.5	9.2
1958	16.9	10.0
1959	16.7	9.3
1960	15.3	9.5
1961	16.0	9.4
1962	16.8	8.5
1963	16.1	8.5
1964	14.6	8.6
1965	14.7	8.5
1966	14.4	8.3
1967	15.7	8.2
1968	NA	7.8
1969	NA	7.5

[a] Data from Statistical Abstract (1970). NA, not available.

[b] Data from Metropolitan Life Statistical Bureau.

than half those experienced by policyholders in the late 1920s and late 1930s, and less than one-quarter that which occurred within the general population. Although the low incidence of suicide in this group may reflect to some extent the selection policies of the Metropolitan Life Insurance Company, it may be attributable, at least in part, to the use of antidepressant drugs.

The evaluation of the social consequences of the antianxiety agents is even more difficult than that of the antidepressant or antipsychotic drugs. Their effect might be apparent from statistics reflecting personal adjustments, but no such tabulations appear to be available at the present time.

V. Potential for Social Damage

The introduction of psychotropic agents has substantially altered the care of the mentally ill and brought about economic and social gains, as well as improvements in the life situations of many individuals. Yet, many people have feared that these agents might reduce human initiative and drives and that this might lead to a society in which people live in chemical straitjackets or, at least, are dependent on such drugs. None of these fears has been realized.

A. Anxiety and Psychotropic Drugs

It is still widely believed that anxiety is an important motivational force in solving everyday problems of living and that it sustains initiative and the creative drive. This fallacy is due, at least in part, to a confusion between the meaning of anxiety and fear. Anxiety, in the scientific sense of the word, is an unpleasant feeling of apprehension occurring in the presence of a threat, that is, by reasonable standards, out of proportion to the emotion it evokes (Lewis, 1967). An anxious person reacts to a trivial danger as if it were a matter of life and death, and such a reaction often leads to inappropriate behavior. Fear, in contrast to anxiety, is an emotional response to a clearly defined danger which is preparatory to appropriate behavior (Berger, 1970).

Modern research in psychology has furnished a more precise understanding of the state of anxiety and has provided reliable and verifiable data describing the structure of this state. Investigations carried out primarily by Cattell and his associate (Cattell and Scheier, 1958, 1961) showed that there is only a single general reaction pattern representing the manifestations of anxiety. It is characterized by behavioral attributes, such as lack of confidence, a sense of guilt, an unwillingness to venture, general tenseness, and a readiness to become fatigued, irritable, and discouraged. It does not include behavioral responses, such as stress, neuroticism, or motivational strength. When measured in a large number of persons of various backgrounds and suffering from a variety of different diseases, anxiety was found to be qualitatively the same and indistinguishable in its characteristics and nature from person to person. Thus, there appears to be no justification in differentiating between neurotic, psychotic, or normal anxiety. They are all the same and they are all abnormal. Anxiety is not a disease but a symptom of disease which may be present in many different conditions.

It has been further shown that anxiety is not a specific drive such as sex, self-assertion, fear, or curiosity. Anxiety, in having a disruptive influence on the mind, is the opposite of a motivational drive. Motivation organizes and initiates behavior; anxiety disorganizes and suppresses initiative. Anxiety interferes with performance—more creative men are less anxious than less creative men (Berelson and Steiner, 1964). Creative men may also possess a higher ability to cope with anxiety-provoking situations than less creative men.

B. Control of the Mind and Antisocial Behavior

Many people believe that drugs used in the treatment of mental diseases could be used to control the minds of normal people. This belief may be based on the mistaken assumption that these drugs exert such an influence on the minds of the mentally sick. This, of course, is not the case. All these drugs can do and all they have done is to affect favorably certain symptoms of mental disease such as excitement, anxiety, delusions, or hallucinations. At the present, there are no known drugs that have any usefulness in the control of the mind which can be used for "brainwashing" (Kety, 1961). We do not even know how to search for a drug that could be used for this purpose (Cole, 1961).

There is no evidence that the psychotropic drugs affect the characteristic ways of thinking and acting which make up our personality. They do not alter the basic attitudes or loyalties of people (Berger and Potterfield, 1969). There is no reliable evidence to support the view that psychotropic drugs are associated with antisocial behavior or crime (Blum, 1967).

C. Habituation and Dependence

Habituation or physical dependence have not been observed after administration of antipsychotic or antidepressant drugs. The antianxiety tranquilizers can produce habituation and physical dependence if administered in excessive doses for prolonged periods of time. Abuse has occurred, with rare exceptions, only in individuals who have previously been habituated to known habit-forming agents, such as alcohol, barbiturates, or the opiates. Although these drugs can be abused, the incidence and prevalence of abuse is very low. No abuse on college campuses or by "hippie" communities has been reported. The antianxiety tranquilizers have neither the euphoriant action of alcohol or opium, nor the hallucinogenic action of the psychedelic substances. Thus, there is little incentive for normal people to take antianxiety drugs.

D. Use in Suicide

Although the incidence of suicide in the United States has not changed significantly over the period from 1953 to 1963, there has been a marked change in the means used to commit it. During this period the number of suicidal deaths due to drugs has increased from 856 in 1954 to 2666 in 1963 (Grove, 1967). In a study of suicides reported for 1963, drugs of all kinds were used in about 12% of all cases. The most frequently used drugs were barbiturates which accounted for over 75% of all the drugs used

TABLE III

Suicide from Poisoning by Drugs in 1963 (Category E 970)[a]

Drug	Alone	Mixtures	Total
Sedatives[b]	84	7	91
Nonbarbiturate hypnotics[c]	133	19	152
Barbiturates	1997	55	2052
Tranquilizers[d]	48	16	64
Neuroleptics[e]	10	5	15
Narcotics	15	3	18
Salicylates	76	7	83
Analgesics	26	8	34
Other and unspecified	8	11	19
Misclassified	40	—	40
Unspecified	98	—	98
Total	2535	131	2666

[a] Data from U.S. Department of Health, Education and Welfare, Office of Vital Statistics.

[b] Chloral hydrate, paraldehyde, carbromal.

[c] Glutethimide, methyprylon, ethinamate, ethchlorvynol.

[d] Meprobamate, chlordiazepoxide.

[e] Chlorpromazine, trifluoperazine.

(Table III). Psychotropic drugs were responsible for only about 3% of all suicides by drugs (Berger, 1967b).

The number of prescriptions written for barbiturates or psychotropic drugs during 1963 was similar (National Prescription Audit, 1965), indicating an equal availability of the two classes of drugs to persons with suicidal intent. One of the reasons for the difference between the number of suicides by these drugs may be the lesser toxicity of psychotropic agents so that suicide attempts with the more toxic barbiturates result in more deaths than suicide attempts with psychotropic drugs. However, psychotropic drugs may suppress suicidal tendencies and thus may be less frequently used for suicidal attempts (Miller *et al.*, 1959; Bell *et al.*, 1959). In a study carried out among New York City adolescents, tranquilizers were used alone or in combination with another drug in 12% of suicidal attempts. Barbiturates were used in suicidal attempts by 35% of this population (Jacobziner, 1965). The available data indicate that the recent increase in the rate of suicide by drugs is not a result of the abuse of tranquilizers or antidepressants but is primarily due to the abuse of barbiturates and of sedative–hypnotic drugs.

VI. Conclusions

The most outstanding contribution achieved by the use of psychotropic drugs has been their effect on the population of mental hospitals. Thousands of persons, who otherwise would have spent many years of their lives in crowded institutions, have been returned to the community. From this society has benefitted in at least two ways. (*1*) The dollar expenditures involved in caring for these people have been substantially reduced. It has been estimated that the cost of mental illness is at least $20 billion a year (Kline, 1968). If the trend that was evident before 1954 had persisted, at least another $6 billion would have been spent just for the construction of additional hospitals for the treatment of mental patients (Conley *et al.*, 1967). (*2*) The twofold or greater increase in the number of patients who have left mental hospitals during this time contributed, at least in some measure, to economic and social productivity that otherwise would have been completely lost to society. Yet, none of the fears and dangers anticipated 15 years ago about the use of psychotropic drugs have been realized. Although measuring social good by dollar savings may not be the most appropriate of criteria, it does suggest that psychotropic drugs have contributed materially to the well-being of our society.

The less tangible benefits that have resulted from the use of psychotropic drugs may be of even greater importance. We have, to some extent, altered our attitudes toward persons with mental illness and now regard these people as suffering from a treatable disease rather than from incurable insanity. Moreover, the introduction of these agents has forced a reappraisal of theories about the origin of mental disease. The psychotropic agents have given new directions to psychiatry and may ultimately lead us to a better understanding of human behavior.

Acknowledgments

I am obliged to Dr. R. D. Grove, Chief of the Division of Vital Statistics, for supplying the breakdown of suicides of classes E970H and M, to Mr. William Holland of the Statistical Bureau of Metropolitan Life for the suicide rates of Standard ordinary policyholders, to Mr. R. A. Gosselin of Dedham, Massachusetts, for permission to use prescription data gathered by his National Prescription Audit Service, and to Dr. M. Roth for permission to use Fig. 4.

References

Barraclough, B. M., Nelson, B., and Sainsbury, P. (1968). *In* "Proceedings of the Fourth International Conference for Suicide Prevention" (N. L. Farberow, ed.), p. 61. Int. Ass. for Suicide Prevention, Los Angeles, California.

Bell, J. L., Tauber, H., Santy, A., and Pulito, F. (1959). *Dis. Nerv. Syst.* **20,** 263.

Berelson, B., and Steiner, G. A. (1964). "Human Behavior—An Inventory of Scientific Findings." Harcourt, New York.

Berger, F. M. (1967a). *In* "Symposium on Suicide" (L. Yochelson, ed.), p. 117. George Washington Univ., Washington, D.C.

Berger, F. M. (1967b). *Clin. Pharmacol. Ther.* **8,** 219.

Berger, F. M. (1970). *In* "Discoveries in Biological Psychiatry" (F. J. Ayd, Jr. and B. Blackwell, eds.), p. 115. Lippincott, Philadelphia, Pennsylvania.

Berger, F. M., and Potterfield, J. (1969). *In* "The Psychopharmacology of the Normal Human" (W. O. Evans and N. S. Kline, eds.), p. 38. Thomas, Springfield, Illinois.

Blum, R. H. (1967). *In* "President's Commission on Law Enforcement and the Administration of Justice. Task Force Report: Narcotics and Drug Abuse" (E. B. Prettyman, Chairman), p. 21. U.S. Govt. Printing Office, Washington, D.C.

Cattell, R. B., and Scheier, I. H. (1958). *Psychological Reports* **4,** 351.

Cattell, R. B., and Scheier, I. H. (1961). "The Meaning and Measurement of Neuroticism and Anxiety." Ronald Press, New York.

Cole, J. O. (1961). *In* "Control of the Mind" (S. M. Farber and R. H. L. Wilson, eds.), p. 110. McGraw-Hill, New York.

Cole, J. O., and Wittenborn, J. R. (1969). "Drug Abuse—Social and Psychopharmacological Aspects." Thomas, Springfield, Illinois.

Conley, R. W., Conwell, M., and Arrill, M. B. (1967). *Amer. J. Psychiat.* **124,** 755.

Goldhamer, H., and Marshall, A. W. (1949). "Psychosis and Civilization." Free Press, Glencoe, Illinois.

Grob, G. N. (1966). "The State and the Mentally Ill." Univ. of North Carolina Press, Chapel Hill, North Carolina.

Grove, R. D. (1967). Personal communication.

Jacobziner, H. (1965). *J. Amer. Med. Ass.* **191,** 7.

Kales, A., Heuser, G., Kales, J. D., Rickles, W. H., Jr., Rubin, R. T., Scharf, M. B., Ungerleider, J. T., and Winters, W. D. (1969). *Ann. Intern. Med.* **70,** 591.

Kass, E. H. (1971). *In* "Antimicrobial Agents and Chemotherapy—1970" (G. L. Hobby, ed.), p. 1. Amer. Soc. Microbiology, Bethesda, Maryland.

Kety, S. S. (1961). *In* "Control of the Mind" (S. M. Farber and R. H. L. Wilson, eds.), p. 79. McGraw-Hill, New York.

Kline, N. S. (1968). *In* "Psychopharmacology—A Review of Progress 1957–1967" (D. H. Efron, ed.), p. 1. U.S. Govt. Printing Office, Washington, D.C.

Lewis, A. (1967). *Israel Annals of Psychiatry* **5,** 105.

Mental Health Statistics (1968). Series MHB–H–12. Dep. Health, Educ. Welfare, U.S. Govt. Printing Office, Washington, D.C.

Miller, M. H., Fellner, C. H., and Greenfield, N. S. (1959). *Ann. Intern. Med.* **51,** 78.

National Prescription Audit (1965). R. A. Gosselin & Co., Inc., Dedham, Massachusetts.

Pasamanick, B., Scarpitti, F. R., Lefton, M., Dinitz, S., Wernert, J. J., and McPheeters, H. (1964). *J. Amer. Med. Ass.* **187,** 177.

Roth, M., and Schapira, K. (1970). *Brit. Med. Bull.* **26,** 197.

Selling, L. S. (1940). "Men Against Madness." Greenberg, New York.

Statistical Abstract of the United States (1970). 91st Ed. U.S. Bur. Census, Washington, D.C.

Statistical Bulletin (1970). Vol. 51. Metropolitan Life Insurance Co., New York.

Wittenborn, J. R., Smith, J. P., and Wittenborn, S. A., eds. (1970). "Communication and Drug Abuse—Proceedings of the Second Rutgers Symposium on Drug Abuse." Thomas, Springfield, Illinois.

Recent Developments in the Pharmacology of the Benzodiazepines*

William Schallek, Walter Schlosser, and Lowell O. Randall

Department of Pharmacology, Research Division
Hoffmann-La Roche Inc.
Nutley, New Jersey

* Dr. Carl L. Scheckel had intended to contribute a section psychopharmacology to this review. We regret that his untimely death made it impossible to carry out this purpose.

I. Introduction

The benzodiazepines are a class of compounds which have been found to show marked antianxiety effects in human subjects. Clinical studies indicate that various members of this series also have anticonvulsant, muscle relaxant, and hypnotic properties. Furthermore, there are reports of psychostimulant activity.

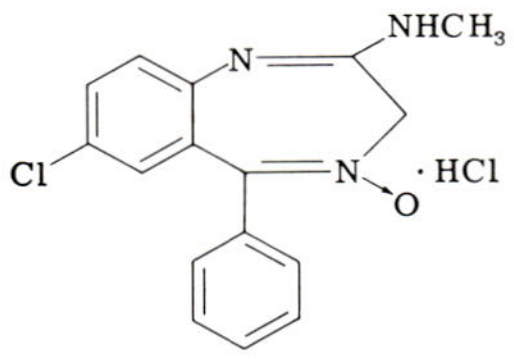

Chlordiazepoxide HCl
Ro 5-0690
Librium (R)

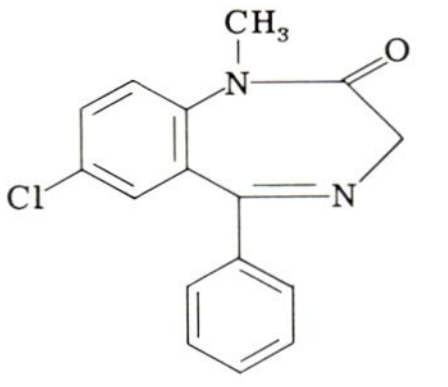

Diazepam
Ro 5-2807
Valium (R)

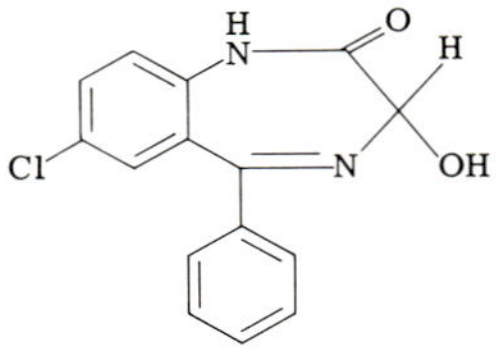

Oxazepam
Ro 5-6789
Serax (R)

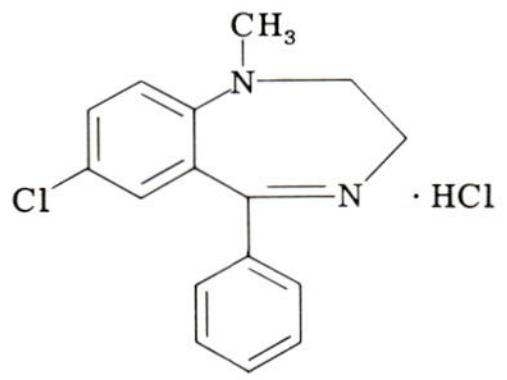

Medazepam HCl
Ro 5-4556
Nobrium (R)

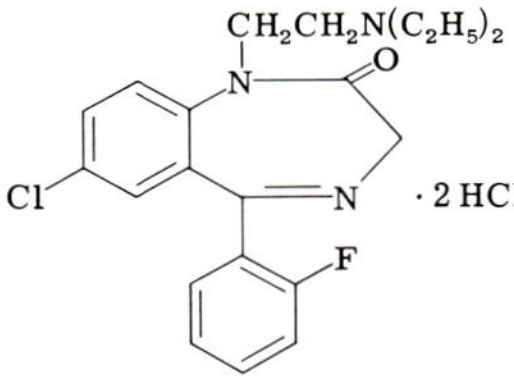

Flurazepam HCl
Ro 5-6901
Dalmane (R)

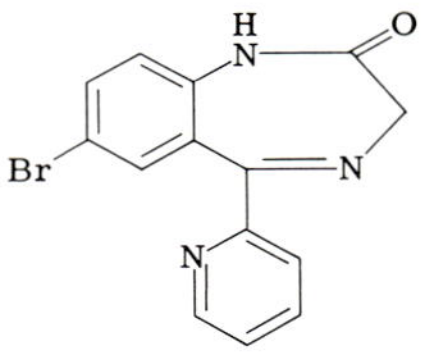

Bromazepam
Ro 5-3350

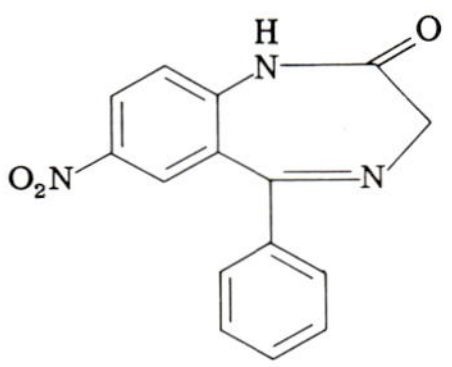

Nitrazepam
Ro 5-3059
Mogadon (R)

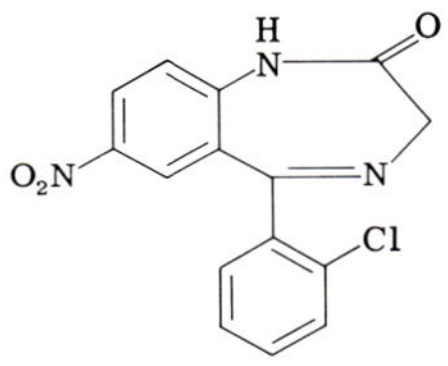

Clonazepam
Ro 5-4023

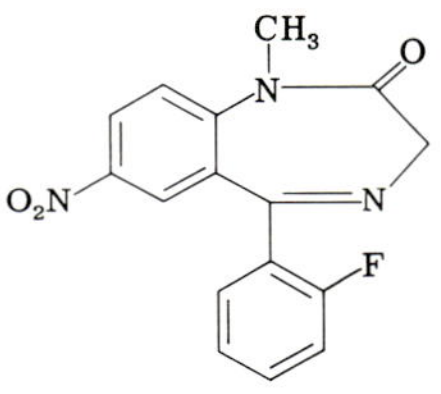

Flunitrazepam
Ro 5-4200

Fig. 1. Structural formulas of some benzodiazepines.

Three previous reviews have covered the pharmacology of the benzodiazepines. Zbinden and Randall (1967) emphasized correlations between laboratory and clinical investigations. Irwin (1968) critically discussed the pharmacology of the minor tranquilizers and sedative hypnotics in animals and humans, whereas Randall and Schallek (1968) concentrated on laboratory studies. References to the older literature will be found in these papers. The present review is based on articles published between 1967 and 1971. Earlier studies are mentioned only when needed to provide background material. The papers selected for review reflect the interests of the authors; no attempt was made to cover the entire literature.

When the previous reviews were published, the benzodiazepines were known to have a variety of depressant effects on the central nervous system (CNS); recent studies indicate that they also have apparent facilitatory actions. Evidence will be presented that these effects may be caused by release from inhibition. Other developments covered in the present review include the mechanism of the muscle relaxant effects, evidence for sites of action in the brain, and studies on the metabolism of these compounds. Structural formulas, generic names, and trade names of some of the benzodiazepines mentioned in this review are shown in Fig. 1.

II. Muscular Relaxant Activity

Early studies of the muscular relaxant properties of the benzodiazepines were based on the ability of mice to hang onto an inclined screen, on the relaxed appearance of cats picked up by the scruff of the neck, and on kymographic studies of spinal reflexes (Randall *et al.*, 1960). From the mid-sixties on, a more detailed analysis of the relaxant properties of these compounds has been made, with an attempt to locate the site or sites of action. This section will be divided into two parts, the first dealing with peripheral effects of benzodiazepines and the second with centrally mediated actions.

A. Peripheral Neuromuscular Action

1. *Nerve Conduction*

Pruett and Williams (1966) reported that the conduction rate of isolated frog sciatic nerves was significantly reduced when the nerves were immersed in solutions of chlordiazepoxide hydrochloride, 3.4×10^{-3} μM/ml. Toman and Sabelli (1968) noted that chlordiazepoxide hydrochloride, in concentrations above 1 mM, first elevated the threshold and then blocked conduction in both earthworm and frog nerves. The amplitude of the action potential in frog nerve was decreased, whereas the earthworm spikes were unaffected or even enhanced. In agreement with Pruett and Williams, the drug reduced conduction velocity in frog nerve. Diazepam (0.5 m*M*) was also observed to elevate nerve threshold, leading to conduction failure. This effect was readily reversed by washing. The diazepam-induced elevation of threshold could be antagonized with strong shocks; this was less commonly seen during treatment with chlordiazepoxide hydrochloride.

2. *Neuromuscular Effects*

High concentrations of chlordiazepoxide hydrochloride (4.15×10^{-4} w/v) and diazepam (8.35×10^{-5} w/v) inhibited contraction in the isolated phrenic nerve–diaphragm preparation of the rat (Hamilton, 1967). This inhibition was often preceded by a potentiation of the twitch. The muscle response to nerve stimulation was generally blocked more readily than the response to direct stimulation; in some instances, however, there was parallel inhibition of direct and indirect stimulation. Diazepam was approximately 5 times as potent as chlordiazepoxide hydrochloride. Hamilton also showed that these drugs, given intravenously in the anesthetized cat, blocked the reflex contraction of the anterior tibialis muscle. Low doses were effective in blocking the reflex but had no significant effect on the twitch response to stimulation of the motor nerve.

An increase in the amplitude of contraction of the indirectly stimulated anterior tibial muscle of the rabbit was noted with diazepam, 5 and 10 mg/kg (Cheymol *et al.*, 1967). Direct stimulation of this muscle in preparations denervated 15 days previously produced identical results. In contrast to these observations, Crankshaw and Raper (1968) reported that diazepam at 0.4 mg/kg i.v. was without effect on the response of the cat anterior tibial muscle to motor nerve stimulation. However, this dose of the drug abolished the polysynaptic reflex contraction produced by stimulation of the homolateral femoral nerve. Similarly, Hudson and Wolpert (1970) found that diazepam at 8 mg/kg i.v. had no effect on the intact neuromuscular preparation of the cat, whereas the patellar reflex was depressed at 0.125 mg/kg.

The interaction of diazepam and neuromuscular blocking agents was studied in the rabbit by Cheymol *et al.* (1967). Diazepam at 5 to 10 mg/kg potentiated the effects of a noncurarizing dose of *d*-tubocurarine, and recurarized the anterior tibial muscle after the effects of a curarizing dose had worn off. Conversely, diazepam produced a rapid resumption of contraction after suppression of transmission by gallamine. Diazepam had no effect in animals treated with succinylcholine.

Dretchen *et al.* (1971) found that recovery rates from neuromuscular blockade induced by *d*-tubocurarine, decamethonium, or gallamine were not affected by therapeutic doses of diazepam (0.3–0.6 mg/kg i.v. in man, 1 mg/kg i.v. in cat, 0.5 μg/ml in superfused nerve muscle preparation of the chick). When 0.5 mg of diazepam was injected intraarterially in the dog, the blockade produced by decamethonium or *d*-tubocurarine was reversed; however, the same action was produced by the solvent system for diazepam.

The studies just reviewed indicate that the peripheral effects of the benzodiazepines are insignificant and probably play little if any role in the muscle-relaxant properties of these compounds. At high dose levels one can see an effect on nerve conduction and on neuromuscular transmission, but this occurs only at concentrations far greater than those needed to block reflex activity. The combined action of benzodiazepines and blockers of neuromuscular transmission requires additional investigation.

B. Central Relaxant Activity

1. *Spinal Cord*

Swinyard and Castellion (1966) tested the effects of benzodiazepines in unanesthetized spinal cats. Reflex responses were elicited by stimulation of a dorsal root and were recorded from the ipsilateral ventral root. Chlordiazepoxide hydrochloride at 0.5 to 32 mg/kg i.v. and Ro 5-4023 at 0.025 to 2.5 mg/kg had no effect on the transmission of isolated impulses in monosynaptic pathways. The drugs were also without effect on posttetanic potentiation. However, they did have significant influences on responses during repetitive stimulation. Under these conditions decreases in synaptic transmission were observed with chlordiazepoxide hydrochloride at 1 mg/kg i.v. and with Ro 5-4023 at 0.05 mg/kg. During stimulation at 30 Hz the monosynaptic spike amplitude was reduced almost to zero by chlordiazepoxide hydrochloride at 4 mg/kg; the pattern could be restored to the control level by injection of pentylenetetrazol, 40 mg/kg.

The effects of diazepam on reflex activity in the spinal cat have been extensively investigated by Schmidt *et al.* (1967). These results have recently been confirmed by Schlosser (1971). In both studies the principal effect of diazepam was a marked enhancement of presynaptic inhibition. This was shown by increases in the amplitude and duration of the dorsal root potential (Schmidt *et al.*, 1967) and the dorsal root reflex (Fig. 2).

The effects of increasing doses of diazepam on presynaptic inhibit on induced through reflex pathways are illustrated in Fig. 3. Additional evidence for an action of the drug at primary afferent terminals was indicated by a prolongation of synaptic recovery, marked by an enhanced depression of the second of two monosynaptic spikes recorded from a ventral root (Fig. 4A). This prolongation of synaptic recovery was not associated with any change in the recovery of the motoneuron, as shown by the lack of effect of diazepam on the depression of a monosynaptic spike conditioned by an antidromic volley (Fig. 4B). These experiments, although showing an effect on presynaptic inhibition, do not indicate whether the drug action was exerted directly on the presynaptic afferent terminals or indirectly through interneurons.

The action of diazepam on presynaptic inhibition was also confirmed by Stratten and Barnes (1971). Furthermore, they observed that diazepam

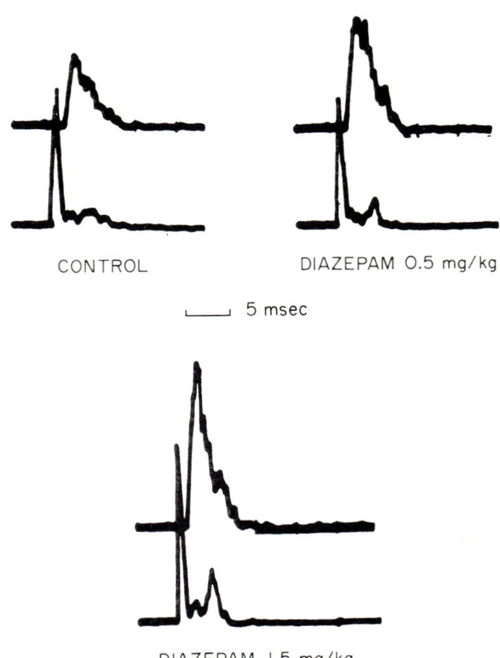

FIG. 2. Effect of diazepam on monosynaptic and dorsal root reflex. Upper trace, dorsal root reflex recorded from rootlet of L_7. Lower trace, monosynaptic and polysynaptic potential recorded from L_7 ventral root on stimulation of L_7 dorsal root. (From Schlosser, 1971, by permission.)

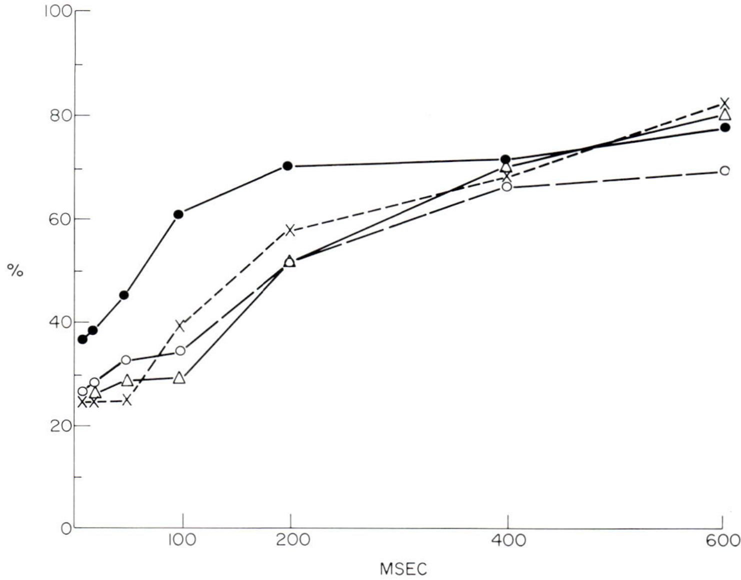

FIG. 3. Effect of diazepam on presynaptic (indirect) inhibition. Ordinate, percent of unconditioned response; abscissa, interval between conditioning train (4 volleys at 250/second) and test stimulus. Test stimulus applied to triceps; conditioning stimuli applied to posterior biceps semitendinosus. Recording electrodes at S_1. Each point represents ten to twenty potentials. ●—control; ○——○0.5 mg/kg diazepam; △— 1.0 mg/kg diazepam; X- - - 1.5 mg/kg diazepam. (From Schlosser, 1971, by permission.)

and picrotoxin act as antagonists at loci responsible for primary afferent depolarization.

Schmidt *et al.* (1967) attribute the muscle-relaxant action of diazepam to increased presynaptic inhibition of proprioceptive and exteroceptive afferents. They believe that this form of inhibition acts as a negative feedback system, whereby an increase in muscle tone produces an increased inhibition of the spinal afferents. This action of the drug may be particularly useful in cases of spasticity.

2. *Brainstem*

The effects of various CNS depressants on polysynaptic reflexes were studied in cats decerebrated at the midcollicular level (Ngai *et al.*, 1966). The ipsilateral or contralateral extensor reflexes were depressed to 50% or less of the control by diazepam (0.05–0.2 mg/kg i.v.), chlordiazepoxide

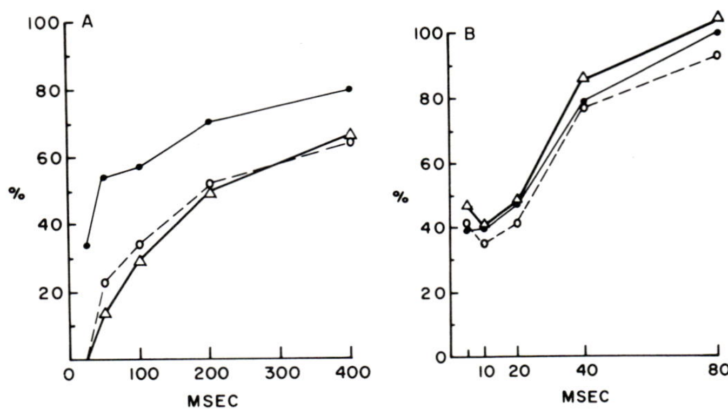

FIG. 4. Effect of diazepam on synaptic recovery in the monosynaptic pathway. (A) Orthodromic conditioning and test stimuli applied to L_7 dorsal root. (B) Test stimulus applied to the dorsal root; antidromic conditioning delivered through sciatic nerve. Recording electrode on sciatic nerve. Ordinates, percent of unconditioned monosynaptic response; abscissas, time interval between conditioning and test stimuli. Each point is an average of ten to twenty potentials. Figures A and B are from different experiments. ●— control; ○— — — 0.5 mg/kg diazepam; △— 1.0 mg/kg diazepam. (From Schlosser, 1971, by permission.)

hydrochloride (10–30 mg/kg), meprobamate (20–40 mg/kg), mephenesin (10–50 mg/kg), and pentobarbital sodium (24 mg/kg). Transection of the spinal cord during diazepam-induced depression resulted in recovery of the ipsilateral extensor reflex, often to a degree greater than in the original control. The contralateral reflex also recovered but remained smaller than in the control. Following spinal transection, diazepam doses ranging from 3 to 10 mg/kg were required to produce substantial polysynaptic blockade, whereas doses of 40 to 120 mg/kg were needed with chlordiazepoxide hydrochloride. The authors conclude that these benzodiazepines block polysynaptic reflexes through an action on reticular facilitatory and inhibitory systems; the facilitatory system is probably more susceptible to depression by the drugs than the inhibitory system.

Przybyla and Wang (1968) have presented strong evidence in favor of the brainstem reticular formation as the major locus of the muscle relaxant action of diazepam. The knee jerk in midcollicular decerebrate cats may be facilitated by electrical stimulation of the mesencephalic reticular formation or depressed by stimulation of the medullary reticular formation. Diazepam reduced both the facilitation and inhibition of the knee jerk. The effective doses were 0.1 mg/kg on injection into the radial vein and

0.01 mg/kg when injected into the vertebral artery. The authors also measured the spontaneous rate of discharge of certain mesencephalic reticular neurons which increased their firing rates on stimulation of the sciatic nerve. These neurons showed a stepwise reduction in their spontaneous rate of discharge following successive injections of diazepam at 0.1 mg/kg i.v. Sciatic nerve stimulation no longer increased the frequency of discharge, and there was a simultaneous reduction of the polysynaptic extensor response. Similar effects followed injection into the vertebral artery, except that the required dose was as little as 0.005 mg/kg, and the latency of drug action was 1 or 2 seconds instead of 10 seconds.

Further support for a brainstem site of action of diazepam was provided by Tseng and Wang (1971a). They found that diazepam at 0.05 mg/kg i.v. caused a 50% reduction in reticular neuronal activity, whereas 0.4 mg/kg was required to reduce the activity of spinal interneurons to the same extent (Fig. 5A). In contrast, tybamate, which depressed contralateral extensor reflexes in both midcollicular and spinal cats, was equally effective in depressing reticular neurons and spinal interneurons (Fig. 5B).

Hudson and Wolpert (1970) compared the effects of diazepam on intact

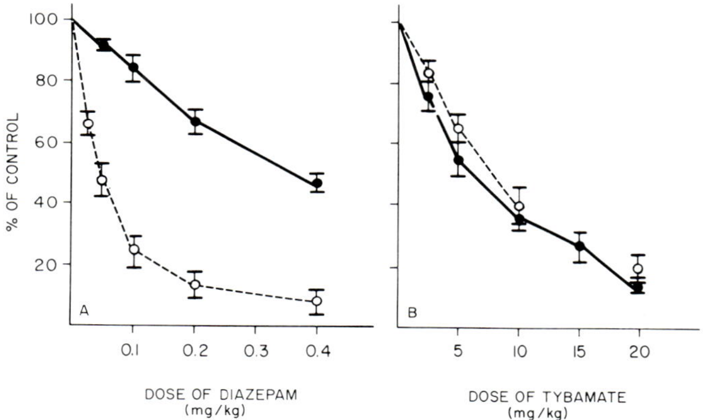

FIG. 5. Comparative effects of diazepam and tybamate on mesencephalic reticular neurons and spinal interneurons; dose–response relationships. Doses are cumulative. Each point represents the mean value of neuronal firing rate represented as a percentage of control value; the vertical line through the point represents the standard error of the mean. For diazepam (A), from 8 to 9 mesencephalic reticular neurons and 4 spinal interneurons; for tybamate (B), from 8 to 11 mesencephalic reticular neurons and 4 to 7 spinal interneurons. ●—● spinal interneurons; ○---○ mesencephalic reticular neurons. (From Tseng and Wang, 1971a, by permission of The Williams & Wilkins Co., Baltimore, Maryland.)

and on spinal cats. In the intact, anesthetized animal the patellar reflex was depressed by 0.125 mg/kg i.v. Electrical stimulation of the mesencephalic facilitatory area produced an increment in the patellar reflex; this increment was reduced by diazepam at 0.125 mg/kg. Stimulation of the medullary inhibitory area produced a decrement in the reflex; the decrement was depressed at 0.25 mg/kg. In the high spinal cat the patellar reflex was not reduced at 16 mg/kg. However, the reflex increment caused by contralateral sciatic nerve stimulation was depressed at 0.125 mg/kg, whereas the reflex decrement produced by ipsilateral sciatic stimulation yielded only to 8 to 16 mg/kg. The authors conclude that "diazepam produces its relaxant effects by a depression of motor systems of both the brainstem reticular formation and the spinal cord."

Additional members of the benzodiazepine group have been tested by other authors. The postural effects of nitrazepam were studied by Ghelarducci *et al.* (1966). A distinct hypotonia was produced in unrestrained cats by 1 mg/kg i.v. The monosynaptic "H" reflex was not changed by this dose of the drug. In spinal cats the monosynaptic reflexes and dorsal root potentials were not affected by several injections of 1.4 mg/kg, whereas a slight depression of polysynaptic reflexes appeared after several injections of the drug. Gamma rigidity, produced by pre- or intercollicular decerebration, was greatly reduced by 1 mg/kg. In contrast, alpha rigidity, produced by deafferentation of the forelimbs and cerebellectomy, was resistant to this dose of the drug. Apparently nitrazepam "acts by depressing a tonic facilitatory influence exerted by the brainstem on the spinal gamma motoneurons."

Tseng and Wang (1971b) found that the contralateral extensor reflex in midcollicular decerebrate cats was abolished by Ro 5-4023 at 0.05 mg/kg i.v., by nitrazepam at 0.1 mg/kg, by Ro 5-3350 at 0.2 mg/kg, and by flurazepam hydrochloride at 1 mg/kg. Transection of the spinal cord produced a return of the reflexes which then became highly resistant to the actions of the drugs. The four agents were found to depress both the reticular facilitatory and inhibitory effects on the knee jerk. The authors conclude that these drugs act mainly on supraspinal structures, most likely in the brainstem reticular formation.

It is apparent that the major muscle relaxant actions of the benzodiazepines occur in the CNS. Two sites have been proposed: one at the spinal level resulting in enhancement of presynaptic inhibition and depression of polysynaptic activity; the other at supraspinal sites, probably in the brainstem reticular formation. The latter area requires very small doses of benzodiazepines to produce depressant effects, suggesting that its cells are extremely sensitive to the action of these drugs.

III. Autonomic and Cardiovascular Responses

A. Effects on Autonomic Nervous System

By the end of 1966 it was evident that the benzodiazepines influenced the central control of autonomic function. Thus, the pressor response to hypothalamic stimulation was blocked by benzodiazepines; the evidence indicated that this action was exerted primarily at the hypothalamic level (Randall and Schallek, 1968). Subsequent studies have examined these relationships in greater detail.

Bolme *et al.* (1967) stimulated the sympathetic vasodilator area in the hypothalamus or mesencephalon of conscious dogs. This resulted in increased behavioral alertness, a rise in blood pressure, and an increase in blood flow to the skeletal musculature. The change in flow was abolished by atropine, indicating its cholinergic nature. Chlordiazepoxide had a selective action on these responses. Following injection of 5 mg/kg i.v., the threshold for the behavioral and pressor effects was elevated, but that for vasodilatation was unchanged. Morphine was also able to block the behavioral but not the vasodilator response. The latter mechanism appears to be resistant to the action of these central depressant agents.

The effects of drugs on the autonomic nervous system of the rat were analyzed by Morpurgo (1968). This author made simultaneous observations of drug actions on pressor responses and on contraction of the eyelids. These effects were elicited centrally (by stimulation of the posterior hypothalamus) and peripherally (by injection of norepinephrine or by stimulation of the cervical sympathetic nerve). The drugs tested were phentolamine, guanethidine, chlorpromazine, and diazepam; each was given at 5 mg/kg i.p. Phentolamine reduced both central and peripheral pressor and eyelid responses. Guanethidine reduced the responses to hypothalamic stimulation and the eyelid contraction to nerve stimulation; the pressor response to norepinephrine was augmented. Chlorpromazine reduced the responses to hypothalamic stimulation and the pressor response to norepinephrine. Diazepam was the only drug to reduce the responses to central stimulation without inhibiting the responses to peripheral stimulation.

Autonomic responses to hypothalamic stimulation were analyzed in immobilized cats by Sigg and Sigg (1969). The central ends of the vagal, sympathetic, and splanchnic nerves were prepared for recording. Stimulation of the posterior hypothalamus increased the discharge rate in each nerve, dilated the pupil, and raised the blood pressure. Chlorpromazine, 0.3–3 mg/kg i.v., reduced both the pupillary and vasopressor responses,

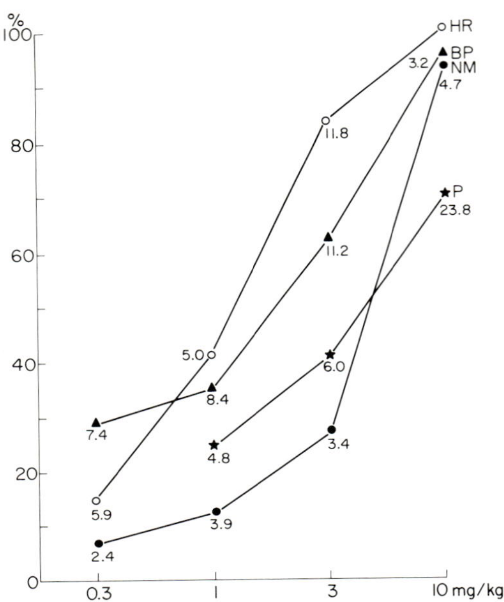

FIG. 6. Effects of pentobarbital on hypothalamically evoked bradycardia (HR), vasopressor response (BP), nictitating membrane contraction (NM), and dilation of pupil (P) in anesthetized cats. The ordinate shows percent inhibition of evoked responses; the abscissa shows doses (mg/kg i.v.) of pentobarbital sodium. Numbers under symbols represent standard errors. (From Sigg *et al.*, 1971, by permission.)

whereas diazepam at the same doses diminished the pressor but not the pupillary response. Although both drugs caused some reduction of activity in the preganglionic cervical sympathetic nerve, they induced a more marked depression of the splanchnic nerve discharges. There were also small reductions in vagal activity. In contrast to these drugs, pentobarbital sodium, 3–10 mg/kg, caused marked depression of evoked potentials in all three nerve preparations. Whereas pentobarbital shows a generalized action, "chlorpromazine and diazepam exert a more discrete depressant effect affecting most consistently the sympathetic vasoconstrictor activity."

A further study of sympathetic reactivity in the immobilized cat was made by Sigg *et al.* (1971). The following "ergotropic" responses were produced by hypothalamic stimulation: rise in blood pressure, compensatory bradycardia, contraction of the nictitating membrane, and dilation of the pupil. Pentobarbital sodium, 0.3–10 mg/kg i.v., caused a dose-related suppression of all these parameters. Chlorpromazine, over the dose range of 0.1 to 3 mg/kg, progressively diminished the pupillary and nictitating membrane responses; the changes in blood pressure and heart rate were only partially blocked. Diazepam at 0.1 to 3 mg/kg showed a highly selective action, blocking the vasopressor response and the reflex slowing of the heart, but dilation of the pupil and contraction of the nictitating membrane were not significantly altered. The effects of pentobarbital and diazepam are compared in Figs. 6 and 7. The authors suggest that "diazepam may prove useful in preventing or delaying the development of 'neurogenic' hypertension, without interfering with other sympathetic reactions."

A new approach to the study of autonomic phenomena involves their changes in controlled behavioral situations. A rise in blood pressure has been observed in squirrel monkeys engaged in lever-pressing experiments (Benson *et al.*, 1970). These authors trained 5 monkeys to press a key in order to avoid an electric shock to the tail. The blood pressure was measured through a cannula implanted in the aorta. The mean arterial pressure before the trials was 135 mm Hg; during the key-pressing sessions it rose

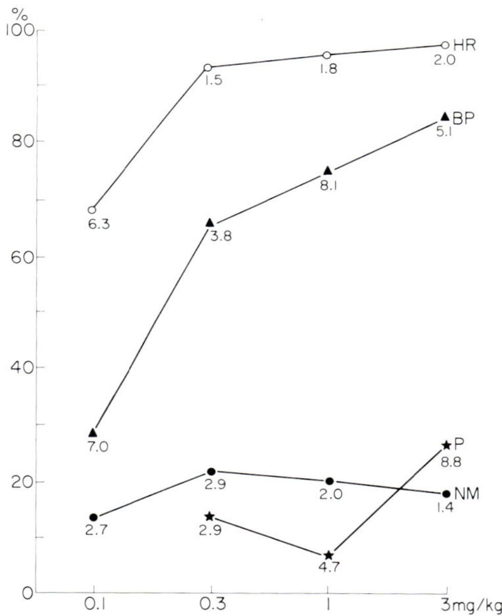

FIG. 7. Influence of diazepam on hypothalamically evoked autonomic responses in anesthetized cats: (HR) bradycardia, (BP) vasopressor response, (NM) nictitating membrane contraction, (P) dilation of pupil. Ordinate, percent inhibition of evoked responses; abscissa, doses (mg/kg i.v.) of diazepam. (From Sigg *et al.*, 1971, by permission.)

to 167 mm Hg. The rise in blood pressure was reduced when the monkeys were pretreated with chlordiazepoxide hydrochloride (3–30 mg/kg i.m.), amobarbital sodium (1–17 mg/kg), or chlorpromazine hydrochloride (0.1–1.0 mg/kg). The drugs also reduced the rate of key-pressing, except for an increase with low doses of amobarbital. These experiments may be relevant to the treatment of those forms of hypertension which are related to environmental circumstances.

B. Cardiovascular Effects

Prindle *et al.* (1970) tested the action of drugs on myocardial contractility. The studies were made on the isolated papillary muscle of the cat. Diazepam, in a wide range of concentrations (0.1–2.5 μg/ml), showed no effect on the development of isometric tension. Chlordiazepoxide hydrochloride had no effect at 1 to 8 μg/ml; these concentrations represent the blood levels found in patients under treatment with the drug. Higher levels 8–24 μg/ml) produced negative inotropic effects. Chlorpromazine was also found to depress myocardial contractility only in concentrations above the therapeutic range.

The effects of diazepam on left ventricular function and on systemic vascular resistance were studied in anesthetized dogs (Abel *et al.*, 1970). A total cardiopulmonary bypass was instituted, using a disk oxygenator, a heat exchanger, and a roller pump. Heart rate and aortic pressure were held constant. When diazepam, 0.1 mg/kg, was injected into the oxygenator, a marked increase both in peak left ventricular isovolumetric pressure and in maximum rate of rise of left ventricular pressure occurred in each of 10 dogs. Improved cardiac performance was demonstrated by the force–velocity and length–tension relations. There were also significant decreases in systemic vascular resistance. The authors point out that patients with inadequate cardiac output often show an increase in vascular resistance. They therefore suggest that diazepam may "have a salutary effect when employed as a sedative or tranquilizer drug in patients with impaired cardiac function."

IV. Anticonvulsant Activity

A review of the literature through 1966 shows that benzodiazepines are active in blocking both chemically and electrically induced seizures in a variety of animal species (Randall and Schallek, 1968). These findings have been extended by more recent publications.

Banziger and Hane (1967) produced convulsions in mice with 2,4-

TABLE I

ANTICONVULSANT ACTIVITY IN MICE[a]

Anticonvulsant	Anticonvulsant $ED_{50} \pm$ S.E. (mg/kg p.o.)			
	Maximal electroshock	Pentylene-tetrazol	TSC[b]	DHMP[c]
Phenobarbital sodium	12.3 ± 1.8	27.4 ± 3.2	63 ± 7	50 ± 4
Diphenylhydantion sodium	10 ± 2	>800	>800	170 ± 37
Trimethadione	>800	400	>800	>800
Chlordiazepoxide hydrochloride	29.9 ± 3	8 ± .9	27 ± 6	16 ± 4
Diazepam	6.4 ± .8	1.37 ± .2	3.4 ± .5	4 ± .7
Clonazepam	400	.16 ± .02	.73 ± .35	3.45 ± 1.22

[a] From Banziger and Hane (1967), by permission.
[b] TSC = Thiosemicarbazide.
[c] DHMP = 2,4-Dimethyl-5-hydroxymethylpyrimidine.

dimethyl-5-hydroxymethyl pyrimidine (DHMP). The effects of benzodiazepines and standard anticonvulsants on seizures produced by this and other techniques are shown in Table I. The benzodiazepines were more active than the standard agents in blocking chemically induced seizures. In the maximal electroshock test, phenobarbital and diphenylhydantoin were more potent than chlordiazepoxide hydrochloride and clonazepam but equal to diazepam.

Motor and electroencephalogram (EEG) manifestations of convulsions were induced in unanesthetized rabbits by topical application of morphine, nicotine, or strychnine to the exposed sensorimotor cortex (Scotti de Carolis and Longo, 1967). The motor phenomena were abolished in 1 to 2 minutes by diazepam at 2 to 5 mg/kg i.v. and by chlordiazepoxide hydrochloride or oxazepam at 5 to 10 mg/kg. Spiking in the EEG disappeared after 5 to 10 minutes; drug effects lasted about 1 hour. Sodium phenobarbital (20 mg/kg) and sodium diphenylhydantoin (30 mg/kg) also blocked the motor and EEG effects of the convulsant agents, but after a delay of about 30 minutes; the duration of action was more than 2–3 hours.

Convulsions induced by local anesthetic agents were antagonized by diazepam (Fenistein *et al.*, 1970). Generalized seizures occurred in each of 28 control cats injected with procaine hydrochloride, 250–300 mg/kg i.p. When 13 cats were pretreated with diazepam, 0.3 mg/kg i.v., the administration of procaine produced convulsions in only 1 animal. In another group of 26 cats, seizures were induced by procaine; diazepam was injected immediately after the appearance of the first convulsion. Seizures ceased completely within 30 seconds in 22 cats and were reduced in intensity and frequency in the remaining 4 animals. Diazepam also abolished seizures in 3 cats given lidocaine at 150 mg/kg i.p.

Other workers have tested the effects of benzodiazepines on seizures induced by pentylenetetrazol. Oxazepam, 10 mg/kg p.o., raised the seizure threshold 7–8 times in chronically prepared cats (Dolce and Kaemmerer, 1967). In immobilized cats the threshold for EEG discharges was significantly increased by chlordiazepoxide hydrochloride (1 mg/kg i.v.), diazepam (0.25 mg/kg), and nitrazepam (0.125 mg/kg), but these drugs did not affect the duration of the seizures (Straw, 1968). Chlordiazepoxide hydrochloride at 1 mg/kg i.v. and diazepam at 0.05 mg/kg prevented pentylenetetrazol seizures in monkeys with chronic irritative foci produced by the injection of alumina cream into the sensorimotor cortex (Kopeloff and Chusid, 1967; Chusid and Kopeloff, 1969). Protection against pentylenetetrazol seizures was also observed in freely moving cats and monkeys following administration of diazepam, 1–3 mg/kg i.v. or i.p. (Guerrero-Figueroa *et al.*, 1969).

A state of recurrent generalized seizures ("status") was induced in freely moving cats by repeated doses of pentylenetetrazol. This status was terminated in 2 to 6 minutes by diazepam, 1 or 2 mg/kg i.m. The animals were mildly ataxic. In contrast, sodium phenobarbital, 30–60 mg/kg, required 4–8 minutes to terminate the seizures and the cats showed marked somnolence or coma (Spehlmann and Colley, 1968). These observations support the clinical opinion that diazepam is "the drug of choice for the emergency treatment of all cases of status epilepticus" (Gastaut *et al.*, 1965).

An extensive study of the mechanism of the anticonvulsant action of diazepam has been made by Guerrero-Figueroa *et al.* (1967, 1968, 1969, 1970). In the first of these investigations, crystals of aluminum oxide or of penicillin were implanted in the intralaminar thalamic nuclei or reticular formation of kittens. These produced irritative lesions, with the appearance of 3-Hz spike and wave discharges in the EEG, as well as facial ticlike contractions, and other signs resembling those of clinical petit mal epilepsy. These effects were suppressed for 1 to 2 hours by diazepam at 4 mg/kg per day i.m. or i.p., and for 6 to 8 hours at 9 mg/kg per day. The authors believe the drug acts by "increasing or producing inhibitory actions in disturbed neuronal populations." They suggest that the drug might be efficacious in the treatment of petit mal epilepsy.

In the second of these studies (Guerrero-Figueroa *et al.*, 1968), primary epileptogenic foci were established in healthy adult cats by implantation of aluminum oxide or penicillin into the olfactory bulb or hippocampus. Secondary epileptiform activity subsequently developed in regions connected by one or more neurons to the primary foci, presumably as the result of continuous abnormal bombardment. Diazepam, 2 mg/kg i.p. daily for 2 to 3 months, suppressed epileptiform discharges in the secondary foci, but had little or no effect on activity in the primary foci. Evidently "different neurochemical changes" are involved in the primary and secondary epileptogenic neuronal populations, with the latter being more susceptible to the action of diazepam.

In the third study (Guerrero-Figueroa *et al.*, 1969) the effects of diazepam (1–3 mg/kg i.v. or i.p.) were tested in adult cats with irritative lesions in the septum, amygdala, and hippocampus. "Local evoked potentials" were induced by single-pulse electrical stimulation applied 200–400 μ from the recording site. Diazepam decreased the amplitude of these potentials in secondary epileptogenic foci, but had little effect on primary foci. When lesions were placed in midline structures (reticular formation, hypothalamus, intralaminar nuclei of thalamus), local evoked potentials in secondary foci were reduced in amplitude by diazepam, while smaller changes occurred in the primary foci. The cortical patterns induced by these lesions were suppressed. Finally, when irritative lesions were placed in the cortex, diazepam suppressed the spread of epileptiform discharges without affecting activity in the primary lesion. These effects of diazepam are attributed to "an increase in subcortical inhibitory mechanisms that arrest or suppress epileptiform activity."

In a fourth paper (Guerrero-Figueroa *et al.*, 1970) the authors investigated the effects of diazepam on alcohol withdrawal states. Cats were first subjected to chronic alcohol administration (18–30 ml, 4 times a day for 2 to 5 months). The EEG was marked by fast activity during this period; after 12 to 30 days the fast activity spread to subcortical areas. The amplitude of local evoked potentials was reduced. On withdrawal from alcohol, there was a general slowing of electrical activity. Sporadic subcortical and cortical seizure patterns were recorded in all animals. These seizures were abolished by diazepam, 1.5 mg/kg i.p. daily for 5 days. Local evoked potentials were augmented during the withdrawal phase and suppressed or reduced by diazepam. The authors suggest that chronic administration of alcohol produces a prolonged potentiation of CNS inhibition. Sudden abstinence removes this inhibition, producing an abnormal excitatory state. Diazepam antagonizes the withdrawal syndrome by increasing the inhibitory action of the reticular formation and limbic system.

A fascinating new approach to the pharmacology of anticonvulsant agents is described by Killam *et al.* (1967). Photosensitive epilepsy was induced in the baboon, *Papio papio*. Stimulation with intermittent light at 25 Hz induced paroxysmal EEG and motor activity in a large number of the animals. The appearance of epileptiform seizures was blocked for 24 hours after diazepam (0.5–2.0 mg/kg i.m.), phenobarbital (15 mg/kg), or trimethadione (50 mg/kg). The last two drugs did not change the background EEG, but bursts of fast activity appeared in the frontal leads after diazepam. In another series of tests, responses were evoked in the cortex by stimulation with light at 1 Hz. Diazepam reduced responses from the frontal and temporal but not from the occipital areas, whereas phenobarbital reduced responses from the parietotemporal but not from the frontal and occipital regions. Trimethadione had no effect on evoked responses. In contrast to these drugs, chlorpromazine (3–6 mg/kg) increased all responses to photic stimulation.

Several authors have tested the anticonvulsant effects of other benzodiazepines. Mille *et al.* (1969) tested 7-chloro-1,3-dihydro-1-methyl-3-hydroxy-5-phenyl-2H-1,4-benzodiazepine-2-one* in unanesthetized rabbits. This drug at 5 mg/kg i.v. shortened the duration of afterdischarge in the hippocampus and increased the threshold in the amygdala. It had no effect on activation thresholds in the reticular formation or medial thalamus. When spiking was induced by application of strychnine to the cortex, the drug prevented the spread of epileptic activity, but had no effect on the focus itself. The potency of the drug is equal to that of diazepam, but its duration of action is longer.

The effects of clonazepam (Ro 5-4023) have been studied by several authors. Guerrero-Figueroa *et al.* (1969) tested this drug at doses of 15–100 mg/kg i.v., i.p., or p.o., in cats with irritative lesions in the septum, amygdala, and hippocampus. Although there was little change in local evoked potentials in primary foci, the amplitude of the potentials in secondary epileptogenic foci was decreased. The drug also suppressed spontaneous epileptiform activity in both primary and secondary foci in these brain areas. However, the drug did not reduce potentials in midline structures or in the cortex. The authors suggest that Ro 5-4023 might be useful in temporal lobe epilepsy.

Vuillon-Cacciuttolo and Issautier (1970) tested Ro 5-4023 against pentylenetetrazol seizures in cats. The effect of this drug at 5 mg/kg i.v. was equal to that of chlordiazepoxide at 12 to 14 mg/kg. In contrast, the anticonvulsant potency of Ro 5-4023 was less than that of diazepam or nitrazepam.

Somewhat different results were obtained when Ro 5-4023 was tested

* Also known as ER 115 or Ro 5–5345.

against the effects of intermittent photic stimulation in the baboon (Stark *et al.*, 1970). In control tests, 12 out of 13 animals showed abnormal motor and EEG responses to this stimulation. Following diphenylhydantoin (15 mg/kg i.m. for 3 days), 3 out of 9 animals showed abnormal responses. Ro 5-4023, 0.1 mg/kg prevented any abnormal response in the 8 animals tested. No change in the behavior of the baboons was noted at this dose level. These effects were comparable to those observed with diazepam at 0.5 mg/kg (Killam *et al.*, 1967).

In a clinical study, Gastaut (1970) compared the effects of Ro 5-4023 with those of Ro 5-4200. Both compounds were 5 times as potent as diazepam or nitrazepam. At a total dose of 1 mg i.v. these drugs antagonized the EEG paroxysms triggered by intermittent photic stimulation as well as those occurring spontaneously in generalized epilepsy. Both drugs blocked status epilepticus at a dose of 1 mg. Although sedative effects were noted with Ro 5-4200, these were not seen with Ro 5-4023. Gastaut concludes that the latter compound is "the drug of the future in the treatment of status epilepticus."

V. Behavioral Effects

A. Aggressive Behavior

The activity of a number of drugs on various forms of aggressive behavior in laboratory animals was reviewed by Valzelli (1967). Chlordiazepoxide hydrochloride was effective in blocking isolation-induced aggression in mice, electrically induced fighting in mice, vicious behavior produced by lesions of the brain in rats, and the spontaneous aggressiveness of killer cats and vicious monkeys. These effects occurred at doses below the muscle relaxant level and, therefore, displayed a degree of specificity not observed with many classes of CNS depressants.

Tedeschi *et al.* (1969) reported that the fighting behavior induced in mice by footshock was inhibited by chlordiazepoxide hydrochloride, 30 mg/kg p.o. This dose also depressed locomotor activity. The depressant effect on fighting behavior was antagonized by pentylenetetrazol, 40 mg/kg s.c., but the depression of motor activity was unchanged. Chlordiazepoxide hydrochloride and pentylenetetrazol could be titrated against each other both for effects on fighting behavior and on convulsions. This suggests that the mechanisms and/or sites of action of these drugs on fighting and on seizures may be interrelated in some manner.

Sofia (1969) tested the effects of chlordiazepoxide hydrochloride and diazepam on four models of aggression (fighting following prolonged isolation in mice, fighting induced in mice by electroshock, rats with lesions in the septal area of the brain, and muricidal rats). Muscle relaxant effects were measured by determining the dose of drug causing the animals to fall off a rotating rod. Only in the case of electroshock-induced fighting was the aggression diminished at doses below those effective in the rotarod test. The effects in the other models can be attributed to muscle relaxant or general depressant actions.

The above results were confirmed and extended by Christmas and Maxwell (1970). Four benzodiazepines (chlordiazepoxide hydrochloride, diazepam, nitrazepam, oxazepam) were compared with amobarbital and meprobamate in the following tests in mice and rats: aggression induced by electroshock; analgesia induced by electroshock; and locomotor activity. The benzodiazepines differed from amobarbital and meprobamate by reducing aggressive behavior at doses well below those affecting locomotor activity. Nitrazepam was approximately twice as potent as diazepam and 4 times as potent as chlordiazepoxide hydrochloride and oxazepam. These effects were not due to analgesia, as the benzodiazepines were inactive in that test.

Three different models of aggression were produced in rats by placing lesions in the septum, the ventromedial hypothalamus (VMH), or the olfactory bulb (OB) (Malick *et al.*, 1969). There were no significant differences among the three preparations after treatment with chlordiazepoxide hydrochloride or phenobarbital. Chlorpromazine was significantly less active in the VMH rat than in the other preparations, whereas diazepam and meprobamate were less active in the OB rat than in the other models. The authors conclude that "further work is necessary to determine the mechanism of these differences."

Bauen and Possanza (1970) reported that the aggressive nature of the mink renders this animal especially suitable for testing psychoactive compounds Following oral administration of the test substance, each animal was scored for the ease with which it could be handled by the experimenter. Chlordiazepoxide hydrochloride, oxazepam, diazepam, and meprobamate were found to be highly active in reducing the aggressiveness of the mink, whereas chlorpromazine and pentobarbital were without effect.

Fox *et al.* (1970) found increased aggression in grouped male mice which were fed a diet containing 0.03% chlordiazepoxide hydrochloride. These were a wild strain of brown mice which had a high level of spontaneous aggression. The increased aggression in mice was observed over a 2-week period with the low dose of the drug. Increased mortality over 2- and 8-week periods was also observed with the treated mice. Mice consuming up to 1.5 mg of chlordiazepoxide per day exhibited no neuromuscular impairment. A similar increase in the aggression of grouped male mice was observed with low doses of diazepam in the diet (Fox and Snyder, 1969).

The increased aggression observed with low doses of benzodiazepines may be related to the disinhibitory effects of these drugs (see below). A second interesting finding with benzodiazepines is the antiaggressive action noted in the electroshock test. Whether this experimental result has any relevance to the clinical effects of these drugs remains to be determined.

B. Suppressed Behavior

This section will consider a group of experiments which demonstrate an interesting behavioral characteristic of the benzodiazepines. This is the phenomenon of disinhibition or the release of previously suppressed responses.

The experiments in this section are based on operant techniques. In this type of test, the response of the animal determines the consequences Thus if a rat presses a lever when a certain tone sounds, it may be rewarded with a food pellet (positive reinforcement). At another signal, an electric shock to the feet (negative reinforcement) may be avoided by a lever press. Various modifications of these procedures will be described below.

Some problems involved in these techniques were discussed by Cook (1965). When chlordiazepoxide hydrochloride, 10 mg/kg p.o., was administered to squirrel monkeys, the effects depended on the following variables.

1. Experimental parameters. The monkeys were placed on a fixed-interval escape schedule, in which the first response after 10 minutes turned off a shock. The rate of responding under the drug was increased at low shock levels (0.8 mA) but decreased at high shock levels (2.5 mA). Furthermore, the predrug rate of responding varied with the shock level. Hence it was not possible to tell from these data whether the shock level or the predrug response rate was the cause of the changes observed in the drug tests.

2. Schedule differences. The monkeys were placed on a fixed-ratio schedule, in which every thirtieth response was reinforced. Under conditions in which the rate of fixed-interval responding was increased by the drug, the rate of fixed-ratio responding was reduced. Once again, the drug effects may depend on different predrug rates of responding to the two schedules.

3. Chronic treatment. When the drug was administered orally for 4 days, there was a progressive reduction in the increased rate of fixed-interval responding. "This may be a tolerance phenomenon or may be due to other mechanisms."

Margules and Stein (1967) used a variety of operant techniques to study the actions of psychodepressant drugs. They divided these agents into two types. The *neuroleptics* include the phenothiazines, butyrophenones, reserpine, and tetrabenazine. These drugs "weaken all operant responses, regardless of the type of reinforcement that maintains the behavior. Thus these compounds reduce, more or less equally, the tendency to perform both approach behaviors maintained by positive reinforcement and avoidance behaviors maintained by negative reinforcement." In contrast to these drugs are the *tranquilizers*, which include benzodiazepines, barbiturates, meprobamate, and possibly ethanol. Their effects "are best demonstrated if a strong tendency to respond is suppressed by electric shock or some other form of punishment. In moderate or optimal doses, the drugs markedly increase the rate of occurrence of the previously suppressed behavior, presumably by releasing the behavior from inhibition."

These authors illustrated the differences between the two classes of drugs by a series of tests in rats in which the effects of oxazepam were compared with those of chlorpromazine.

1. In a punishment situation, in which every response was simultaneously rewarded with milk and punished by an electric shock, the rate of responding was increased by oxazepam but not by chlorpromazine.
2. When operant behavior was suppressed by nonreinforcement (withdrawal of the milk reward), responding was restored by oxazepam but not by chlorpromazine.
3. Oxazepam restored operant responses which had been suppressed by aversive brain stimulation.
4. Drinking behavior was inhibited by the bitter taste of quinine which had been added to the milk. This inhibition was eliminated by oxazepam but not by chlorpromazine.
5. Oxazepam increased milk-drinking in satiated rats; chlorpromazine did not do so.

The authors conclude that "the disinhibitory effect of tranquilizers is clearly a general action." Later experiments (Margules and Stein, 1968) indicated that there was no development of tolerance to the disinhibitory action of oxazepam during chronic administration of the drug to rats. In contrast, the animals rapidly became tolerant to the depressant effects of the drug (which were measured by a decrease in the rate of unpunished behavior).

Further evidence for the disinhibitory effect of benzodiazepines is provided by other authors. Davidson and Cook (1969) trained rats to press a lever for food. In addition to unpunished reinforcement, a punishment contingency was added in which every tenth response resulted in the simultaneous delivery of a food pellet and an electric footshock. Responding was suppressed during the punishment periods. Chlordiazepoxide hydrochloride caused a dose-related increase of punished responses at doses between 1.25 and 10 mg/kg p.o. Higher doses decreased the rate of responding.

Wedeking (1969) trained rats in a two-lever situation. A press on the lever illuminated by a signal light was rewarded with food, whereas a press on the other lever was not rewarded. Each reward was followed by a "time-out" period. After the administration of chlordiazepoxide hydrochloride, 5–10 mg/kg i.p., there were significant increases in the number of unrewarded responses and of time-out responses. Wedeking attributes this effect to "a general breakdown of inhibition."

In a different type of experiment, rats were trained to press a lever for water reinforcement (Heise *et al.*, 1970). When the water was withdrawn, responding was reduced. However, responding during the withdrawal period was increased by chlordiazepoxide hydrochloride, 7.5 mg/kg i.p. The same effect was produced by scopolamine hydrobromide, 0.3 mg/kg,

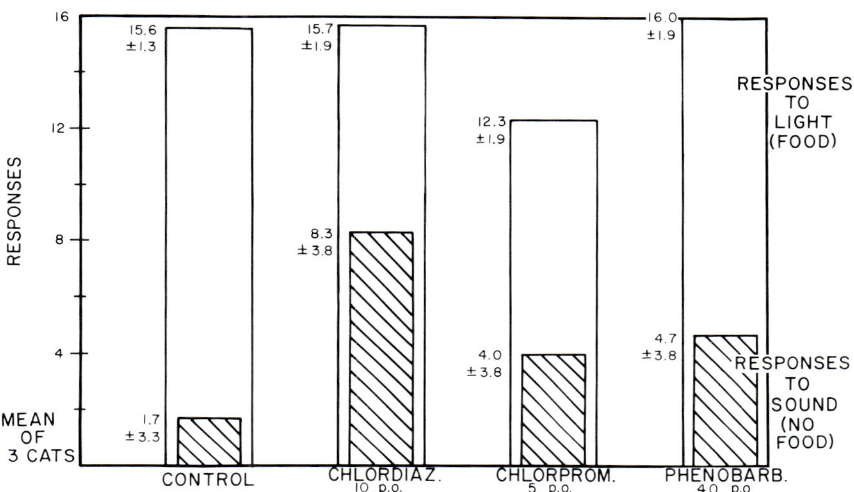

FIG. 8. Effects of psychotropic drugs on behavior of cats trained to distinguish between a light signal (rewarded) and a sound signal (nonrewarded). Responses to the rewarded signal are shown by open bars, whereas those to the nonrewarded signal are shown by lined bars. Each cat received 16 light and 16 sound signals per day; figures show mean number of responses with standard errors. Treatments from left to right are control; chlordiazepoxide hydrochloride, 10 mg/kg p.o.; chlorpromazine hydrochloride, 5 mg/kg p.o.; sodium phenobarbital, 40 mg/kg p.o.

and by atropine sulfate, 5 mg/kg. (Some possible relationships between benzodiazepines and cholinergic systems will be mentioned in Sections VI and VII.)

In another series of tests, freely moving cats were trained to distinguish between a light signal and a sound signal (Schallek *et al.*, 1972). Following the light, the cat could open a door with its paw in order to receive a milk reward. The door could not be opened after the sound signal. Drugs were given at the minimum doses causing distinct changes in the gross behavior of the animals.

The results are shown in Fig. 8. Chlordiazepoxide hydrochloride, 10 mg/kg p.o., had no effect on the number of responses to the rewarding signal. However, the drug significantly increased the number of attempts to open the door following the nonrewarding signal. Chlorpromazine at 5 mg/kg p.o. had quite different effects: the number of responses to the rewarding signal was significantly reduced, whereas there was no change in the responses to the nonrewarding signal. Phenobarbital at 40 mg/kg had no significant effects in these experiments. The authors believe that the increased responding to the nonrewarding signal under the action of chlordiazepoxide hydrochloride is an example of the disinhibiting effect described by Margules and Stein (1967).

C. Sleep and Wakefulness

Only a few studies on the effects of benzodiazepines on the sleep cycle of laboratory animals appeared before 1967, but several interesting papers have been published since that time.

The mechanism of the induction of sleep by nitrazepam was analyzed by Zattoni and Rossi (1967). Sleep might be caused by general depression of the entire brain, by selective depression of activating systems, or by selective excitation of hypnogenic mechanisms. The following experimental procedures were designed to distinguish between these possibilities: (*1*) intravenous injection to allow a drug to be distributed to the entire brain; (*2*) intracarotid injection to permit selective distribution to the diencephalic and rostral mesencephalic structures where important arousing systems are located; (*3*) injection into the vertebral artery to afford a selective distribution to the caudal mesencephalic and rhombencephalic structures containing hypnogenic systems.

The experiments were conducted in rabbits. Injection of 1 to 2 mg of nitrazepam into the femoral vein resulted in synchronization of the EEG, and the rabbit assumed a sleeping posture. However, sensory stimuli sufficient to arouse the animal from natural sleep were not effective for a period of 10 to 15 minutes. When 0.2–1 mg of nitrazepam was injected into the carotid artery, a synchronized pattern appeared in the EEG, and the animal assumed a sleeplike attitude. These effects lasted 3–8 minutes. Injection of 0.1 to 0.8 mg of nitrazepam into the vertebral artery produced an activation pattern in the EEG and behavioral alertness was observed. This action lasted for over 1 minute. All the above phenomena are attributed by the authors to depressant actions of nitrazepam. EEG and behavioral alertness following intravertebral injection correlates with a depression of sleep-inducing neurons in the caudal brainstem. The signs of sleep following intracarotid injection correlate with depression of arousal mechanisms at or in front of the mesodiencephalic junction. The induction of a sleeplike state by intravenous injection indicates that "in the rabbit at least, the functional tone of the arousing neurons is prevalent on that of the hypnogenic ones."

Lanoir and Killam (1968) tested the effects of acute administration of diazepam and nitrazepam on the sleep–wakefulness patterns of cats with chronically implanted electrodes. Observations were made over 24-hour periods. Diazepam, 0.25–2.0 mg/kg i.m., changed the spontaneous electrical activity, producing fast waves of moderate amplitude in the frontal cortex and hippocampus. There was a sharp drop in muscle tone, with transient abolition of rapid eye movements. Total wakefulness was increased, particularly at the expense of rapid eye movement (REM) sleep. Although drug effects were maximal during the first 6 hours, changes could still be detected after 24 hours. Nitrazepam showed similar effects, but at somewhat lower doses; changes could be detected as long as 72 hours after drug administration. The authors note that the increased wakefulness observed with these drugs in the cat contrasts with hypnogenic effects described for the same drugs in man.

The fast neocortical activity observed in cats under the action of nitrazepam was investigated by Vieth *et al.* (1968). They inquired whether this fast activity is equivalent to that found in the desynchronized (REM) phase of sleep. This sleep phase has been linked to the nucleus reticularis pontis caudalis. Six cats were prepared with transections at the midpontine level, thus separating the cortex from the nucleus. Nitrazepam, 2.5 mg/kg i.v., still produced fast neocortical activity. This experiment indicates that the fast activity observed with nitrazepam is not equivalent to that found in desynchronized sleep. The authors suggest that this fast activity, which they observed with pentobarbital as well as nitrazepam, might "be due to depression of ascending inhibitory influences."

The action of medazepam on the sleep–wakefulness cycle of the cat was studied by Heinemann *et al.* (1968). These authors administered the drug by continuous infusion through a cannula implanted in the jugular vein. Nine control and 9 drug experiments lasted 10 hours each. The following doses were used to keep the blood concentration of medazepam at 3 to 5 μg/ml; initial injection, 10 mg; infusion for first hour, 1.67 mg; for the next 2 hours, 1.67 mg; for the next 5 hours, 0.83 mg. Under these conditions waking time decreased from 2.8 hours in control tests to 2.2 hours in drug tests; dozing time decreased from 2.7 to 1.7 hours. But slow wave sleep increased from 3.6 to 4.7 hours, and desynchronized sleep increased from 0.8 to 1.3 hours. The cats were fully awake at the end of the experiment.

The effects of chronic administration of benzodiazepines on the sleep cycle of the cat have been studied by two groups. Dolce and Kaemmerer (1967) found that daily dosing with oxazepam, 10 mg/kg p.o., increased total sleeping time by 5.5%. This increase occurred entirely in the slow wave phase of sleep, since time spent in REM sleep was reduced. Schallek *et al.* (1972) tested chlordiazepoxide hydrochloride at 10 mg/kg p.o., which was the minimum dose causing distinct ataxia when the cats were placed on the laboratory floor. Four cats received this dose for 4 successive days; the drug was administered 30 minutes before the start of the 6-hour observation period. On the first day, time awake was greater than in control tests, whereas time in slow wave and REM sleep was decreased. This situation was reversed on the subsequent days of drug administration. Waking time was less than in control tests, whereas both phases of sleep were longer than in the controls.

The authors suggest several mechanisms which might account for this shift from increased wakefulness to increased sleep. One possibility is a change in the metabolism of the drug during chronic administration. Another is the progressive accumulation of a metabolite with more depressant effect than chlordiazepoxide hydrochloride. It is interesting to note that in the experiments of Heinemann *et al.* (1968), in which medazepam was administered by slow intravenous infusion, no phase of increased wakefulness was noted. If the action of medazepam resembles that of chlordiazepoxide hydrochloride, the slow infusion might have permitted some critical metabolic change to take place.

VI. Effects on Different Areas of the Brain

A number of authors have compared the effects of benzodiazepines with those of other drugs on various areas of the brain. One aim of this work has been to determine whether benzodiazepines have a pattern of action on the brain which distinguishes them from other classes of drugs. Some of these studies were based on electrophysiological techniques, others used behavioral methods, and a small group used radiochemical procedures.

A. Electrophysiological Studies

1. *Cortex; Visual Pathways*

Several workers have found that certain benzodiazepines tend to produce fast frequency patterns in the electrocorticogram (ECoG). Studies before 1967 were reviewed by Randall and Schallek (1968). Low doses of oxazepam (1–5 mg/kg i.v.) produce spindle patterns in the ECoG of the curarized cat, whereas higher doses (5–10 mg/kg) produce a fast frequency, high amplitude rhythm (Dolce and Kaemmerer, 1967). An electronic analysis of the EEG of the rabbit was made by Vatter (1967). He found that nitrazepam, 4 mg/kg i.v., decreased activity at 4 to 5 Hz, but caused a fivefold increase in activity at 16 Hz.

The technique of power spectrum analysis was used to evaluate the effects of drugs on the ECoG of the immobilized cat (Schallek *et al.*, 1968). This technique provides two measurements of the effects of drugs on the electrical activity of the brain: (*1*) changes in "total power," which is proportional to the mean squared amplitude of the trace; and (*2*) changes in the power spectrum or distribution of power over a given frequency range (in this case, 1–32 Hz). To facilitate comparisons between spectra, the power at each frequency is expressed as a fraction of the total power. Hence these spectra show distribution of "relative power."

The compounds tested were chlorpromazine, pentobarbital, and several benzodiazepines. Each drug was tested at 5, 10, and 20 mg/kg i.v., with intervals of 1 hour between doses. Pentobarbital was the only compound to have a significant effect on total power; this was increased at all dose levels. Drug effects on the power spectra fell into three groups: (*1*) chlorpromazine, pentobarbital, and Ro 5-2092 increased power at 9 to 12 Hz and decreased it at 22 to 30 Hz; (*2*) diazepam increased power at 9 to 23 Hz, whereas medazepam hydrochloride (Ro 5-4556) increased it at 14 to 30 Hz—this groups of drugs showed no significant decreases in power; (*3*) flurazepam hydrochloride (Ro 5-6901) decreased power at 9 to 32 Hz—this compound caused no significant increase in power.

The fact that different benzodiazepines affect the ECoG in different ways suggests that all benzodiazepines may not have the same mode of action. The authors also suggest that differences between the effects of drugs on the ECoG might depend on their actions on subcortical centers. These actions were explored in a subsequent paper (see Section VI, A, 2).

The power spectrum technique was used to study the effects of benzodiazepines on *Macaca nemestrina* monkeys seated in restraining chairs (Joy *et al.*, 1971). Electrodes were placed in the frontal cortex, parietal cortex, and in the ventral hippocampus. Spectral peaks at 12 Hz appeared in all control recordings. Following diazepam at 0.1 mg/kg i.m., there was no change in gross behavior, but significant increases in density at 15 to 30 Hz occurred in all cortical leads. At 1 mg/kg the monkeys appeared to be calmer and less aggressive; the dominant spectral peak was 20 Hz in the frontal cortex, 14 Hz in the parietal cortex, and 10 Hz in the hippocampus. At 2 mg/kg the animals were depressed and ataxic but did not sleep; spectra from all leads showed a shift toward lower frequencies.

Several compounds listed in Fig. 1 were compared by Joy *et al.* The lowest dose producing EEG changes was 0.1 mg/kg i.m. with diazepam, Ro 5-4023, and Ro 5-4200; 1 mg/kg with nitrazepam and Ro 5-4556; and 15 mg/kg with chlordiazepoxide hydrochloride. Compound Ro 5-4556 differed from the other benzodiazepines by producing greater sedation and EEG slowing; the EEG slowing observed with this compound in the monkey contrasts with the fast activity observed with the same compound in the cat.

The effects of diazepam were studied on slabs of neuronally isolated cortex in the decerebrate cat (Frank and Jhamandas, 1970). The surface of the slab was stimulated every 15 seconds, producing a surface negative response following by a positive response. Diazepam at 1 mg/kg i.v. reduced both responses for about 2 hours. Similar effects were obtained with meprobamate at 20 mg/kg. The authors had previously observed actions of this type with general anesthetic agents. They suggest "that these depressant effects are a generalized but weak form of anesthetic depression."

Several authors have studied the effects of benzodiazepines on visual pathways. Dolce and Kaemmerer (1967) found that evoked potentials in the visual pathway of the cat were depressed by oxazepam, 3 mg/kg i.v. Heiss *et al.* (1969a) studied the spontaneous activity of retinal neurons in the cat. Before drug administration the interval histogram showed a two-peak pattern; after diazepam, 4.5 mg/kg i.v., the histogram showed multiple peaks. The authors suggest that the drug alters transmission to retinal ganglion cells. In a further study (Heiss *et al.*, 1969b) the effects of diazepam were tested on visually evoked potentials in the cortex of the cat. As the dose was increased from 4 to 44 mg/kg i.v., there was increasing latency of the first positive component; the amplitude was also decreased. The authors suggest that these changes may be caused by inhibition of synaptic activity.

A comprehensive study of the effects of diazepam on evoked cerebral responses was made by Sherwin (1971). The tests were conducted in unanesthetized immobilized cats; the drug was injected in doses of 0.5 to 5 mg/kg i.v. Diazepam showed common actions on a variety of responses (visual evoked response in occipital cortex; augmenting response induced in motor cortex by stimulation of ventral lateral thalamus; pyramidal tract response to stimulation of motor cortex). In each case the initial phases of the response were relatively unchanged, but the later components were diminished. These late components probably represent the activity of cortical interneurons. The author concludes "that in the cerebrum, the depressant effects of diazepam are exerted principally on polysynaptic substrates, possibly at the inter-neuronal level." He suggests that this action may account for the beneficial effects of diazepam in myoclonic disorders.

A possible parallelism in the actions of diazepam on visual pathways and on the spinal cord is suggested by Barnes and Moolenaar (1971). These authors studied responses evoked in the visual cortex by stimulation of the optic tract in midpontine pretrigeminal cats. When the animals were dark-adapted, these responses were potentiated by flashes of light. Diazepam, 1 mg/kg i.v., caused a further facilitation which lasted more than 1500 msec. The authors suggest that this facilitation results from presynaptic inhibition of inhibitory inteneurons in the lateral geniculate nucleus. An enhancement of presynaptic inhibition by diazepam has already been described in the spinal cord (Section II).

2. *Limbic System*

The effects of nitrazepam and sodium phenobarbital were compared on the activity of single neurons in the brains of anesthetized cats (Steiner and Hummel, 1968). The brain areas studied were the hippocampus and the lateral geniculate body. When drugs were applied directly to the neurons by microelectrophoresis, nitrazepam caused the cells to fire rhythmically rather than continuously, whereas phenobarbital slowed the rate of discharge. On systemic application, nitrazepam (0.15–2.5 mg/kg i.v.) depressed spontaneous discharge for 2 minutes, whereas phenobarbital (0.3–20 mg/kg) depressed activity for 60 minutes; the actions of the drugs were similar in both brain areas.

A striking difference between the effects of these drugs was found when the neurons were activated by visual stimulation. Nitrazepam at 0.15 mg/kg completely blocked visually evoked responses in the hippocampus for as long as 5 hours. The cells continued to discharge spontaneously during this period. Phenobarbital at doses up to 20 mg/kg failed to block visually evoked potentials, although spontaneous activity was reduced. Neither drug blocked the responses of lateral geniculate units to photic stimulation.

The experiments on direct application of drugs suggest that phenobarbital has a general depressant effect which is not shown by nitrazepam. On systemic application, nitrazepam differs from phenobarbital by blocking visually evoked responses in the hippocampus. Since nitrazepam has little direct action on hippocampal neurons, the evidence indicates that afferent systems are involved. The lack of effect on the lateral geniculate body shows that the classic visual projection system is not disturbed. "Post-visual connections with and within the limbic cortex" may be involved.

Another study of the effects of drugs on the spontaneous discharges of single neurons was made by Olds and Olds (1969). Microelectrodes were chronically implanted in the hippocampus, preoptic area, and reticular midbrain of freely moving rats. Fifteen recordings, each 200 msec in length, were made before drug injection, and 12 recordings were made after the drug. The data consist of the mean number of spike discharges; postdrug values are presented as percentage of control values (Table II).

Every dose of chlordiazepoxide hydrochloride and diazepam depressed

TABLE II

EFFECTS OF DRUGS ON SPONTANEOUS FIRING OF NEURONS IN THREE AREAS OF RAT BRAIN[a]

Drug	Dose (mg/kg i.p.)	Mean percentage of control values[b]		
		Hippocampus	Preoptic area	Reticular area
Chlordiazepoxide hydrochloride	5	76	86	94
	10	64	77	78
	20	49	50	60
	40	60	64	60
Diazepam	5	60	86	81
	10	45	78	90
	20	51	93	91
Meprobamate	80	88	102	67
	100	70	77	86
	120	97	59	48
Sodium pentobarbital	5	82	102	85
	10	86	81	64
	20	91	81	52

[a] Reprinted by permission from M. E. Olds and J. Olds, 1969, Pergamon, Oxford.

[b] Data based on mean number of spikes in twelve periods of 200 msec each, recorded 15–90 minutes after drug administration.

the activity of hippocampal neurons, whereas meprobamate and sodium pentobarbital had comparatively minor effects. In the preoptic area the most effective depressants were chlordiazepoxide hydrochloride and meprobamate; these actions were most evident at the higher dose levels. The greatest depression in the reticular area was produced by meprobamate, closely followed by sodium pentobarbital. Chlordiazepoxide hydrochloride was active only at higher doses, and diazepam showed little effect on this part of the brain.

The authors note that "the most interesting and least expected result was the selective inhibition in hippocampus after chlordiazepoxide and diazepam." This selective action is evident with low doses of the former and with all doses of the latter compound. Low doses of meprobamate and sodium pentobarbital show no selective depression of the hippocampus. Sodium pentobarbital at higher doses shows a selective inhibition of the reticular area, whereas the highest dose of meprobamate depresses both the reticular and preoptic areas.

Olds and Olds (1969) propose some behavioral consequences of the action of benzodiazepines on the hippocampus. If this brain area normally exerts an inhibitory action on the hypothalamus, depression of the hippocampus would release the hypothalamus from inhibition. Such an action might be involved in some of the increased behavioral responding under the action of benzodiazepines which is described in the next section of this review. It might also be involved in some of the increased ECoG frequencies which have been observed with these drugs.

Further evidence for a selective action of chlordiazepoxide hydrochloride on the hippocampus is provided by Schallek and Thomas (1971). These workers tested the effects of drugs on the spontaneous electrical activity of seven subcortical areas in the brain of the immobilized cat. The areas studied were the caudate nucleus, basolateral amygdala, posterior hippocampus, septum, lateral hypothalamus, medial hypothalamus, and mesencephalic reticular formation. The effects of chlordiazepoxide hydrochloride and diazepam were compared with those of chlorpromazine and pentobarbital. Each drug was tested at 5, 10, and 20 mg/kg i.v.; doses were given at hourly intervals. The data were evaluated by the power spectrum technique (for a description, see Schallek *et al.*, 1968, in Section VI,A,1).

Chlordiazepoxide hydrochloride had little effect on total power (mean squared amplitude) but caused considerable change in distribution of relative power. The largest changes were in the hippocampus. Following the 10-mg/kg dose, relative power was significantly greater than control over all frequency bands from 10 to 20 Hz (Fig. 9).

Chlorpromazine increased total power in all brain areas except the

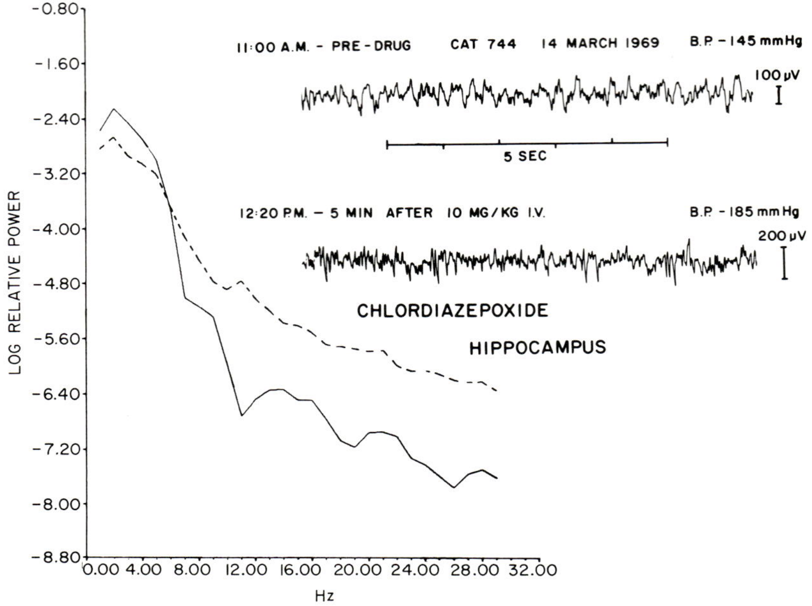

FIG. 9. Effects of chlordiazepoxide hydrochloride, 10 mg/kg i.v., on spontaneous electrical activity of hippocampus in immobilized cats. Sample recordings are upper right. (B.P.) Peripheral blood pressure. Power spectra are lower left. Solid line is predrug spectrum, dashed line post-drug spectrum; each spectrum represents mean of 5 cats. Change in total power (mean squared amplitude, post-drug/pre-drug) is 1.06. (From Schallek and Thomas, 1971, by permission.)

hippocampus; the largest increase was in the caudate nucleus. In contrast to chlordiazepoxide hydrochloride, relative power at the upper part of the frequency span was decreased by chlorpromazine; this change occurred in all areas except the hippocampus and reticular formation. The largest shift was in the medial hypothalamus (Fig. 10).

Pentobarbital was the only drug to increase total power in all brain areas. Relative power distribution was decreased at the higher frequency bands in the caudate nucleus, septum, lateral hypothalamus, and reticular formation; the largest shift occurred in the reticular area (Fig. 11). The effects of pentobarbital on the reticular formation were greater than those of any other drug.

Diazepam had only small and scattered effects in this group of experiments.

Control tests indicated that the changes in the electrical activity of the brain were not correlated with changes in peripheral blood pressure.

The observation that chlordiazepoxide hydrochloride acts predominantly on the hippocampus confirms the findings of Olds and Olds (1969). This confirmation is particularly interesting because these authors worked on the rat, whereas Schallek and Thomas (1971) used the cat. However, the effects of diazepam differed sharply in the two groups of experiments. Although this compound showed marked activity in the freely moving rat, it had little effect on the immobilized cat. Diazepam has effects on the sensory inflow to the brain (Olds and Baldrighi, 1968) and we believe that this sensory inflow is greatly reduced in the immobilized preparation. Further studies with this drug should avoid conditions of reduced afferent input to the brain.

What is the relationship between the action of chlordiazepoxide hydrochloride on the hippocampus and the psychotropic effects of the drug? Nauta and Haymaker (1969) point out that the fornix system, which is the main efferent pathway of the hippocampus, distributes fibers to the septum, hypothalamus, and midbrain. The circuit of Papez connects the hippocampus with the mammillary bodies, anterior thalamus, and cingulate

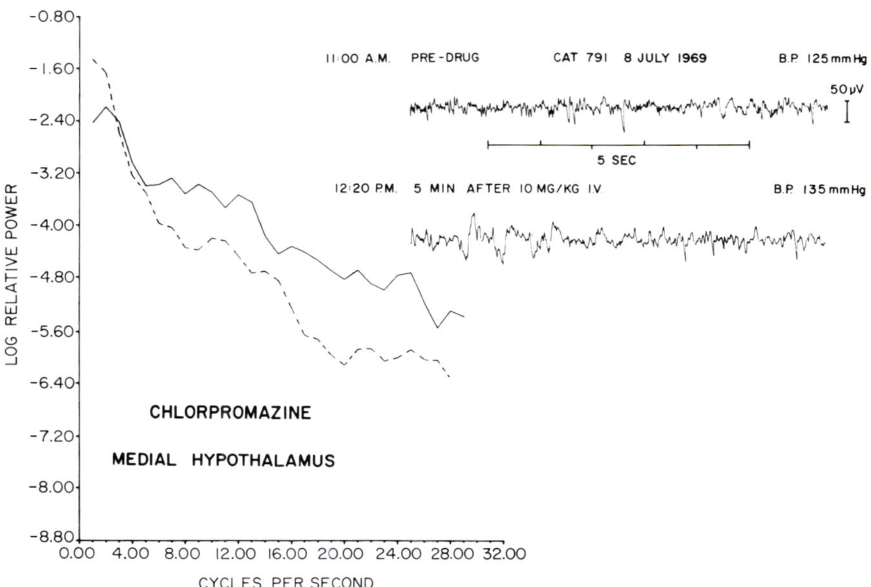

FIG. 10. Effects of chlorpromazine hydrochloride, 10 mg/kg i.v., on medial hypothalamus of immobilized cats. Arrangement as in Fig. 9. Upper right—sample recordings; lower left—power spectra. (B.P.) Peripheral blood pressure. Change in total power (mean square amplitude, post-drug/pre-drug) is 1.51.

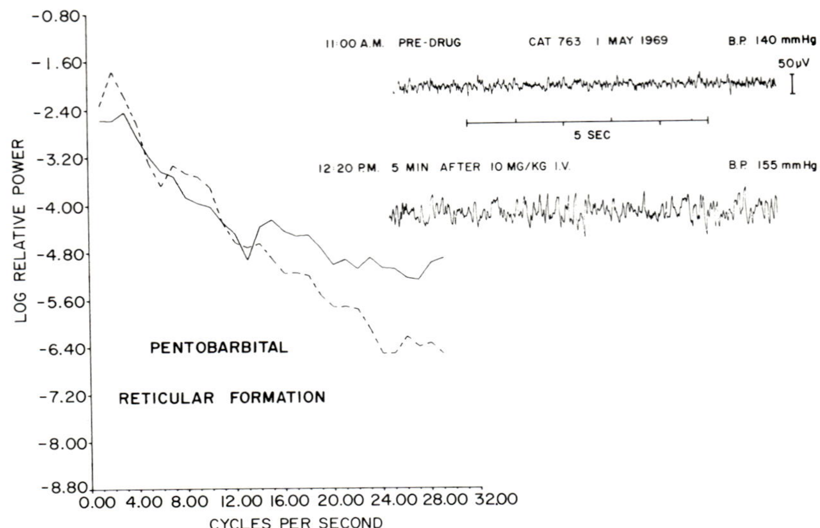

FIG. 11. Effects of sodium pentobarbital, 10 mg/kg i.v., on mesencephalic reticular formation of immobilized cats. Upper right—sample recordings; lower left—power spectra. (B.P.) Peripheral blood pressure. Change in total power (mean square amplitude, post-drug/pre-drug) is 3.07. (From Schallek and Thomas, 1971, by permission.)

gyrus; association fibers from the cingulate reach a large portion of the cerebral cortex. The action of a drug on the hippocampus might modulate activity in one or more of these brain areas; hence the drug might display a variety of psychotropic effects.

Two groups of workers have tested the effects of medazepam or medazepam hydrochloride on the limbic system of the cat. Heinemann *et al.* (1970) placed electrodes in the central nucleus of the amygdala, ventral hippocampus, dorsomedial thalamus, and the septum of freely moving cats. Each electrode was used for both stimulation and recording. Medazepam was administered by continuous infusion through a cannula implanted in the jugular vein; blood concentrations of 6 to 8 μg/ml were maintained over a 5-hour period. Thresholds for the following pathways were lowered under the action of the drug: responses evoked in the amygdala by stimulation of the thalamus and septum and responses evoked in the thalamus and septum by stimulation of the amygdala. Thresholds for the remaining eight pathways were elevated, including all responses to or from the hippocampus. The authors suggest that the lowered reactivity of the hippocampus may be involved in the sleep-inducing action of medazepam observed by Heinemann *et al.* (1968).

The increased responsiveness of the amygdala does not agree with studies made in freely moving cats by Schallek *et al.* (1970). These authors found that medazepam hydrochloride, 12 mg/kg p.o., elevated the threshold for behavioral arousal induced by electrical stimulation of the basolateral or anterior amygdala. They also observed that fast activity appeared in the ECoG 4 hours after administration of the drug. Shifts toward faster frequencies have been noted with this drug in the cortex, caudate nucleus, and hippocampus of immobilized cats (Schallek *et al.*, 1968, 1970).

3. *Brainstem*

Vieth *et al.* (1968) tested the effects of nitrazepam in acute experiments on *encéphale isolé* cats. Bipolar stainless-steel electrodes were placed in the amygdala, hippocampus, septum, thalamus, hypothalamus, and reticular formation. Each electrode was used for both stimulation and recording. Following administration of nitrazepam, 20–80 mg/kg p.o., the largest increases in threshold occurred in the responses evoked in the amygdala, hippocampus, and septum by stimulation of the reticular formation. The results suggest that nitrazepam produces "a selective attenuation of limbic inputs from the brainstem."

Olds and Baldrighi (1968) tested the effects of drugs on visually evoked responses in the tectotegmental area of the rat. This area is at the dorsal boundary of the reticular activating system. The tests were conducted in unanesthetized animals with chronically implanted electrodes. Stimuli consisted of single flashes of white light at an average interval of 48 seconds. The responses to each set of twenty stimuli were summated by a computer of average transients.

The results are summarized in Table III. Chlordiazepoxide hydrochloride and diazepam reduced the amplitude of the evoked responses. Meprobamate increased the amplitude at low doses and reduced it at a higher dose; sodium pentobarbital facilitated the response at all doses tested. It is evident that at low doses the effects of the benzodiazepines are opposite to those of meprobamate and sodium pentobarbital.

The authors point out that the reticular formation is usually considered to have an inhibitory influence on sensory inflow. Hence a drug that facilitates this formation might reduce the size of sensory evoked responses, whereas one that depresses the formation might potentiate the responses. If this view is correct, then low doses of benzodiazepines facilitate the reticular formation, and low doses of meprobamate and sodium pentobarbital depress it.

TABLE III

EFFECTS OF DRUGS ON AMPLITUDE OF VISUAL EVOKED RESPONSES IN TEGMENTUM OF RAT[a]

	Mean percentage of control values[b]					
	Dose (mg/kg i.p.)					
Drug	5	10	20	40	80	120
Chlordiazepoxide hydrochloride	93	95	81	—	—	—
Diazepam	92	92	70	—	—	—
Meprobamate	—	—	—	112	107	93
Sodium pentobarbital	113	108	106	—	—	—

[a] Reprinted by permission of M. E. Olds and G. Baldrighi, 1968, Pergamon, Oxford.

[b] Each figure is mean value for seven or eight observations made between 25 and 200 minutes after drug administration. Each observation consists of the summated responses to twenty photic stimuli.

The importance of studying drug effects at low doses is emphasized by Olds and Baldrighi (1968). High doses of many compounds cause a general depression of the CNS; "the question is therefore one of differentiating compounds at the low doses effective on behavior, in order to determine not merely particular sensitivity of a structure to a given compound, but also the pattern of action."

That benzodiazepines activate the reticular formation could explain not only the reduction of evoked potentials but also some other observations. Behavioral restlessness and increased ECoG frequencies in cats after acute administration of benzodiazepines were reported previously (Randall and Schallek, 1968). Increased behavioral responding and reduced sleep under acute treatment with benzodiazepines are described in the present review. Effects of low doses on the reticular formation might provide an important distinction between benzodiazepines and other centrally active drugs.

The effects of drugs on the red nucleus were studied by Gogolak *et al.* (1969). Hypnotic barbiturates such as pentobarbital (30 mg/kg i.v.) elicit a very regular rhythm in this nucleus in the rabbit. Similar regular rhythms were observed with meprobamate (100–150 mg/kg) and with chlordiazepoxide hydrochloride (50 mg/kg), but not with chlorpromazine (10–20 mg/kg). The authors suggest that elicitation of a regular red nucleus rhythm is a property common to a group of drugs which are, or could be, used for induction of general anesthesia. However, it should be noted that the dose of chlordiazepoxide hydrochloride used by these authors is 10 times that shown to be effective in rat brain (Olds and Baldrighi, 1968; Olds and Olds, 1969).

B. Behavioral Studies

An increasing number of workers are using behavioral techniques to determine the parts of the brain involved in the actions of psychotropic drugs. The studies may be divided into those based on general observation of the animal's response and those using operant techniques.

1. *Observations of Responses*

Kido *et al.* (1967) described behavioral responses to stimulation of various parts of the brain in cats with chronically indwelling electrodes. Four different drugs produced rises in threshold, but the patterns of activity fell into three groups (Table IV).

1. The largest rise in threshold produced by chlordiazepoxide hydrochloride was for the hissing response caused by stimulation of the central gray matter of the mesencephalon. Meprobamate also produced its largest threshold rise in this area.

2. Following administration of chlorpromazine, the greatest rise in threshold was for the searching response induced by stimulation of the anterior hypothalamus.

3. Phenobarbital produced its greatest threshold rise for the somatic movement caused by stimulation of the reticular formation. This selective action of a barbiturate on the reticular formation agrees with the electrophysiological data described in the previous section. In contrast to the action of phenobarbital, chlordiazepoxide hydrochloride had no effect on the reticular threshold.

Two workers have studied the action of benzodiazepines on the hissing response induced in cats by stimulation of the perifornical area of the anterior hypothalamus. Malick (1970) obtained threshold rises of 1.9 to 2.0 V with chlordiazepoxide hydrochloride (10 mg/kg i.p.), diazepam (4 mg/kg), oxazepam (12 mg/kg), and phenobarbital (40 mg/kg). In contrast to these drugs, chlorpromazine (7.5 mg/kg) lowered the hiss threshold. Similar results were obtained by Funderburk *et al.* (1970). A 30% elevation in threshold voltage was produced by chlordiazepoxide hydrochloride, 10 mg/kg i.p. Pentobarbital sodium, 10 mg/kg, produced a threshold rise of approximately 85%. Effective doses of the latter drug produced ataxia. In agreement with the previous study, chlorpromazine at 2.5 mg/kg consistently lowered the threshold for hissing.

Several authors have tested the effects of psychoactive drugs on the

TABLE IV

EFFECTS OF DRUGS ON BEHAVIOR INDUCED BY BRAIN STIMULATION IN THE CAT WITH CHRONICALLY INDWELLING ELECTRODES[a]

Brain area	Response	Mean % rise in threshold[b]			
		Chlordiazepoxide hydrochloride (20 mg/kg p.o.)	Chlorpromazine (3 mg/kg i.v.)	Meprobamate (30 mg/kg i.v.)	Phenobarbital (30 mg/kg i.v.)
Anterior hypothalamus	Searching	46	80	50	67
Posterior hypothalamus	Rage	35	4	65	60
Reticular formation	Somatic movement	0	38	32	75
Central gray matter	Hissing	59	8	83	40
Septum	Feeding	12	5	5	37
Amygdala	Feeding	10	7	30	63

[a] Reproduced by permission from R. Kido, K. Hirose, K. Yamamoto, and A. Matsushita (1967). *In* "Progress in Brain Research, Structure and Function of the Limbic System" (W. R. Adey and T. Tokizane, eds.), Volume 27, p. 377. Elsevier, Amsterdam.

[b] The experiments were performed on 15 cats, using a Latin square design for drug administration at 2-week intervals.

hyperreactivity produced in rats by lesions in various areas of the brain. Stark and Henderson (1966) used rats with septal lesions. The hyperreactivity was attenuated by chlordiazepoxide hydrochloride (20 mg/kg i.p.) and by chlorpromazine (5 mg/kg). However, meprobamate (100 mg/kg), phenobarbital (20 mg/kg), and pentobarbital (10 mg/kg) produced varying degrees of ataxia but failed to decrease the reactivity of the rats. Slightly different results were obtained in the same preparation by Beattie *et al.* (1969). Chlordiazepoxide hydrochloride at 15 mg/kg i.p. produced a 60% taming effect with no neurological deficit, whereas pentobarbital at 10 mg/kg had a 50% taming effect and a 26% neurological deficit. Both groups of workers agree that the action of chlordiazepoxide hydrochloride on septal hyperreactivity is more specific than that of pentobarbital.

The classification of psychotropic drugs depends very much on the procedure being used. Thus in various tests described in this section, chlordiazepoxide hydrochloride was classified with meprobamate, with phenobarbital, and with chlorpromazine. Each of these drugs has a variety of central effects; a single test can measure only one of these actions.

2. *Operant Procedures*

Margules and Stein (1969) attempted to determine which brain areas are involved in the disinhibitory effects of benzodiazepines. There is evidence that a periventricular system, which extends from the forebrain through the medial hypothalamus to the midbrain, may be involved in the suppression of behavior. They tested the role of this system in rats trained to press a lever for milk reward. In addition to this unpunished schedule, the presence of a tone indicated that every response would be rewarded with milk and also punished with a shock to the feet.

When cannulas were implanted so as to produce bilateral lesions in the medial hypothalamus, a marked increase occurred in the rate of punished responses. Unpunished responses were not affected. Crystalline drugs were now applied directly to the hypothalamus by forcing them through the cannulas. Cholinergic agents such as carbachol restored the suppression of punished responses.

In another group of rats, in which the cannulas had produced smaller lesions in the medial hypothalamus, response rates were suppressed during the punishment schedule. Implantation of atropine or scopolamine released the punished behavior from suppression. Implantation of chlordiazepoxide hydrochloride or other benzodiazepines was without effect.

The authors interpret these results in the following manner. The restoration of punished behavior by midline diencephalic lesions indicates that this brain area is involved in mediating the suppressant effects of punishment. The suppression of the punished behavior by cholinergic agents indicates that cholinergic synapses are involved. This indication is supported by the opposing effects of cholinergic blocking agents.

Benzodiazepines were shown (Margules and Stein, 1967) to restore punished responses when administered systemically. Their failure to do so when applied directly to the hypothalamus suggests that they act "at a non-hypothalamic level of the punishment system."

Margules and Stein (1967) activated the ventromedial hypothalamus (VMH) by direct application of carbachol. The resulting suppression of response was antagonized by systemic injection of oxazepam, 2.5 mg/kg i.p. "Since such direct activation of the VMH presumably would override any effects on input, this observation suggests that benzodiazepines act on the efferent side of the VMH."

C. Radiochemical Studies

Several authors have used biochemical techniques to localize the action of benzodiazepines on the brain. Placidi and Cassano (1968) injected chlordiazepoxide-^{14}C into mice at a dose of 11 mg/kg i.v. Radioautographic techniques showed that the drug or its metabolites easily passed the blood–brain barrier. The highest brain concentrations appeared 1 minute after injection. At this time activity was concentrated in the choroid plexuses and in the gray matter, particularly in the thalamic nuclei and in the cortex of the cerebrum and cerebellum. After 10 minutes, activity was lower and was evenly distributed within both gray and white matter. From 20 minutes to 12 hours after drug administration, there was a progressive decrease in radioactivity in the gray matter, whereas the white matter retained higher levels. Only traces of radioactivity were found after 24 hours. The authors suggest that the initial brain distribution depends on vascularity and blood flow. The decrease in radioactivity during the next 12 hours indicates that "^{14}C-chlordiazepoxide was not retained selectively in any portion of the gray matter."

Similar findings were obtained by van der Kleijn (1969a), who studied chlordiazepoxide-^{14}C and diazepam-^{14}C. Both drugs were injected into mice at a dose of 15 mg/kg i.v. There was a rapid uptake in the gray matter, especially in the colliculi, in the thalamic and medullary nuclei, and in the cerebral and cerebellar cortex. The maximum uptake of diazepam was at 1 minute, whereas chlordiazepoxide showed a maximum at 5 minutes. After 30 minutes, retention appeared in the white matter, particularly in the corpus callosum, midbrain, cerebellum, and spinal cord. The patterns of distribution were similar for both compounds, although the loss of radioactivity was faster with chlordiazepoxide than with diazepam.

Two studies used radioautographic techniques to describe the distribution of diazepam in monkey brain. van der Kleijn and Wijffels (1971), using newborn rhesus monkeys, observed high concentrations of the drug in the cerebrum, cerebellum, brainstem, and spinal cord. Accumulation of the drug in myelinated tissues was noteworthy. Idänpään-Heikkilä *et al.* (1971b), using cynomolgus monkeys, also observed that diazepam had a high affinity for white matter. The highest uptake was in the cerebral white matter, optic tract, corpus callosum, dentate nucleus, pons, and medulla. Relatively low amounts of radioactivity were found in cerebral gray matter, caudate nucleus, hippocampus, and hypothalamus.

The areas in which diazepam was concentrated in the radioautographic studies differ markedly from the areas in which the drug showed activity in electrophysiological tests (Section VI,A). The reviewers suggest that benzodiazepines which are absorbed by lipids of the myelin sheath may be in storage. Pharmacological activity may be attributed to a few molecules reaching key sites in gray matter.

The effects of benzodiazepines on catecholamine metabolism in various regions of the rat brain were studied by Taylor and Laverty (1969). Chlordiazepoxide, diazepam, and nitrazepam were each given at a dose of 10 mg/kg s.c. The drugs had little effect on the endogenous levels of catecholamines. However, radioisotopic experiments revealed that the drugs increased the concentrations of tritiated norepinephrine in the thalamus, midbrain, cortex, and cerebellum, but not in the brainstem. Tritiated dopamine levels were increased in the corpus striatum. The benzodiazepines also prevented increase in norepinephrine turnover induced by the stress of electroshock to the feet; this effect was maximal in the regions in which the drugs affected catecholamine metabolism in unstressed rats. The authors suggest that benzodiazepines "act by decreasing catecholamine turnover in specific regions of the rat brain." (See also Corrodi *et al.*, 1971 in Section IX.)

It is evident that the use of radioisotopes to localize the action of these drugs is still in its infancy. An intriguing possibility for the future is the combination of radiochemical techniques with electron microscopy. This might make it possible to determine the sites of action of drugs at the subcellular level.

VII. Discussion of Neuropharmacology and Behavior

Recent studies indicate that the CNS displays a balance of excitatory and inhibitory influences. Examples of such antagonistic effects on spinal reflexes are presented in Section II. Some opposing actions on cortical activity are described by Moruzzi (1964). In addition to the reticular activating system in the rostral part of the brainstem, there is a deactivating (or hypnogenic) system in the medulla. These systems can be separated pharmacologically. Injection of thiopental into the carotid artery, reaching the rostral brainstem, synchronizes the EEG, whereas injection into the vertebral artery, reaching the caudal brainstem, produces EEG activation (Magni *et al.*, 1959).

The actions of benzodiazepines may be considered in relation to these dual aspects of central nervous function. The present review shows that whereas under certain conditions these agents exhibit depressant effects, under other circumstances they show signs of facilitation.

Among the depressant actions of these drugs are the following: depression of polysynaptic reflexes in spinal cord of cat; reduced behavioral and pressor responses to hypothalamic stimulation; suppression of chemically or electrically induced seizure discharges; taming effect in rats with septal lesions; induction of sleep by injection into femoral vein or carotid artery; depression of visually evoked potentials in hippocampus and cortex; blocking of unit activity in hippocampus.

The following responses demonstrate apparent facilitatory actions of benzodiazepines: activation response following injection into vertebral artery; shift toward faster frequencies in spontaneous electrical activity of cortex and hippocampus; lowered threshold of evoked potentials in amygdala; increased rate of fixed-interval responding in monkeys; restoration of suppressed behavior in rats and cats.

A key to the problem of how one group of drugs can have both facilitatory and depressant effects is provided by the experiments of Zattoni and Rossi (1967). When nitrazepam is injected into the activating areas of the brainstem, the rabbits show signs of sleep; when the drug is injected into hypnogenic areas, the animals become alert. Both the depressant and the facilitatory effects of benzodiazepines may be caused by suppressant actions of the drugs; the net result will depend on whether excitatory or inhibitory areas of the brain are affected.

There are two cases in which the actions of the benzodiazepines have been attributed to increased inhibition. These situations involve depression of spinal reflexes (Schmidt *et al.*, 1967) and anticonvulsant activity (Guerrero-Figueroa *et al.*, 1967, 1968, 1969, 1970). We would like to suggest that these actions are caused primarily by depression of facilitatory influences, thereby shifting the balance of activity toward increased inhibition. Further research, possibly involving the use of microelectrodes, is needed in this area.

An important question is whether the benzodiazepines show a unique type of action. Examples of distinct differences between the actions of benzodiazepines and phenothiazines have been mentioned throughout this review. Diazepam blocks seizure responses to photic stimulation in the baboon, whereas chlorpromazine potentiates the response (Killam *et al.*, 1967). Chlordiazepoxide hydrochloride causes a shift toward faster frequencies in various areas of the cat brain, but chlorpromazine shifts activity toward slower frequencies (Schallek and Thomas, 1971). Oxazepam releases a variety of behaviors from suppression, but chlorpromazine lacks this effect (Margules and Stein, 1967).

Different mechanisms of action of benzodiazepines and phenothiazines are proposed by Stein (in Buser *et al.*, 1970). He suggests that there are dual systems for behavioral reward and punishment:

1. The medial forebrain bundle (passing through the lateral hypothalamus) is the reward system. This has adrenergic mediation and is blocked by phenothiazines and other neuroleptics.
2. The periventricular system, which generates the punishment reaction, is cholinergic. These neurons are influenced not only by anticholinergic drugs, but are also "specifically inhibited" by benzodiazepines and other tranquilizers.

Both benzodiazepines and barbiturates have been classified as tranquilizers (Margules and Stein, 1967). Several situations have been cited in the present review in which drugs of these two classes show similar actions.

Pentobarbital, diazepam, and chlordiazepoxide hydrochloride depress polysynaptic reflexes in the spinal cord of the cat; amobarbital and chlordiazepoxide hydrochloride prevent blood pressure rises in lever-pressing monkeys; fast activity in the ECoG of the sleeping cat has been noted with nitrazepam and with pentobarbital; both chlordiazepoxide hydrochloride and phenobarbital raise the "hiss threshold" induced by hypothalamic stimulation in the cat.

Nevertheless, distinct differences have been noted between the actions of the benzodiazepines and those of the barbiturates: diazepam reduces traffic in the splanchnic nerve to a greater extent than in the cervical sympathetic or vagus, whereas pentobarbital causes marked depression in all three nerves; pentobarbital reduces the pressor, cardiac, pupillary, and nictitating membrane responses to hypothalamic stimulation, whereas diazepam shows a selective block of the vasopressor and cardiac responses; visually evoked potentials in the hippocampus are blocked by nitrazepam but not by phenobarbital; unit activity in the hippocampus is selectively inhibited by chlordiazepoxide hydrochloride and diazepam, whereas pentobarbital shows a selective inhibition of the reticular formation; chlordiazepoxide hydrochloride and diazepam reduce the amplitude of visually evoked responses in the brainstem of the rat, but pentobarbital increases the amplitude.

Olds and Olds (1969) observe that "there now appears to be general agreement that there are drug receptors in the mesencephalic reticular formation which are directly acted upon by barbiturates before action on other structures occurs, and that such action is largely responsible for the behavioral and EEG effects noted with these compounds." In contrast to the barbiturates, their findings support the likelihood of a selective action of benzodiazepines on hippocampal neurons. They conjecture that the hippocampus may have an inhibitory action on the hypothalamus. Release of the hypothalamus from inhibition could, in turn, stimulate the reticular activating system. Olds and Baldrighi (1968) propose that stimulation of the reticular formation might account for the increased behavioral responses and EEG activation sometimes observed with benzodiazepines.

If some behavioral effects of benzodiazepines involve depression of the hippocampus, we would expect similar effects to follow lesions in this area. Behavioral results of hippocampal lesions were reviewed by two authors. Douglas (1967) found that these lesions produce a deficit consisting of "an inability to withhold a response." Kimble (1968) concluded that animals with hippocampal damage differ from normals by being less able to inhibit previously learned responses. Thus the number of trials needed to reach extinction in a maze test was 24 in control rats, 22 in rats with cortical lesions, and 88 in rats with hippocampal lesions. These results provide an interesting parallel to the disinhibitory effects of benzodiazepines described in Section V,B.

Summary

The benzodiazepines show both depressant and facilitatory effects in laboratory experiments. The depressant actions include depression of spinal reflexes, suppression of seizure discharges, reduction of responses to hypothalamic stimulation and blocking of unit activity in the hippocampus. Among the facilitatory effects are a shift toward faster frequencies in the ECoG, a lowered threshold of evoked responses in the amygdala, and restoration of suppressed behaviors in rats and cats. It is suggested that depressant actions are caused by direct suppression of hyperactive neurons, whereas facilitation is due to release from inhibition. There may be a shift from excitatory to depressant effects during chronic administration of these drugs.

There are distinct differences between the activities of benzodiazepines and of phenothiazines (e.g., the latter drugs do not release suppressed behaviors). Although the actions of the benzodiazepines and the barbiturates overlap, somewhat, there are also differences. The primary site of action of the barbiturates seems to be in the reticular formation, whereas that of the benzodiazepines may be in the hippocampus. Since the hippocampus has neural connections with many parts of the brain, a drug acting on this area might display a variety of psychotropic effects.

VIII. Metabolism

The metabolism of benzodiazepines by the drug metabolizing enzymes of the liver follows the classic rules outlined by Brodie *et al.* (1958). The benzodiazepines may be oxidized, reduced, demethylated, deaminated, hydroxylated, acetylated, glucuronidated, or sulfated during the processes of detoxification and excretion. Since most benzodiazepines are fat-soluble, they are stored in fat depots and slowly released. This accounts for the relatively long half-lives of certain members of the series. Some of the metabolic products originating in the liver may retain equal, greater, or lesser activity than the parent compound and may have different durations of action. A problem exists as to how much of the CNS effect of a benzodiazepine may be accounted for by active metabolites. This is of primary concern when the potency or duration of action of the metabolite is greater than that of the parent substance.

A. Metabolites of Chlordiazepoxide Hydrochloride

The major metabolites of chlordiazepoxide hydrochloride in man, dog, and rat were shown to be demoxepam (Ro 5-2092, lactam) by Koechlin *et al.* (1965), and *N*-desmethylchlordiazepoxide (Ro 5-0883) in dog and man by Schwartz and Postma (1966) (Fig. 12). After administration of demoxepam to dogs, Schwartz *et al.* (1971) found the additional metabolites desmethyldiazepam, oxazepam, and other hydroxylated products which are also metabolites of diazepam. These will be discussed in Section VIII,B. Demoxepam and the *N*-desmethyl metabolite had the same order of activity as chlordiazepoxide hydrochloride in tests for muscle relaxant, anticonvulsant, and antifighting activity in mice and muscle relaxant activity in cats but showed less activity in conditioned avoidance behavior in rats and in taming of monkeys (Randall *et al.*, 1965, 1969).

Chlordiazepoxide-2-^{14}C given orally to mice (20 mg/kg) showed rapid absorption and protected against metrazole convulsions for 0.5 to 4 hours (Coutinho *et al.*, 1969). The metabolite *N*-desmethylchlordiazepoxide (Ro

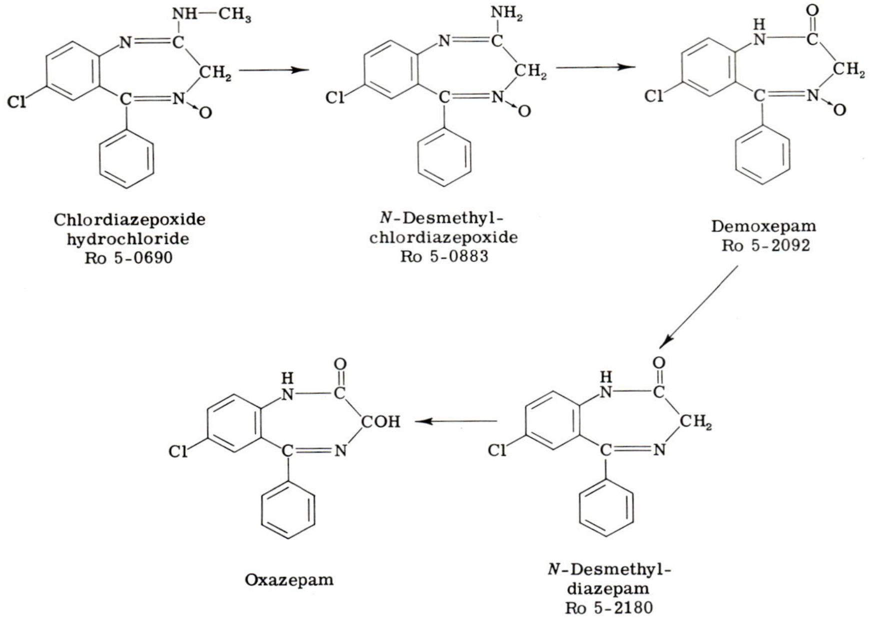

Chlordiazepoxide hydrochloride
Ro 5-0690

N-Desmethyl-chlordiazepoxide
Ro 5-0883

Demoxepam
Ro 5-2092

Oxazepam

N-Desmethyl-diazepam
Ro 5-2180

FIG. 12. Metabolic pathway of chlordiazepoxide hydrochloride.

5-0883) was the major constituent in blood, brain, and muscle. It was present in brain and blood in higher concentration than chlordiazepoxide hydrochloride for 0.5 to 6 hours. Demoxepam (Ro 5-2092) was present in blood and brain at lower concentrations than chlordiazepoxide hydrochloride for 6 hours. The *N*-desmethyl metabolite, Ro 5-0883, most closely paralleled the antimetrazole activity in onset and duration and probably accounted for the anticonvulsant action.

Kaplan *et al.* (1970) presented a six-compartment open-system model to elucidate the physiological disposition of chlordiazepoxide hydrochloride and its two pharmacologically active biotransformation products, Ro 5-0883 and demoxepam. The tests were made in dogs following the intravenous administration of 10 mg/kg chlordiazepoxide hydrochloride. The pharmacokinetic parameters used in the model were obtained by administering each of the three compounds separately. After administration of chlordiazepoxide hydrochloride, excellent agreement was obtained between the plasma levels of the intact drug and the *N*-desmethyl metabolite and the calculated levels of each generated from the model. The main features of chlordiazepoxide hydrochloride disposition were (*a*) its complete biotransformation to the desmethyl metabolite (Ro 5-0883), (*b*) elimination of the desmethyl metabolite almost entirely by biotransformation with up to 50% proceeding to demoxepam by oxidative deamination, and (*c*) elimination of demoxepam by urinary excretion and further biotransformation.

B. Major Metabolites of Diazepam

The major metabolites of diazepam in man, dogs, and rats were identified by Schwartz *et al.* (1965, 1967) and by Ruelius *et al.* (1965) as *N*-desmethyl-

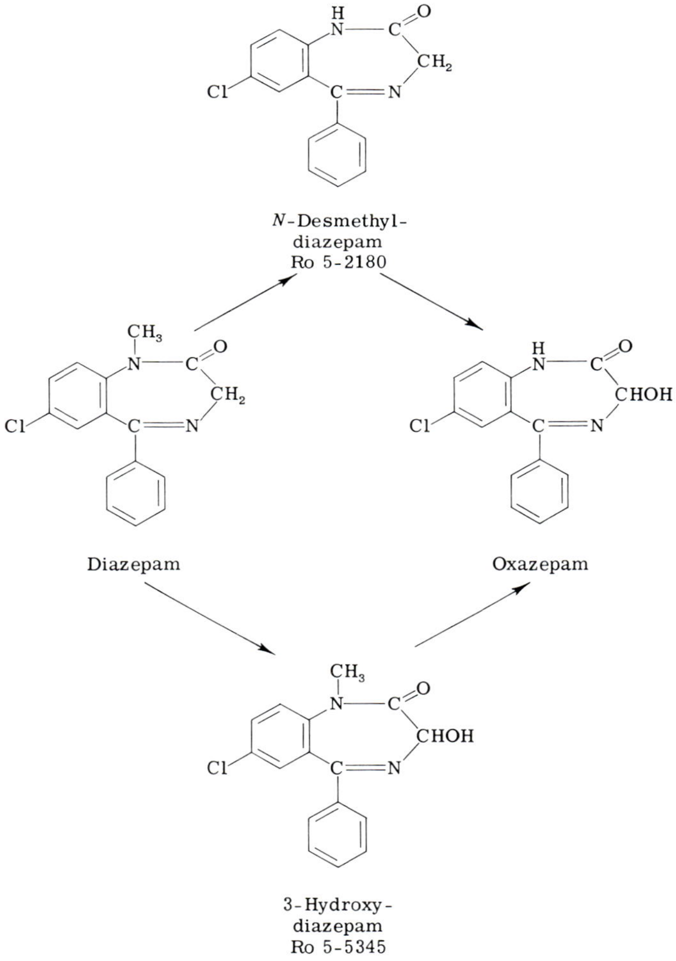

N-Desmethyl-
diazepam
Ro 5-2180

Diazepam

Oxazepam

3-Hydroxy-
diazepam
Ro 5-5345

FIG. 13. Metabolic pathway of diazepam.

diazepam, 3-hydroxydiazepam, and oxazepam (Fig. 13). Minor metabolites included various hydroxylated products.

DeSilva *et al.* (1966) observed that single doses of diazepam given to man produced diazepam blood levels which declined in 24 hours, whereas repeated daily doses produced gradually rising levels. *N*-Desmethyldiazepam was the major metabolite which appeared in blood 24 hours after a single dose. It accumulated with daily doses and, on discontinuing the treatment, persisted longer in the blood than diazepam. Only traces of the urinary metabolites, 3-hydroxydiazepam and oxazepam, were found in blood.

Pharmacological studies showed that 3-hydroxydiazepam resembled diazepam in muscle relaxant, anticonvulsant, and sedative effects and also in depression of conditioned avoidance responding in rats and monkeys. The *N*-desmethyl analog was weaker than diazepam in most of the pharmacological tests, and oxazepam (3-hydroxy-*N*-desmethyldiazepam) showed further reduction in most pharmacological activities (Randall *et al.*, 1965; 1970).

Gluckman (1965) pointed out the potent antimetrazole activity together with the low toxicity of oxazepam. Owen *et al.* (1970) also described the low acute toxicity of oxazepam in various species and its good tolerance on chronic administration in dogs, rats, and rabbits and in pregnant animals.

Marcucci *et al.* (1968) reported that after administration of diazepam, 5 mg/kg i.v., the drug accumulated in brain and disappeared from blood at similar rates in mice and rats. The *N*-desmethyl metabolites were present in higher concentration in the blood and brain of mice than of rats. The anticonvulsant activity of diazepam was stronger and of longer duration in mice than rats. In rats the antimetrazole activity paralleled the concentration of diazepam; in mice the antimetrazole activity paralleled the concentration of the *N*-desmethyl metabolites.

The preceding study used methods which could not distinguish *N*-desmethyldiazepam from oxazepam. The effects of the latter compound were compared with diazepam by Marcucci *et al.* (1970a). Administration of diazepam, 5 mg/kg i.v., to mice gave brain levels of 0.17 μg/gm of oxazepam and about 80% protection against metrazole convulsions at 20 hours. Administration of oxazepam, 5 mg/kg i.v., to mice also gave brain levels of 0.15 μg/gm of oxazepam and 80% protection against metrazole at 18 hours and levels of 0.11 μg/gm and 60% protection at 24 hours. *N*-Desmethyldiazepam and *N*-methyloxazepan were not present in brain at 20 hours. Therefore the long duration of action of diazepam in mice was due to accumulation of oxazepan in the brain.

In studies on species differences, *N*-desmethyldiazepam, one of the principal metabolites of diazepam in mice but not in rats, disappeared from the bloodstream and accumulated in the brain and adipose tissue similarly in mice and rats (Marcucci *et al.*, 1970b). 3-Hydroxydiazepam also disappeared from the bloodstream and accumulated in the brain of rats and mice at about the same rate. However, the pattern of accumulation in the adipose tissue was different in the two species because 3-hydroxydiazepam entered this tissue more slowly in the mouse than in the rat. In rats there was no accumulation of oxazepam from *N*-desmethyldiazepam, and only limited concentrations were present in blood, brain, or adipose tissue when 3-hydroxydiazepam was given. In contrast, high concentrations of oxazepam were formed in mice and accumulated for several hours from both *N*-desmethyldiazepam and 3-hydroxydiazepam. The reason for the accumulation of oxazepam in mice and not in rats may be related to different rates of disappearance of this metabolite from plasma and tissues in these two species. In fact, when oxazepam was injected into rats, it disappeared in about 3 hours, whereas in mice the same dose of oxazepam was still present in blood and tissues after 10 hours.

Coutinho *et al.* (1970) reported that diazepam-^{3}H, administered to mice at 2.5 mg/kg p.o., gave maximum protection against metrazole seizures for 30 minutes to 2 hours after dosing, with 50% protection from 4 to 6 hours. The anticonvulsant activity was compared with the tissue concentrations of diazepam and its major metabolites. Measurable levels of diazepam and its *N*-demethylated and 3-hydroxylated derivatives were obtained in blood, brain, and muscle as early as 1 minute after oral administration of diazepam. Peak values were reached in 5 minutes. Diazepam fell to unmeasurable levels in 2 hours, and its hydroxylation product in 4 hours. The concentration of *N*-desmethyldiazepam reached unmeasurable levels in 6 to 12 hours. In contrast, oxazepam showed a peak value 30 minutes after administration of diazepam. The concentration remained relatively constant for 12 hours and showed a slight fall at 24 hours. The authors suggest that the antimetrazole activity in mice is more closely related to the presence of the *N*-demethylated derivative than to the other biotransformation products.

Van der Kleijn (1969b) compared the distribution and metabolism of diazepam in animals and humans. The tests involved administration of diazepam-$^{14}C_2$ or -*N*-$^{14}CH_3$. The half-life of diazepam ranged from 40 minutes in mice and dogs to 9 to 24 hours in humans. The half-life of desmethyldiazepam was 6 hours in mice, 9 hours in dogs, and 25–50 hours in man. The great species differences are believed to be controlled by differences in disposition rates owing to differences in circulation and behavioral activity rather than to differences in rates of metabolism.

Idänpään-Heikkilä *et al.* (1971a) studied the crossing of placental barriers by diazepam. They injected 25 mice (13 in early pregnancy and 12 in late pregnancy), 8 hamsters in late pregnancy, and 4 third trimester pregnant *Cynomolgus iris* monkeys with diazepam-^{14}C. The animals were sacrificed at various time intervals. Diazepam-^{14}C and its metabolites crossed the placental barrier and accumulated in the fetal tissue in all three species. In mice, diazepam-^{14}C and its metabolites accumulated in the fetuses more rapidly in late than in early pregnancy. Fetal hamsters had a high uptake of radioactivity in the peripheral nerves, liver, spinal cord, kidney, lung, fat, cerebellum, and plasma. There was a pronounced uptake and long retention of diazepam and its metabolites in the fetal monkey cerebellum, spinal cord, and peripheral nerves.

C. Metabolites of Nitrazepam

Rieder (1965) showed that orally administered nitrazepam was absorbed by the human with maximum blood levels at 4 hours. The half-life for elimination of an intravenous dose of the radioactive drug was 6 hours. The 7-nitro group of nitrazepam was reduced in human subjects to the

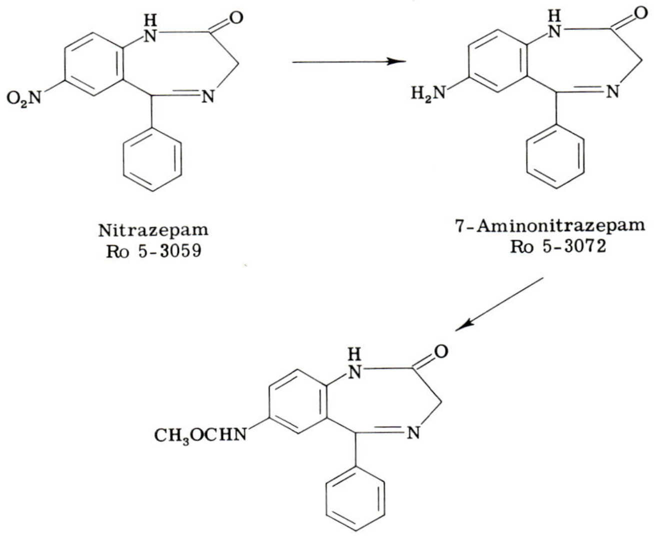

O_2N H N O N

Nitrazepam
Ro 5-3059

H_2N H N O N

7-Aminonitrazepam
Ro 5-3072

CH_3OCHN H N O N

7-Acetylaminonitrazepam
Ro 5-3308

Fig. 14. Metabolic pathway of nitrazepam.

7-amino derivative and this was acetylated to the 7-acetylamino derivative (Randall *et al.*, 1965) (Fig. 14). In the rat, the half-life was 4 hours after oral administration. The radioactive compound was eliminated in the urine and feces over 5 days.

Bartosek *et al.* (1970a) observed that during perfusion of the isolated rat liver, the 7-nitro group of nitrazepam was reduced to the 7-amino derivative and then acetylated to the 7-acetylamino derivative. These compounds were present mainly in perfusion fluid; only small amounts were found in bile or liver tissue. Similar results were found with livers of guinea pigs and rabbits. In contrast, the 7-amino derivative was the final product of nitrazepam metabolism in perfused mouse livers. Bartosek *et al.* (1970b) further reported that the reduction of nitrazepam to the 7-amino compound in rat liver homogenates was much higher than in homogenates of muscle, kidney, heart, lung, and spleen and was not apparent in brain homogenate. Nitrazepam reduction was also demonstrated in guinea pig, rabbit, and mouse liver homogenates. The rate of reduction in rat liver was modified by very high concentrations of diazepam, chlorpromazine, and imipramine. Much lower concentrations of SKF 525A were effective in inhibiting the reduction of nitrazepam.

The pharmacological profile of nitrazepam in mice was similar to that of diazepam as a sedative, muscle relaxant, and anticonvulsant. The drug was also similar to diazepam as a muscle relaxant in cats. However, it was stronger than diazepam in taming of vicious monkeys and in depressing rats in conditioned avoidance procedures (Randall *et al.*, 1965). The 7-amino and 7-acetylamino derivatives were inactive in the tests for sedative, muscle relaxant, and anticonvulsant activity.

D. Major Metabolites of Medazepam

The major metabolites of medazepam were identified in man by Rieder and Rentsch (1968), and in man, dog, and rat by Schwartz and Carbone (1970), as represented in Fig. 15. When administered to human subjects in single or multiple doses, deSilva and Puglisi (1970) found measurable blood levels of medazepam, diazepam, and desmethyldiazepam, whereas the urine contained oxazepam as the major excretion product. Multiple daily doses to the human resulted in medazepam blood levels reaching measurable amounts in an hour and declining to nonmeasurable levels by 24 hours, whereas diazepam remained at measurable levels throughout the period of drug administration; the *N*-desmethyldiazepam levels increased steadily, indicating accumulation.

Pharmacological studies (Randall *et al.*, 1970) showed that *N*-demethylation and dehydrogenation of medazepam did not change the sedative,

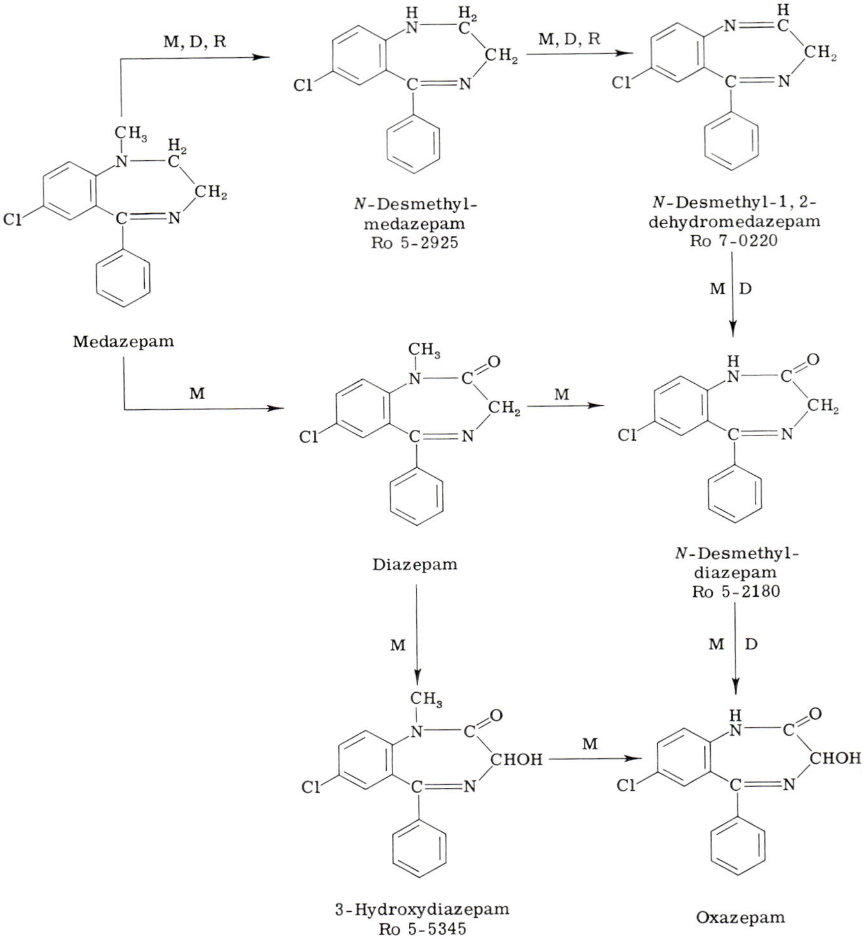

Medazepam

M, D, R

N-Desmethyl-medazepam
Ro 5-2925

M, D, R

N-Desmethyl-1, 2-dehydromedazepam
Ro 7-0220

M | D

M

Diazepam

M

N-Desmethyl-diazepam
Ro 5-2180

M

M | D

3-Hydroxydiazepam
Ro 5-5345

M

Oxazepam

FIG. 15. Metabolic pathway of medazepam in man (M), dog (D), and rat (R). (From Randall *et al.*, 1970, by permission.)

muscle relaxant, and anticonvulsant properties of the drug. However, diazepam, the major metabolite in humans and rats, showed greater potency in the same pharmacological tests and much stronger effects in taming and in modifying avoidance behavior in squirrel monkeys. The conditioning tests in rats and monkeys indicate that medazepam and its metabolites may be divided into two categories: (*1*) medazepam and its dehydrogenated and demethylated metabolites showing only sedative properties; and (2) diazepam and its metabolites showing stimulant effects at low doses and sedative effects at higher doses.

E. Metabolism of Prazepam

Robichaud *et al.* (1970) reported on the pharmacology of prazepam, the cyclopropyl analog of diazepam. It was found to possess pharmacological properties similar to other benzodiazepines. It was more potent than chlordiazepoxide hydrochloride as an anticonvulsant in mice. It was about half as potent as chlordiazepoxide hydrochloride in a conflict test in rats and was also less effective in temporal discrimination tests in cats. It was more potent in antagonizing reserpine excitation in mice pretreated with a monoamine oxidase inhibitor, resembling the action of chlorpromazine in this respect. It did not cause loss of the righting reflex at high doses in mice and so was not a hypnotic. It caused convulsions by the intravenous route in dogs, cats, and rabbits. It was suggested that this convulsant effect, unusual for the benzodiazepines, may be the result of cleavage of the cyclopropyl group.

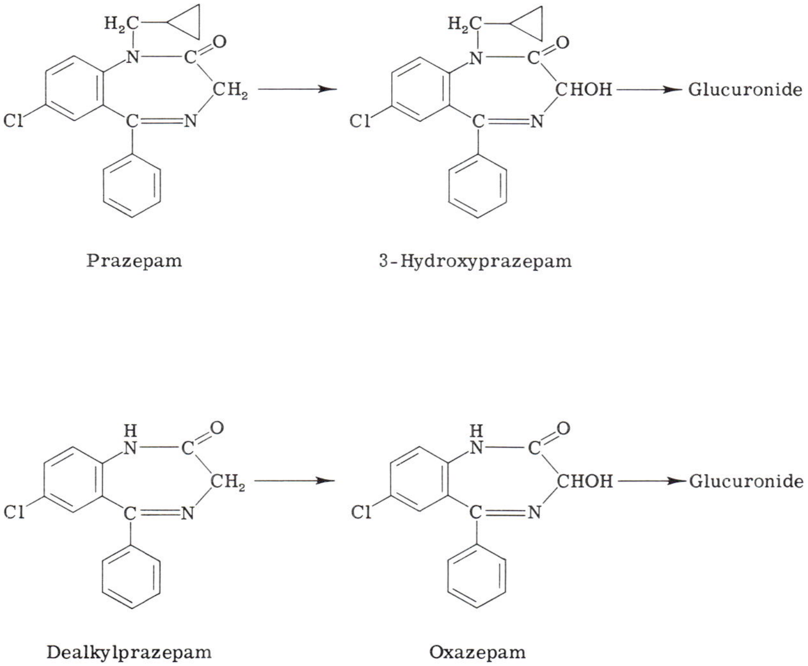

Fig. 16. Metabolic pathway of prazepam.

Prazepam metabolism in man was studied by DiCarlo *et al.* (1970). Prazepam labeled with ^{14}C showed slow absorption in man with a maximum blood level at 6 hours and a slow clearance process with a half-life of 78 hours. The primary metabolite in the blood is 3-hydroxyprazepam which is excreted in the urine as the glucuronide (Fig. 16). The dealkylation to dealkylprazepam is a slower process than the hydroxylation but in time oxazepam glucuronide is excreted in increasing quantities in the urine. Prazepam does not appear in the urine but is completely metabolized to products which appear as glucuronides. Prazepam appears to be hydroxylated in the human before it is dealkylated in contrast to diazepam which is demethylated followed by hydroxylation. This indicates that the cyclopropyl methyl group of prazepam is more resistant to metabolism than the methyl group of diazepam.

DiCarlo and Viau (1970) reported on prazepam metabolites in dog urine. In the dog, the major metabolite of prazepam (10 mg/kg p.o.) was oxazepam glucuronide. Small quantities of prazepam, dealkylprazepam, oxazepam, 3-hydroxyprazepam glucuronide, and 4′-hydroxyoxazepam glucuronide were identified.

F. Pharmacology of Flurazepam and Metabolites

The pharmacological properties of flurazepam were described by Randall *et al.* (1969). Flurazepam was stronger than chlordiazepoxide hydrochloride as a sedative, muscle relaxant, and anticonvulsant in mice and in producing sedation and muscle relaxation in cats. It was less potent than chlordiazepoxide hydrochloride in modifying conditioned behavior in rats and monkeys. In contrast to chlordiazepoxide hydrochloride, a stimulant effect at low doses was observed in behavioral tests in rats and monkeys.

The metabolic products of flurazepam in man and dog were identified by Schwartz and Postma (1970) as shown in Fig. 17. In both species, flurazepam was rapidly absorbed and eliminated from the plasma. Transformation to metabolites was rapid and complete. In man the major metabolite was the N_1-ethanol (Ro 7-2750) and in the dog the analogous N_1-acetic acid (Ro 7-5096).

G. Summary of Metabolism

Chlordiazepoxide hydrochloride may be demethylated and deaminated to give metabolic products which are equal to chlordiazepoxide hydrochloride in some tests and weaker in others. Hydroxylation leads to weaker products.

Diazepam may be demethylated or hydroxylated to yield products

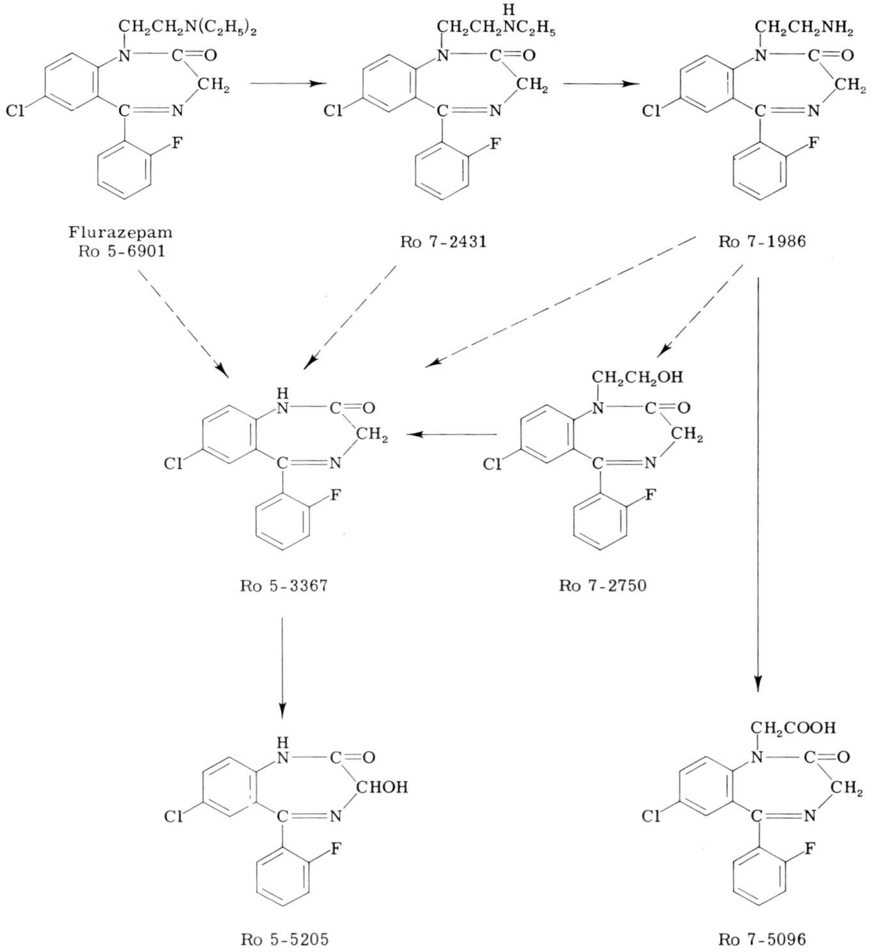

Flurazepam
Ro 5-6901

Ro 7-2431

Ro 7-1986

Ro 5-3367

Ro 7-2750

Ro 5-5205

Ro 7-5096

FIG. 17. Postulated pathways of flurazepam metabolism in man and dog.

equal to diazepam in some tests and weaker in others. The metabolites may account for some of the activity of the parent compound.

Medazepam may be demethylated, oxidized, or hydroxylated to give some of the same metabolites as diazepam with similar variability of activity in various pharmacological tests.

Flurazepam undergoes metabolic degradation of the N_1 side chain and also hydroxylation of the benzazepine ring to give a variety of products.

The 7-nitro group of nitrazepam is reduced to a 7-amino group which is acetylated for excretion. These products are essentially inactive.

Prazepam undergoes the same metabolism as chlordiazepoxide hydrochloride.

IX. Biochemical Effects

The actions of benzodiazepines on the metabolism, transport, and storage of neurohumoral transmitters were studied by Pletscher (1969). Isolated blood platelets were used as a model for measuring the membrane effects of tranquilizers. Chlordiazepoxide hydrochloride and diazepam did not affect the uptake of radioactive serotonin, whereas chlorpromazine and imipramine caused inhibition. The liberation of serotonin from rabbit platelets *in vitro* was partially induced by chlordiazepoxide hydrochloride only at the high concentration of 10^{-3} M, whereas chlorpromazine caused complete liberation. Chlordiazepoxide hydrochloride (50 mg/kg i.p.) and diazepam (5 mg/kg i.p.) had insignificant effects on brain serotonin levels in rats and only slightly increased the content of the primary metabolite, 5-hydroxyindoleacetic acid. Chlordiazepoxide hydrochloride and diazepam did not markedly affect the content of catecholamines in the brain and induced no significant changes in the primary metabolite, homovanillic acid. This work indicates that the turnover of catecholamines is not accelerated by these drugs as it is by chlorpromazine.

Taylor and Laverty (1969) confirmed the above study by finding that chlordiazepoxide hydrochloride, diazepam, and nitrazepam at doses of 10 mg/kg s.c. had no effect on the endogenous levels of norepinephrine in various areas of the rat brain. However, when dopamine-^{3}H was injected into the lateral ventricles of rats pretreated with these drugs, the radioactive norepinephrine concentration was increased in the thalamus, midbrain, cortex, and cerebellum but not in the brainstem, whereas dopamine-^{3}H was increased in the striate region. The increase in radioactive catecholamines in the brain was interpreted as a decreased rate of turnover.

Histochemical and biochemical evidence for decreased catecholamine turnover in rat brain under the action of benzodiazepines was provided by Corrodi *et al.* (1971.). Chlordiazepoxide hydrochloride (10 and 25 mg/kg i.p.) and diazepam (10 mg/kg) decreased norepinephrine turnover in the cerebral and cerebellar cortex and in the hippocampus, but not in the hypothalamus or lower brainstem. There was also a decrease in dopamine turnover in neurons ascending to the neostriatum and limbic forebrain. These effects were observed only at doses which produced sedation and EEG slowing.

Chase *et al.* (1970) investigated the influence of diazepam on the disposition of intracisternally injected serotonin-^{14}C in the rat. Pretreatment with diazepam, 20 mg/kg i.p., failed to affect the uptake of this monoamine into the brain. In contrast, whole brain levels of serotonin-^{14}C and 5-hydroxyindoleacetic acid-^{14}C were substantially above control levels when diazepam was injected 10 minutes after serotonin-^{14}C administration. Diazepam markedly retarded the efflux of intracisternally administered 5-hydroxyindoleacetic acid-^{14}C but had no effect on the efflux of metaraminol-^{3}H, a monoamine which is not metabolized in brain. These findings suggest that diazepam may act either on mechanisms subserving the transport of 5-hydroxyindoleacetic acid from brain or on the cerebral metabolism of serotonin.

Young *et al.* (1969) suggested that the neuropharmacological responses elicited by diazepam might result from quantitative differences in the effects of the drug on the metabolism of different regions of the CNS. They studied the action of diazepam on levels of glucose and malate in various areas of the CNS of mice. The results indicated that there were regional differences in the metabolic response to diazepam, with malate appearing as the more sensitive indicator of its action. Diazepam, 20 mg/kg i.p., produced muscle relaxation in mice and caused increased concentrations of glucose in the forebrain and decreased concentrations of malate and lactate while glutamate remained unchanged. Doses of 1, 2, and 5 mg/kg i.p. of diazepam depressed malate in the cortex, brainstem, and spinal cord whereas glucose increased only after 5 mg/kg i.p. Plasma glucose was not altered by this dose.

Martelli and Corsico (1969) observed that, in rats, chlordiazepoxide hydrochloride, 40 mg/kg i.p., produced a sustained elevation of the plasma, free, fatty acid levels; a similar effect was elicited by theophylline, 20 mg/kg i.p. The lipid-mobilizing effect of norepinephrine was potentiated by pretreatment of rats with chlordiazepoxide hydrochloride or with theophylline. The lipid-mobilizing effect of chlordiazepoxide hydrochloride was almost doubled in rats pretreated with theophylline and vice versa. The similarity of the effects of chlordiazepoxide hydrochloride and theophylline on plasma free fatty acid levels suggests that these two drugs act through a similar mechanism.

X. Discussion of Metabolism and Biochemistry

It is evident that the benzodiazepines do not affect basic levels of serotonin and catecholamines in the brain but that the turnover of these biogenic amines may be inhibited. These findings correlate with certain pharmacological results after using drugs that modify biogenic amines in the brain. If tetrabenazine, which releases biogenic amines, and iproniazid, which blocks destruction of the amines, are injected into rats there is behavioral stimulation as measured by a continuous avoidance procedure. This stimulant effect of the tetrabenazine–iproniazid combination is attenuated by extremely small doses of benzodiazepines (Randall *et al.*, 1965). Chlordiazepoxide hydrochloride blocks stimulation at a dose of 0.45 mg/kg i.p., but it requires 13.7 mg/kg to decrease avoidance rates in nonpretreated rats. Likewise, diazepam prevents stimulation by tetrabenazine–iproniazid at 0.05 mg/kg i.p. and decreases avoidance only at 13.0 mg/kg i.p. Thus the pharmacological effect of releasing biogenic amines in the brain is extremely sensitive to attenuation by benzodiazepines.

Further evidence that chlordiazepoxide hydrochloride interferes with the central effects of released biogenic amines was obtained by Mennear and Rudzik (1966). They found that the anticonvulsant properties of chlordiazepoxide hydrochloride in mice were antagonized by the biogenic amine depleters, reserpine, and Ro 4-1284 (2-hydroxy-2-ethyl-3-isobutyl-9,10-dimethoxy-1,2,3,4,6,7-hexahydro-11*bH*-benzo[*a*]quinolizine hydrochloride). Chlordiazepoxide hydrochloride resembled diphenylhydantoin in its anticonvulsant properties which are antagonized by reserpine and Ro 4-1284. In addition, the antagonism of the anticonvulsant properties of chlordiazepoxide hydrochloride and diphenylhydantoin by reserpine could be reversed by the usual antagonists of reserpine, amphetamine, 5-hydroxytryptophan, α-methyldopa, and dopa (3,4-dihydroxyphenylalanine).

Additional evidence that chlordiazepoxide hydrochloride may modify the effects of the release of biogenic amines is the antagonism by chlordiazepoxide hydrochloride of morphine analgesia in mice (Weis, 1969). This result is analogous to the antagonism of morphine analgesia by reserpine which is attributed to modifications of adrenergic and tryptaminergic mechanisms (Fennessy and Lee, 1970). The antagonism of morphine analgesia by chlordiazepoxide hydrochloride was confirmed by Randall *et al.* (1970) and extended to diazepam, medazepam, and other benzodiazepines.

Possible differences in the actions of various benzodiazepines on the effects of biogenic amines have been reported. Thus flurazepam hydrochloride, at the very low doses of 0.5 to 0.7 mg/kg i.p., potentiated the stimulation induced in rats by *d*-amphetamine or cocaine, and produced stimulation when combined with an inactive dose of tetrabenazine. In contrast, chlordiazepoxide hydrochloride at 4 mg/kg had none of these effects (Randall *et al.*, 1969). Thus flurazepam hydrochloride in rats may differ from chlordiazepoxide hydrochloride by potentiating the effects of catecholamines which are released in the brain by *d*-amphetamine or tetrabenazine and by potentiating the increased responsiveness to catecholamines which is induced by cocaine.

The above discussion suggests that the general sedative properties of the benzodiazepines may be related to the modification of adrenergic and serotonergic neurons in the nervous system. However, these general depressant properties in no way account for the specific antianxiety, anticonvulsant, muscle relaxant, and antidepressant properties of various benzodiazepines in man. Most of the studies on biogenic amine metabolism have been done on rats, and this species has very little usefulness in predicting the specific antianxiety activity of the benzodiazepines in humans (Zbinden and Randall, 1967). If the specific CNS activity of benzodiazepines is to be related to biogenic amine metabolism, the studies should be extended to cats and monkeys in which some specificity of action may be obtained.

XI. Future Developments

Reviewers usually confine themselves to a survey of research done in the recent past. However, a fascinating article by Lehmann (1969) gives us a glimpse into some possible characteristics of drugs of the future.

Lehmann classifies the benzodiazepines among the anxiolytic sedatives. He points out that there are certain clinical insufficiencies in this group of drugs.

1. "Ideally, the effect of an anxiolytic sedative should be a pure reduction of excessive anxiety or tension without producing drowsiness or any other decrease in performance." However, larger doses of all available agents produce drowsiness, sleep, ataxia, and slurred speech.

2. The ideal agent should not produce disinhibition. Available drugs "induce cortical disinhibition before they produce behavioral or emotional inhibition." Such disinhibition might be displayed as a phase of increased hostility. In unpublished studies, Lehmann and Ban gave a fingerpainting test to student volunteers. Disinhibition was measured by reduction in realism and clarity, with an increase in affect and energy output. Chlordiazepoxide hydrochloride had a stronger disinhibiting effect than an equivalent dose of amobarbital.

3. In animal experiments, conflict behavior is increased by anxiolytic sedatives. In an experiment on human subjects, Lehmann and Ban set up a conflict situation with the simultaneous presentation of monetary

rewards and a possible electric shock. Conflict responding was increased by chlordiazepoxide hydrochloride (30 mg) but not by chlorpromazine (75 mg). This indicates a changed balance in the appreciation of positive and negative stimuli. "This balance, however, is often critically important . . . as a guide for appropriate biological and social behavior."

4. Reduction in REM sleep, with decreased dreaming time, "may have unsettling effects on the person's adaptation to daily life stresses." Clinical trials indicate that both secobarbital and nitrazepam decrease REM time.

5. Other aspects of drug action on which further information is needed are possible changes in stimulus input, in habituation to sensory stimuli, in responses of the autonomic nervous system, in learning and memory, in weakening of the ego, and in defense mechanisms.

Lehmann concludes his discussion by painting a picture of the ideal tranquilizer of the future:

> It should be a drug which is completely safe and has a built-in automatic cut-off device which makes dangerous overdosage impossible and makes the drug suicide proof. It will produce just sufficient side effects to prevent unnecessary self-medication, but not so many side effects as to reduce the patient's willingness to take the drug as prescribed. It will not be habit-forming. It will selectively reduce tension and anxiety without reducing alertness beyond the optimal level on the arousal continuum and will, therefore, not just be a hypnotic used at lower dosage. It will not be ego-weakening by producing disinhibition of higher nervous functions, or inducing increase of conflict behavior, unless specially designed for it. It will not impair discrimination, memory and learning . . .Finally, to conclude this dream of the ideal tranquilizer or tranquilizers of the future, they will induce or eliminate specific psychodynamic defense mechanisms and will provide substitutions for flaws in the patient's basic character structure, according to the clinician's therapeutic choice. (From Lehmann, 1969, by permission of the author and of Excerpta Medica Found., Amsterdam.)

XII. Conclusions

New insights into the mechanism of action of the benzodiazepines have been provided by research published during the period 1967–1971. Some of the principal findings are the following:

The major muscle relaxant actions occur in the central nervous system. The primary effect seems to be a reduction in the facilitatory influence of the reticular formation on spinal reflexes. A direct action on the spinal cord may also occur.

Central modulation of autonomic responses may involve a discrete depressant effect on sympathetic vasoconstrictor activity.

Primary epileptogenic foci can be established by implantation of irritating substances in the brain of the cat; secondary foci develop in regions connected by one or more neurons to the primary foci. While benzodiazepines suppress discharges in secondary foci, they have less effect on primary foci.

A behavioral characteristic of benzodiazepines is the release of previously suppressed responses. Thus, before drug treatment rats learn to press a lever which produces a food reward, while ignoring a lever which produces no reward. During the action of chlordiazepoxide hydrochloride, the number of unrewarded responses is increased. This action is attributed to a breakdown of inhibition.

Electrophysiological studies in rats and cats indicate that a major action of benzodiazepines is on the hippocampus. This finding is in contrast to the action of barbiturates, which seem to act primarily on the brainstem reticular formation.

Metabolic studies show that benzodiazepines may be demethylated, deaminated, hydroxylated, oxidized, reduced, or acetylated. Some metabolites are equal to the parent compound in pharmacological activity, while others are less active.

Studies with radioactive catecholamines indicate that benzodiazepines may decrease the rate of catecholamine turnover in rat brain. Cerebral metabolism of serotonin may also be depressed. The relationship of these findings to the antianxiety activity of the benzodiazepines is still unclear.

Acknowledgment

The authors wish to thank Mrs. Wendy Fordi for excellent secretarial assistance.

References

Abel, R. M., Staroscik, R. N., and Reis, R. L. (1970). *J. Pharmacol. Exp. Ther.* **173,** 364.

Banziger, R., and Hane, D. (1967). *Arch. Int. Pharmacodyn. Ther.* **167,** 245.

Barnes, C. D., and Moolenaar, G. M. (1971). *Neuropharmacology* **10,** 193.

Bartosek, I., Kvetina, J., Guaitani, A., and Garattini, S. (1970a). *Eur. J. Pharmacol.* **11,** 378.

Bartosek, I., Mussini, E., Saronio, C., and Garattini, S. (1970b). *Eur. J. Pharmacol.* **11,** 249.

Bauen, A., and Possanza, G. J. (1970). *Arch. Int. Pharmacodyn. Ther.* **186,** 133.

Beattie, C. W., Chernov, H. I., Bernard, P. S., and Glenny, F. H. (1969). *Int. J. Neuropharmacol.* **8,** 365.

Benson, H., Herd, J. A., Morse, W. H., and Kelleher, R. T. (1970). *J. Pharmacol. Exp. Ther.* **173,** 399.

Bolme, P., Ngai, S. H., Uvnäs, B., and Wallenberg, L. R. (1967). *Acta Physiol. Scand.* **70,** 334.

Brodie, B. B., Gillette, J. R., and LaDu, B. N. (1958). *Annu. Rev. Biochem.* **27,** 427.

Buser, P., Cook, L., Giurgea, C., Jacobsen, E., Ray, O. S., Richelle, M., Silverman, A. P., Stein, L., and Votava, Z. (1970). *Mod. Probl. Pharmacopsychiat.* **5,** 85.

Chase, T. N., Katz, R. I., and Kopin, I. J. (1970). *Neuropharmacology* **9,** 103.
Cheymol, J., van den Driessche, J., Allain, P., and Eben-Moussi, E. (1967). *Anesth. Anal. Rean.* **24,** 329.
Christmas, A. J., and Maxwell, D. R. (1970). *Neuropharmacology* **9,** 17.
Chusid, J. G., and Kopeloff, L. M. (1969). *Epilepsia* **10,** 239.
Cook, L. (1965). *In* "Neuropsychopharmacology" (D. Bente and P. B. Bradley, eds.), Vol. 4, pp. 91–99. Elsevier, Amsterdam.
Corrodi, H., Fuxe, K., Lidbrink, P., and Olson, L. (1971). *Brain Res.* **29,** 1.
Coutinho, C. B., Cheripko, J. A., and Carbone, J. J. (1969). *Biochem. Pharmacol.* **18,** 303.
Coutinho, C. B., Cheripko, J. A., and Carbone, J. J. (1970). *Biochem. Pharmacol.* **19,** 363.
Crankshaw, D. P., and Raper, C. (1968). *Brit. J. Pharmacol.* **34,** 579.
Davidson, A. B., and Cook, L. (1969). *Psychopharmacologia* **15,** 159.
deSilva, J. A. F., and Puglisi, C. V. (1970). *Anal. Chem.* **42,** 1725.
deSilva, J. A. F., Koechlin, B. A., and Bader, G. (1966). *J. Pharm. Sci.* **55,** 692.
DiCarlo, F. J., and Viau, J. P. (1970). *J. Pharm. Sci.* **59,** 322.
DiCarlo, F. J., Viau, J. P., Epps, J. E., and Haynes, L. J. (1970). *Clin. Pharmacol. Ther.* **11,** 890.
Dolce, G., and Kaemmerer, E. (1967). *Arzneim.-Forsch.* **17,** 1057.
Douglas, R. J. (1967). *Psychological Bulletin* **67,** 416.
Dretchen, K., Ghoneim, M. M., and Long, J. P. (1971). *Anesthesiology* **34,** 463.
Feinstein, M. B., Lenard, W., and Mathias, J. (1970). *Arch. Int. Pharmacodyn. Ther.* **187,** 144.
Fennessy, M. R., and Lee, J. R. (1970). *J. Pharm. Pharmacol.* **22,** 930.
Fox, K. A., and Snyder, R. L. (1969). *J. Comp. Physiol. Psychol.* **69,** 663.
Fox, K. A., Tuckosh, J. R., and Wilcox, A. H. (1970). *Eur. J. Pharmacol.* **11,** 119.
Frank, G. B., and Jhamandas, K. (1970). *Brit. J. Pharmacol.* **39,** 707.
Funderburk, W. H., Foxwell, M. H., and Hakala, M. W. (1970). *Neuropharmacology* **9,** 1.
Gastaut, H. (1970). *Mod. Probl. Pharmacopsychiat.* **4,** 261.
Gastaut, H., Naquet, R., Poiré, R., and Tassinari, C. A. (1965). *Epilepsia* **6,** 167.
Ghelarducci, B., Lenzi, G., and Pompeiano, O. (1966). *Arch. Int. Pharmacodyn. Ther.* **163,** 403.
Gluckman, M. I. (1965). *Curr. Ther. Res., Clin. Exp.* **7,** 721.
Gogolak, G., Liebeswar, G., and Stumpf, C. (1969). *Electroencephalogr. Clin. Neurophysiol.* **27,** 296.
Guerrero-Figueroa, R., Rye, M. M., and Gallant, D. M. (1967). *Curr. Ther. Res., Clin. Exp.* **9,** 522.
Guerrero-Figueroa, R., Rye, M. M., and Guerrero-Figueroa, C. (1968). *Curr. Ther. Res., Clin. Exp.* **10,** 150.
Guerrero-Figueroa, R., Rye, M. M., and Heath, R. G. (1969). *Curr. Ther. Res., Clin. Exp.* **11,** 27.
Guerrero-Figueroa, R., Rye, M. M., Gallant, D. M., and Bishop, M. P. (1970). *Neuropharmacology* **9,** 143.
Hamilton, J. T. (1967). *Can. J. Physiol. Pharmacol.* **45,** 191.
Heinemann, H., Hartmann, A., and Sturm, V. (1968). *Arzneim.-Forsch.* **18,** 1557.
Heinemann, H., Hartmann, A., Stock, G., and Sturm, V. (1970). *Arzneim.-Forsch.* **20,** 413.
Heise, G. A., Laughlin, N., and Keller, C. (1970). *Psychopharmacologia* **16,** 345.
Heiss, W. D., Heilig, P., and Hoyer, J. (1969a). *Vision Res.* **9,** 493.

Heiss, W. D., Hoyer, J., and Heilig, P. (1969b). *Vision Res.* **9,** 507.
Hudson, R. D., and Wolpert, M. K. (1970). *Neuropharmacology* **9,** 481.
Idänpään-Heikkilä, J. E., Taska, R. J., Allen, H. A., and Schoolar, J. C. (1971a). *J. Pharmacol. Exp. Ther.* **176,** 752.
Idänpään–Heikkilä, J. E., Taska, R. J., Allen, H. A., and Schoolar, J. C. (1971b). *Arch. Int. Pharmacodyn.* **194,** 68.
Irwin, S. (1968). *In* "Psychopharmacology: A Review of Progress 1957–1967" (D. Efron, ed.), Publ. No. 1836, pp. 185–204. U.S. Pub. Health Serv., Washington, D.C.
Joy, R. M., Hance, A. J., and Killam, K. F., Jr. (1971). *Neuropharmacology* **10,** 483.
Kaplan, S. A., Lewis, M., Schwartz, M. A., Postma, E., Cotler, S., Abruzzo, C. W., Lee, T. L., and Weinfeld, R. E. (1970). *J. Pharm. Sci.* **59,** 1569.
Kido, R., Hirose, K., Yamamoto, K., and Matsushita, A. (1967). *Progr. Brain Res.* **27,** 365.
Killam, K. F., Killam, E. K., and Naquet, R. (1967). *Electroencephalogr. Clin. Neurophysiol.* **22,** 497.
Kimble, D. P. (1968). *Psychological Bulletin* **70,** 285.
Koechlin, B. A., Schwartz, M. A., Krol, G., and Oberhansli, W. (1965). *J. Pharmacol. Exp. Ther.* **148,** 399.
Kopeloff, L. M., and Chusid, J. G. (1967). *Int. J. Neuropsychiat.* **3,** 469.
Lanoir, J., and Killam, E. K. (1968). *Electroencephalogr. Clin. Neurophysiol.* **25,** 530.
Lehmann, H. E. (1969). *In* "The Present Status of Psychotropic Drugs" (A. Cerletti and F. J. Bové, eds.), pp. 168–175. Excerpta Med. Found., Amsterdam.
Magni, F., Moruzzi, G., Rossi, G. F., and Zanchetti, A. (1959). *Arch. Ital. Biol.* **97,** 33.
Malick, J. B. (1970). *Arch. Int. Pharmacodyn. Ther.* **186,** 137.
Malick, J. B., Sofia, R. D., and Goldberg, M. E. (1969). *Arch. Int. Pharmacodyn. Ther.* **181,** 459.
Marcucci, F., Guaitani, A., Kvetina, J., Mussini, E., and Garattini, S. (1968). *Eur. J. Pharmacol.* **4,** 467.
Marcucci, F., Fanelli, R., Mussini, E., and Garattini, S. (1970a). *Eur. J. Pharmacol.* **11,** 115.
Marcucci, F., Mussini, E., Fanelli, R., and Garattini, S. (1970b). *Biochem. Pharmacol.* **19,** 1847.
Margules, D. L., and Stein, L. (1967). *In* "Neuropsychopharmacology" (H. Brill, J. O. Cole, P. Deniker, H. Hippius, and P. B. Bradley, eds.), Vol. 5, pp. 108–120. Excerpta Med. Found., Amsterdam.
Margules, D. L., and Stein, L. (1968). *Psychopharmacologia* **13,** 74.
Margules, D. L., and Stein, L. (1969). *Amer. J. Physiol.* **217,** 475.
Martelli, E. A., and Corsico, N. (1969). *J. Pharm. Pharmacol.* **21,** 59.
Mennear, J. H., and Rudzik, A. D. (1966). *J. Pharm. Sci.* **55,** 640.
Mille, T., Pastorino, G., and Arrigo, A. (1969). *Arzneim.-Forsch.* **19,** 730.
Morpurgo, C. (1968). *Brit. J. Pharmacol.* **34,** 532.
Moruzzi, G. (1964). *Electroencephalogr. Clin. Neurophysiol.* **16,** 2.
Nauta, W. J. H., and Haymaker, W. (1969). *In* "The Hypothalamus" (W. Haymaker, E. Anderson, and W. J. H. Nauta, eds.), pp. 136–209. Thomas, Springfield, Illinois.
Ngai, S. H., Tseng, T. C., and Wang, S. C. (1966). *J. Pharmacol. Exp. Ther.* **153,** 344.
Olds, M. E., and Baldrighi, G. (1968). *Int. J. Neuropharmacol.* **7,** 231.
Olds, M. E., and Olds, J. (1969). *Int. J. Neuropharmacol.* **8,** 87.
Owen, G., Smith, T. H. F., and Agersborg, H. P. K., Jr. (1970). *Toxicol. Appl. Pharmacol.* **16,** 556.
Placidi, G. F., and Cassano, G. B. (1968). *Int. J. Neuropharmacol.* **7,** 383.

Pletscher, A. (1969). *In* "Psychotropic Drugs in Internal Medicine" (A. Pletscher and A. Marino, eds.), Int. Congr. Ser. No. 182, pp. 1–15. Excerpta Med. Found., Amsterdam.

Prindle, K. H., Jr., Gold, H. K., Cardon, P. V., and Epstein, S. E. (1970). *J. Pharmacol. Exp. Ther.* **173,** 133.

Pruett, J. K., and Williams, B. B. (1966). *J. Pharm. Sci.* **55,** 1139.

Przybyla, A. C., and Wang, S. C. (1968). *J. Pharmacol. Exp. Ther.* **163,** 439.

Randall, L. O., and Schallek, W. (1968). *In* "Psychopharmacology: A Review of Progress 1957–1967" (D. Efron, ed.), Publ. No. 1836, pp. 153–184. U.S. Pub. Health Serv., Washington, D.C.

Randall, L. O., Schallek, W., Heise, G. A., Keith, E. F., and Bagdon, R. E. (1960). *J. Pharmacol. Exp. Ther.* **129,** 163.

Randall, L. O., Scheckel, C. L., and Banziger, R. F. (1965). *Curr. Ther. Res., Clin. Exp.* **7,** 590.

Randall, L. O., Schallek, W., Scheckel, C. L., Stefko, P. L., Banziger, R. F., Pool, W., and Moe, R. A. (1969). *Arch. Int. Pharmacodyn. Ther.* **178,** 216.

Randall, L. O., Scheckel, C. L., and Pool, W. (1970). *Arch. Int. Pharmacodyn. Ther.* **185,** 135.

Rieder, J. (1965). *Arzneim.-Forsch.* **15,** 1134.

Rieder, J., and Rentsch, G. (1968). *Arzneim.-Forsch.* **18,** 1545.

Robichaud, R. C., Gylys, J. A., Sledge, K. L., and Hillyard, I. W. (1970). *Arch. Int. Pharmacodyn. Ther.* **185,** 213.

Ruelius, H. W., Lee, J. M., and Alburn, H. E. (1965). *Arch. Biochem. Biophys.* **111,** 376.

Schallek, W., and Thomas, J. (1971). *Arch. Int. Pharmacodyn. Ther.* **192,** 321.

Schallek, W., Lewinson, T., and Thomas, J. (1968). *Int. J. Neuropharmacol.* **7,** 35.

Schallek, W., Kovacs, J., Kuehn, A., and Thomas, J. (1970). *Arch. Int. Pharmacodyn. Ther.* **185,** 149.

Schallek, W., Kuehn, A., and Kovacs, J. (1972). *Neuropharmacology* **11,** 69.

Schlosser, W. (1971). *Arch. Int. Pharmacodyn. Ther.* **194,** 93.

Schmidt, R. F., Vogel, M. E., and Zimmermann, M. (1967). *Naunyn-Schmiedebergs Arch. Pharmakol. Exp. Pathol.* **258,** 69.

Schwartz, M. A., and Carbone, J. J. (1970). *Biochem. Pharmacol.* **19,** 343.

Schwartz, M. A., and Postma, E. (1966). *J. Pharm. Sci.* **55,** 1358.

Schwartz, M. A., and Postma, E. (1970). *J. Pharm. Sci.* **59,** 1800.

Schwartz, M. A., Koechlin, B. A., Postma, E., Palmer, S., and Krol, G. (1965). *J. Pharmacol. Exp. Ther.* **149,** 423.

Schwartz, M. A., Bommer, P., and Vane, F. M. (1967). *Arch. Biochem. Biophys.* **121,** 508.

Schwartz, M. A., Postma, E., and Kolis, S. J. (1971). *J. Pharm. Sci.* **60,** 438.

Scotti de Carolis, A., and Longo, V. G. (1967). *Arzneim.-Forsch.* **17,** 1580.

Sherwin, I. (1971). *Electroencephalogr. Clin. Neurophysiol.* **30,** 445.

Sigg, E. B., and Sigg, T. D. (1969). *Int. J. Neuropharmacol.* **8,** 567.

Sigg, E. B., Keim, K. L., and Kepner, K. (1971). *Neuropharmacology* **10,** 621.

Sofia, R. D. (1969). *Life Sci.* **8,** pt. 1, 705.

Spehlmann, R., and Colley, B. (1968). *Neurology* **18,** 52.

Stark, L. G., Killam, K. F., and Killam, E. K. (1970). *J. Pharmacol. Exp. Ther.* **173,** 125.

Stark, P., and Henderson, J. K. (1966). *Int. J. Neuropharmacol.* **5,** 385.

Steiner, F. A., and Hummel, P. (1968). *Int. J. Neuropharmacol.* **7,** 61.

Straw, R. N. (1968). *Arch. Int. Pharmacodyn. Ther.* **175**, 464.
Stratten, W. P. and Barnes, C. D. (1971). *Neuropharmacology* **10**, 685.
Swinyard, E. A., and Castellion, A. W. (1966). *J. Pharmacol. Exp. Ther.* **151**, 369.
Taylor, K. M., and Laverty, R. (1969). *Eur. J. Pharmacol.* **8**, 296.
Tedeschi, D. H., Fowler, P. J., Miller, R. B., and Macko, E. (1969). *In* "Aggressive Behaviour" (S. Garattini and E. B. Sigg, eds.), pp. 245–252. Wiley, New York; Excerpta Med. Found., Amsterdam.
Toman, J. E. P., and Sabelli, H. C. (1968). *Int. J. Neuropharmacol.* **7**, 543.
Tseng, T. C., and Wang, S. C. (1971a). *J. Pharmacol. Exp. Ther.* **178**, 350.
Tseng, T. C., and Wang, S. C. (1971b). *Proc. Soc. Exp. Biol. Med.* **137**, 526.
Valzelli, L. (1967). *Advan. Pharmacol.* **5**, 79.
van der Kleijn, E. (1969a). "Pharmacokinetics of Ataractic Drugs," pp. 33–58. St. Catherines Press, Bruges, Belgium.
van der Kleijn, E. (1969b). *Arch. Int. Pharmacodyn. Ther.* **182**, 433.
van der Kleijn, E., and Wijffels, C. C. G. (1971). *Arch. Int. Pharmacodyn.* **192**, 255.
Vatter, O. (1967). *Arzneim.-Forsch.* **17**, 1363.
Vieth, J. B., Holm, E., and Knopp, P. R. (1968). *Arch. Int. Pharmacodyn. Ther.* **171**, 323.
Vuillon-Cacciuttolo, G., and Issautier, G. (1970). *C. R. Soc. Biol.* **164**, 572.
Wedeking, P. W. (1969). *Psychonomic Science* **15**, 232.
Weis, J. (1969). *Experientia* **25**, 381.
Young, R. L., Albano, R. F., Charnecki, A. M., and Demcsak, G. (1969). *Fed. Proc. Fed. Amer. Soc. Exp. Biol.* **28**, 444.
Zattoni, J., and Rossi, G. F. (1967). *Physiol. Behav.* **2**, 277.
Zbinden, G., and Randall, L. O. (1967). *Advan. Pharmacol.* **5**, 213.

Effect of Drugs upon Axoplasmic Transport

WILLIAM O. MCCLURE

Department of Biochemistry
University of Illinois
Urbana, Illinois

I. Introduction

During the past two decades the phenomenon of axoplasmic transport has progressed from an interesting suggestion to a clearly defined fact of great importance in the metabolic economy and physiological function of the neuron. Indeed, maintaining a properly functioning transport system probably ranks in importance with the more commonly considered properties of the neuron, such as basal cellular metabolism and the propagation of action potentials. A number of arguments support the importance of axoplasmic transport. For example, several enzymes important in the metabolism of neurotransmitters are transported from the cell body to the synapse. Furthermore, the axon seems able to synthesize little, if any, protein (for discussion, see Barondes, 1967; Lasek, 1970b). This would require that all, or certainly most, of those proteins necessary to maintain the axonal membrane, to carry out metabolic functions in the axoplasm, and to interact with surrounding cells, as well as those required to control these functions, must be supplied to the extremities of the cell from the perikaryon (Gerard, 1932). More detailed discussion of the function of transported molecules is presented in later sections of this article (see Section II,C).

In view of the importance of axoplasmic transport, it seems reasonable to assume that any interference with axoplasmic flow will ultimately lead to an alteration in some aspect of axonal metabolism. Several hypothetical actions can be considered. For example, compounds that inhibit axoplasmic flow would prevent the arrival at the synapse of enzymes and enzyme systems necessary for the metabolism and release of neurotransmitters. Since the synapse could continue to function, using enzymes which had arrived prior to inhibition of transport, synthesis and release of neurotransmitters might be maintained for some time before eventual failure. This type of action may be involved in the peripheral neuritis induced by long-term treatment with colchicine and the *Vinca* alkaloids, which are efficient in blocking transport (Section III,B). It is also possible to consider more immediate effects, which could be produced by preventing the arrival of regulatory molecules. These effects could be brought about in any of a number of ways by drugs that interact with the transport system. Although most attention has been paid to agents which are believed to interact with the microtubules (Sections II,F and III,B), other mechanisms of action are possible. Compounds that interrupt the synthesis of high-energy phosphates will provide an apparent block of transport by preventing the necessary supply of metabolic energy. Agents that damage the perikaryal mechanism by which synthesized proteins are committed to the transport system (the "loading" reactions) could also appear to block transport. Irrespective of the molecular action, drugs that block transport of material to the synapse will probably interfere with normal synaptic function, with the resultant possibility of neurological disturbance.

Arguments such as those presented above suggest that a study of the effects of drugs upon transport could be extremely valuable. In considering the drugs as experimental tools, information can be gained concerning the mechanism of the transport process, as well as the interaction of the transported material with the cell. Alternatively, one can consider an effect upon axoplasmic transport as a means of explaining the molecular action of a given drug.

In this article a number of drugs are considered. In order to orient the reader, the following section contains a general discussion of axoplasmic transport. This discussion is not intended to serve as an exhaustive review of the literature concerning axoplasmic transport, but rather as an introduction to those aspects of the phenomenon that are deemed of particular relevance with respect to the action of drugs. For more detailed reviews of specific aspects, the reader is referred to Lubińska (1964), Ochs (1966), Barondes (1967, 1969), Grafstein (1969), and Lasek (1970b).

Finally, one further important consideration should be noted. There is no reason to believe that intracellular transport of metabolites is limited to the neuron. Rather, it may well be true that all cells, particularly large ones, have specific mechanisms with which to move material from a site of synthesis to a site of utilization. If so, the use of nerves as objects in which to study transport provides a physically convenient model system which may yield results of much wider applicability. Several general aspects of intracellular transport are considered by Porter (1966) and in the text edited by Allen and Kamiya (1964).

II. A General Consideration of Axoplasmic Transport

A. History

In 1932, Ralph Gerard stated that communication between the neuronal perikaryon and the further reaches of the cell processes must involve the physical movement of material along the axon toward the synapse (Gerard, 1932). This suggestion was strengthened by indirect experiments from several laboratories before finally being clearly demonstrated by the classic work of Weiss and Hiscoe (1948). These workers partially obstructed peripheral nerves and observed the gross morphological alterations that ensued. On the side of the "dam" toward the cell body (the *proximal* side), axons became turgid and enlarged, often assuming strange and bizarre shapes. In contrast, the nerve on the peripheral side of the dam (the *distal* side) contained fibers of less than usual diameters. Upon release of the obstruction, the axoplasm which had accumulated began to move along the fibers at rates estimated at 1 to 3 mm/day. These observations defined the phenomenon now termed axoplasmic transport. Furthermore, a useful and long-lived hypothesis was put forth: since the rate of movement seen in the system agreed very well with the rate at which these same nerves regenerated after peripheral section, it was suggested that the rate of 1 to 3 mm/day represented a regrowth of the axon cylinder, with concomitant renewal of all the axonal contents. Although probably not correct, this thesis served to guide research through two decades of work which defined the properties of axoplasmic transport much more clearly. It is the purpose of this review to discuss briefly our current knowledge concerning axoplasmic flow and, then, to consider the effects of several drugs and antimetabolites both upon the material carried by axoplasmic transport and upon the transport mechanism itself.

Interfering with transport by damming or ligating a nerve has proven of great value in many studies. The technique produces results which are, of necessity, indirect. Much more satisfying data were obtained after radioactive tracers were introduced into the study of axoplasmic transport by Samuels *et al.* (1951), who used systemic administration of phosphate-^{32}P to produce labeled phosphorylated compounds in nervous tissue. Several days after the injection, radioactive material could be seen moving along nerve trunks. The radioactivity of a "phosphoprotein" fraction varied with distance along the nerve, being highest near the cells of origin and decreasing at progressively greater distances. Such a distribution agreed well with the hypothesis that material synthesized in the cell body was moving through the nerve to the periphery.

Later studies by Droz and Leblond (1963) utilized radioautographic techniques after systemic injections of ^{32}P- and ^{3}H-labeled precursors to demonstrate a clear-cut "plug" of radioactive material which moved through the interior of axons at a rate of about 3 mm/day. These studies established unequivocally the presence of axoplasmic flow. Furthermore, the radioautographic localization demonstrated that this material was transported within the axon. This conclusion had been suggested earlier on the basis of indirect evidence (Weiss *et al.*, 1945) but had not been completely accepted. At the present time several radioautographic studies have confirmed the intra-axonal nature of the transport system (Ochs, 1966; Lasek, 1968a,b; Hendrickson, 1969; Sjöstrand, 1969).

The use of radioisotopes was further developed by Ochs and his colleagues, who injected radioactive precursors into specific regions of the central and peripheral nervous systems (Ochs and Burger, 1958; Ochs *et al.*, 1962). Unhampered by high levels of "background" incorporation, the movement of material along the nerve was easily demonstrated. Lower levels of background also allowed work on the chemical characterization of the transported material to be initiated (Ochs *et al.*, 1967; McEwen and Grafstein, 1968; Bray and Austin, 1969; Kidwai and Ochs, 1969; Sjöstrand and Karlsson, 1969; Anderson *et al.*,1970; Karlsson and Sjöstrand, 1971b; Norström and Sjöstrand, 1971).

A number of workers have described experimental systems in which localized introduction of isotopes can be utilized (Table I). These techniques have allowed a much easier study of axoplasmic flow. In addition, they have provided several experimental systems with which the effects of drugs can be measured. Of the available systems, the optic pathways of rodents seem the easiest to use. In this case, a radioactive precursor is

TABLE I

METHODS USED TO INTRODUCE PRECURSORS INTO LOCALIZED AREAS

Region	Technique	Ref.
Motor fibers, sciatic nerve[a]	Injection into the ventral horn	Ochs and Burger (1958), Ochs *et al.* (1962)
Ulnar nerve (cat)	Injection into the subarachnoid space	Koenig (1958)
Hypoglossal nerve (rabbit); vagus nerve (rabbit)	Topical application to the ala cinerea	Miani (1962, 1963, 1964)
Optic nerve[a]	Intraocular injections	Taylor and Weiss (1965)
CNS–nerve–muscle (snail, frog)[b]	Bathe CNS, isolated preparation[b]	Kerkut *et al*: (1967)
Olfactory nerve (toad)	Topical application	Weiss and Holland (1967)
Splenic nerve (cat)	Injection of the celiac ganglion	Livett *et al.* (1968b)
Septal neurons (rat)	Inject caudate nucleus	Routtenberg *et al.* (1968)
Ventral nerve cord (crayfish)	Inject abdominal ganglion	Fernandez and Davison (1969)
Sensory fibers, sciatic nerve[a]	Injection into the dorsal root ganglion	Ochs *et al.* (1969)
Individual anterior horn cells (cat)	Intracellular iontophoresis	Lux *et al.* (1970)
Thoracic sympathetic nerves (mice)	Injection of the lowest thoracic sympathetic ganglion	Almon and McClure (unpublished data)

[a] Used with several species by various workers.
[b] CNS, central nervous system.

introduced into the vitreous humor by intraocular injection. Radioactively labeled molecules are synthesized by the retinal ganglion cells and transported through the axons of these cells to terminals in relay nuclei in the brain.

B. RATES OF FLOW

1. *Slow Flow*

Most of the results obtained prior to 1960 measured a rate of 1 to 3 mm/day. Of the several rates now known to exist, the rate of 1 to 3 mm/day is perhaps the easiest to observe. Material moving at this rate is labeled more heavily than is more rapidly moving material. Furthermore, the times involved are long enough that background labeling becomes less of a problem. This point is particularly important when considering systemic administration of precursors (cf. Droz and Leblond, 1963).

2. *Fast Flow*

In the 1960s, several groups described the presence in nerves of material which moved at rates much faster than those seen earlier (Miani, 1962, 1964; Burdwood, 1965; Kerkut *et al.*, 1967; McEwen and Grafstein, 1968; Lasek, 1968a,b; Bray and Austin, 1969; Ochs and Johnson, 1969). These faster rates ranged from about 40 mm/day (Miani, 1962) to 700–1000 mm/day (Kerkut *et al.*, 1967). Ochs *et al.* (1969) have described the movement of an actual wave of material along the sciatic nerve following injections into the dorsal root ganglion or the ventral horn (Ochs and Ranish 1969), and these results have been reproduced by others (Anderson *et al.*, 1970; Kennedy *et al.*, 1971; Fink *et al.*, 1971). The rate of movement of the wave was independent of the time of observation, and averaged 400 mm/day in adult cats, dogs, goats, monkeys, and other species. "Waves" of moving material can also be observed in other experimental systems. By examining the movement of a front of radioactivity, a rate of 400 mm/day has been observed in the optic pathway of rats (Anderson *et al.*, 1970; Schlichter and McClure, unpublished) and in the vagus nerve of the rabbit (Sjöstrand, 1969; Fink *et al.*, 1971). Due to the unambiguous manner in which rates of movement can be measured when a defined wave is present, such data are preferable to rates obtained by other, more indirect, means.

3. *Intermediate Flow Rates*

Rates other than the often-mentioned slow and fast transport have been observed. Miani (1962, 1964) measured rates of 40 to 70 mm/day for the movement of ^{32}P-labeled compounds from the ala cinerea through the hypoglossal and vagus nerves. Similar rates have been observed, employing the movement of a front of material, when $^{32}P_i$ is used to label the optic pathway (Siegel and McClure, unpublished data) or L-leucine-^{3}H is used to label the sympathetic fibers in the mouse (Almon and McClure, unpublished data). Indirect means of measuring the rate of flow have given rates which are similar, although often slightly slower. Intermediate rates of flow have been reported by Karlsson and Sjöstrand (1971b). Lasek has also observed (Lasek, 1968a,b) and discussed (Lasek, 1970b) these rates. It is the opinion of this reviewer that such rates represent a third component of axoplasmic flow. The following evidence supports this suggestion.

(*1*) The rates of measured transport probably do not vary, either from experimental error or physiological factors, by more than a factor of about 2 to 5 (Section II,B,4). Nevertheless, the slow flow (about 2 mm/day), intermediate flow (about 60 mm/day), and fast flow (about 500 mm/day) are separated by more than this margin. (*2*) Different precursors label the various flows in a differential manner. Thus, phosphate-^{32}P labels the intermediate flow very well (Miani, 1962, 1964), but labels the fast flow only to a small extent, if at all (Ochs and Ranish, 1969; Siegel and McClure, unpublished data). (*3*) The different flows respond to treatment with drugs in different ways. These effects will be discussed below (Section III,B,5).

4. *Factors Affecting the Rates of Flow*

The rates measured in a given system depend upon a number of experimental variables. In practice, varying the times of observation allows the experimental separation of the fast and slow flows. Furthermore, different precursors label the two flows differentially. These experimental manipulations can be used to allow the study of any desired phase of transport.

In addition to the preceding variables, a number of physiological factors influence the rate of flow. The rates of the slow and fast flows vary with the age of experimental animals. As animals age from birth to adulthood, fast axoplasmic flow increases in rate and slow axoplasmic flow decreases (Droz and Leblond, 1963; Barondes, 1968; Lasek, 1970a; Hendrickson and Cowan, 1971). Similar changes are seen after injection of mice with the protein nerve growth factor (Levi-Montalcini and Angeletti, 1968) prior to measurement of the rate of transport (Almon and McClure, unpublished). The rate of slow axoplasmic flow increases during regeneration following section of the optic nerve in the goldfish (Grafstein and Murray, 1969). In some cases a given system yields different rates of flow in different species. For example, catecholamine storage granules move at rates of about 3 mm/hour in rabbits (Dahlström and Häggendal, 1967), about 5 mm/hour in rats, and about 10 mm/hour in cats (Dahlström and Häggendal, 1966). Different nerves in a given animal often transport material at different rates. Droz and Leblond (1963) report that the rate of slow transport is 3 mm/day in the trigeminal nerves, but only 0.8 mm/day in the sciatic nerve. Held and Young (1969) find that material is transported through the hypoglossal nerve at a lower rate (6.3 mm/day) than that seen in the vagus nerve (16 mm/day). Sjöstrand (1969) has reported that fast transport proceeds at a rate of 300 mm/day in the hypoglossal nerve, but at 400 mm/day in the vagus. Finally, treatment with drugs can affect both the amount of material transported and the rate of transport (see Section III).

All the changes in rate noted above are relatively small. It is rare to find a change which exceeds a factor of 3 or 4 times, when considering either slow or fast flow. It is possible that physiological or anatomical changes serve only to modulate the fundamental rates of underlying transport processes. This result supplies further evidence that the intermediate flow is a separate physiological entity rather than just an extreme case of either fast or slow flow.

C. Functions of the Transported Material

In order to consider axoplasmic transport in its proper relation to other physiological processes in the neuron, it is necessary to inquire into the function of the transported material. Five hypotheses have been put forth concerning the use of these molecules.

1. *Replenishment*

It has been suggested that the transported material is used to replenish metabolites, enzymes, and other molecules needed to support normal synaptic function (cf. Barondes, 1967). An extension of this hypothesis would state that transport is also necessary to maintain the membrane and the subcellular structures which exist along the length of the axon.

In support of this function, a number of proteins known to be involved in the biosynthesis of neurotransmitters are carried by axoplasmic transport. Among such proteins are dopamine β-hydroxylase and chromogranin A, both of which are believed associated with storage granules for catecholamines (Laduron, 1968; Livett *et al.*, 1969; Geffen *et al.*, 1969, 1970), dopa decarboxylase (Dahlström and Jonason, 1968), acetylcholinesterase (Lubińska, 1964; Johnson, 1970), choline acetylase (Lubińska *et al.*, 1961; Frizell *et al.*, 1970), and adenyl cyclase (Bray *et al.*, 1971). To verify the hypothesis, it will be necessary to observe the replenishment of other components of the axon. In particular, a study of the movement of proteins associated with the axon membrane should prove rewarding. As our understanding of the chemistry of membranes becomes greater, these types of studies should be possible.

2. *Regeneration*

The regeneration of normal axons after section of the nerve probably involves material carried by axoplasmic flow. The findings of altered rates of flow in regenerating neurons (Grafstein and Murray, 1969) and in sympathetic neurons of mice treated with nerve growth factor (Almon and McClure, unpublished data) support this suggestion. Since both regenerating neurons and nerves in immature animals exhibit increased rates of slow flow, it is likely that regeneration of neurons will use material supplied preferentially by the slow component of transport. For a further discussion of the relationship between transport and regeneration, see Grafstein and Murray (1969).

3. *Trophic Factors*

It is likely that trophic factors will be carried to the synapse by axoplasmic flow. Two considerations support this hypothesis. First, intercellular regulatory phenomena in other systems are well controlled by genetic factors. In order for intracellular contacts such as the myoneural junction to come under genetic control, information, probably in the form of macromolecules, must come from the nucleus and be transported to the points of contact. A second line of evidence concerns experiments in which various degenerative changes in muscle are produced by severing the innervating nerves. Several workers have examined the time course of degeneration as a function of the length of the nerve stump which remains attached to the muscle (Parker, 1932; Gutmann *et al.*, 1955; Luco and Eyzaguirre, 1955; Emmelin *et al.*, 1966; Slater, 1966). Longer nerves produce a longer delay in the onset of degenerative changes, suggesting movement of material through the nerve to the muscle. Slater (1966) has used nerves of varying length to estimate a rate of movement of 360 mm/day for a factor that affects the frequency of miniature end-plate potentials. The agreement between this number and the value of about 400 mm/day reported for fast transport in motor fibers further supports the hypothesis that trophic factors are supplied to the muscle by axoplasmic transport.

4. *Electrical Activity and Transport*

A question of central importance to neurologists concerns the relationship between axoplasmic transport and the propagation of action potentials by the nerve. At the present time it seems likely that the presence or absence of electrical activity has little or no effect upon axoplasmic transport. For example, Geffen and Rush (1968) found that sectioning the fibers caused no significant change in norepinephrine accumulated at a constriction placed upon the postganglionic nerves innervating the spleen. If a given sympathetic nerve is ligated simultaneously at two points, norepinephrine accumulates equally at both ligations, despite the fact that the interrupted segment will not be conducting action potentials (cf. Dahlström, 1967a; Mayor and Kapeller, 1967). Similar observations have been made in other systems (Lubińska, 1964). Ochs and Smith (1971a) report that direct stimulation of isolated segments of the cat sciatic nerve produces only a small decrease in the rate at which radioactively labeled proteins are carried by fast transport. The authors state that the decrease seen may be due to a lowered supply of metabolic energy (see Section III). Finally, levels of either tetrodotoxin or procaine which prevent propagation of action potentials have no effect upon fast transport through sections of the cat sciatic nerve (Ochs and Hollingsworth, 1971; Sections III,D,2 and E,2).

The converse experiments with drugs have also been carried out. Colchiicne can effectively block both fast and slow transport at doses which have no effect upon the electrical activity of nerves (Hinkley and Green, 1971).

These results suggest strongly that little or no short-term relationship exists in mammals between axoplasmic transport and the propagation of action potentials by a nerve. A relationship should exist at longer times, however. If axoplasmic transport is completely inhibited, the axon and synapse should be altered in activity and should eventually become nonfunctional. Such an effect may be the basis of the neuropathy induced over a period of several days by the *Vinca* or *Colchicum* alkaloids (see Section III,B).

5. *Regulation of the Synapse*

To the preceding functions for axoplasmic transport should be added a provocative final candidate. It seems clear that most cells operate under a mutually beneficial cooperation between the cytoplasm and the nucleus. For this to be true in the neuron, a transfer of material containing information must take place between the nerve cell body and the periphery, as well as in the opposite direction (Lubińska, 1964; Lasek, 1967). It is quite tempting to believe that informational macromolecules, such as proteins, are carried to the axon terminals in order to modify ongoing chemical events in the nerve endings. Barondes (1967) has suggested that transported molecules may provide a means for synaptic modification in the storing of memory.

It is the feeling of this reviewer that informational macromolecules would be preferentially consigned to the fast flow. Two arguments support this hypothesis. First, movement of molecules by fast transport would allow communication with the synapse in times on the order of 1% of those which would be required if slow flow were utilized. A second argument rests upon the hypothesis that the amount of energy expended by the cell, per molecule transported, is probably greater for molecules transported at the higher rates characteristic of fast axoplasmic flow than at the lower rates characteristic of slow flow. If so, it is clearly in the best interests of the neurons involved to transport at these high-energy-requiring rates only the minimum number of molecules necessary. Presumably, these molecules would then be responsible for controlling the activity of other enzymes or macromolecular structures such as the cell membrane; i.e., the molecules transported would be controlling or modulating macromolecules. If trophic factors are considered informational molecules, as seems probable, the rate of movement of 360 mm/day measured by Slater (1966) provides experimental evidence for the use of the fast phase of transport.

D. Mechanism of Transport

The mechanism by means of which material is moved by any rate of axoplasmic flow is currently little understood. Experiments in which nerves are interrupted have shown that material continues to move at undiminished rates on the distal side of the section, requiring that transport be carried on by local forces within the axon (Lubińska, 1964; Dahlström, 1967a; Ochs and Ranish, 1969; Kennedy and Fink, 1971). Transport is known to be active, being strongly inhibited by anoxia (Ochs, 1971) or by injection into the nerve of a number of antimetabolites such as cyanide, dinitrophenol, or iodoacetic acid (Ochs and Hollingsworth, 1971; Ochs and Smith, 1971b). Transport through the sciatic nerve of the cat can be completely blocked by the application to the nerve of a layer of lanolin, which excludes oxygen from the axons (Ochs, 1971). Nerves so blocked show a sharp piling up of material on the proximal side of the lanolin barrier, with very little diffusion of material away from the site of the block. These results require that the transported material not only be moved by forces generated locally but that the mechanism responsible for generating mechanical movement be localized in very short segments, probably microscopic in length, along the axon. The transport mechanism must also be highly resistant to diffusion, suggesting binding to some subcellular particle.

Material carried by fast axoplasmic transport has been subjected to subcellular fractionation by several groups (Ochs *et al.*, 1967; McEwen and Grafstein, 1968; Kidwai and Ochs, 1969; Sjöstrand and Karlsson, 1969; Anderson *et al.*, 1970; Karlsson and Sjöstrand, 1971a; Norström and Sjöstrand, 1971). It is clear that most of the material carried by fast axoplasmic transport is highly insoluble, presumably reflecting the subcellular structure of the transporting system. Radioactively labeled material carried by slow axoplasmic flow contains much more soluble protein. Further biochemical characterization of the transported material should help our understanding of the transport system.

E. Sources of Energy for Transport

At the present time the energy source responsible for mechanical movement in transport is not known. Recent studies in the laboratory of Ochs have shown that the necessary energy can be provided by respiration, presumably through the synthesis of high-energy phosphate-containing compounds (Ochs, 1971; Ochs and Hollingsworth, 1971; Ochs and Smith, 1971b). Although both adenosine triphosphate (ATP) and guanosine triphosphate (GTP) have been suggested as possible candidates for the primary energy donor, no firm conclusion can be reached until the transducing system is isolated chemically and subjected to further study. Nevertheless, the known involvement of ATP and GTP in other systems involving transduction of chemical into mechanical energy lends credence to the hypothesis that these two nucleotides may be similarly involved in axoplasmic flow.

F. Relation of Axonal Organelles to Transport

The transport mechanism has been associated with subcellular structures in the nerve axon (Schmitt, 1968). If transport is, indeed, linked to some "railroad track" which runs through the axonal length, it seems wise to consider the involvement of all the possible candidates. The components of the axon which could be involved are five in number.

1. *Endoplasmic Reticulum*

The endoplasmic reticulum, which sends branches throughout the axons to the tips of some, but apparently not all, fibers, may be involved in transport. The possible involvement of this structure is strengthened by its assumed connection with the flattened sacs of the Golgi apparatus (Peters *et al.*, 1970), which is associated both with secretion of zymogen granules from the pancreas and with the material destined for transport through axons (Droz, 1967). At the present time no further evidence can be found to support these structures.

2. *Microtubules*

More popular in the last few years have been fibrous structures composed of protein subunits: microtubules, neurofilaments, and microfilaments. Of these, microtubules have been most persistently linked with transport. These structures are made up of subunits of two nonidentical globular proteins of molecular weight about 55,000, joined together by, apparently, noncovalent bonds (Bryan and Wilson, 1971; Olmsted *et al.*, 1971). The microtubule is about 240 Å in diameter and has an open central lumen of about 100 to 150 Å. In cross section, electron microscopy shows thirteen protein subunits arranged as a single turn of a helix which is repeated to form the fiber. Microtubules are straight or only gently curved, suggesting high mechanical strength. The fibers are unbranched and run for very long distances through cells; indeed, it is possible, although presently unproven, that these structures run as a continuous fiber from the neuronal perikaryon to the synapse. Microtubules in nerves often have associated "sidearms" of unknown function.

Arguments favoring the involvement of microtubules in transport include their favorable subcellular localization and known participation in other physiological processes in which movement is seen. For example, the spindle fiber, which is largely composed of microtubules, not only moves the chromosomes at metaphase but also serves as a pathway along which particulate material moves to and fro during cell division (Allen and Kamiya, 1964). Microtubule protein is similar to actin in amino acid composition and by the presence in each of bound nucleotides (Renaud *et al.*, 1968; Shelanski and Taylor, 1968; Stephens, 1968). Actin, however, possesses 3-methyl histidine, which is not present in microtubule protein. Furthermore, Stephens (1970) has reported that the peptide maps of the two proteins differ. If the microtubules do prove to be similar in chemistry or function to actin, their participation in processes such as transport is more likely.

Microtubules specifically bind colchicine (Taylor, 1965)—a fact used to advantage by Taylor and his colleagues to purify the protein subunits (Borisy and Taylor, 1967; Shelanski and Taylor, 1967; Weisenberg *et al.*, 1968). Colchicine interferes with the action of many cellular functions believed associated with microtubules, including the intracellular movement of material in plant cells (Newcomb, 1969). Finally, it should be mentioned that microtubules have other functions. They are believed active in supplying physical strength to some structures, such as the axopods of *Actinosphaerium*, and are probably involved in the motility of flagella and sperm (Porter, 1966). Recent experiments of Yamada *et al.* (1970) suggest that one of the primary functions of microtubules in axons is to provide mechanical support. These latter functions need not necessarily be carried on at the expense of transport; there seems no reason to believe that a given microtubule cannot carry out two functions simultaneously. For more details concerning the structure and function of microtubules, see Porter (1966) and Schmitt and Samson (1968).

These arguments suggest that microtubules may be involved in axoplasmic transport. This view, however, is almost certainly too simple. It seems most likely that both microtubules and other filamentous structures will be required (see Section III,B,5). Furthermore, it should be realized that alternative explanations can be found for each of the lines of evidence associating microtubules and transport. Despite strong circumstantial evidence, it is still possible that these structures are not involved at all. The role of microtubules in transport is discussed in more detail in Section III,B.

3. *Neurofilaments*

The neuron contains large numbers of neurofilaments (Schmitt and Samson, 1968). These structures are smaller than microtubules, being only about 100 Å in diameter. Like microtubules, they are a polymeric structure composed of repeating globular protein subunits. The neurofilaments are unbranched and appear to run in nearly straight lines approximately parallel to the axis of the axon. They also possess sidearms, which often join two neurofilaments together. Although it has been suggested that neurofilaments and microtubules exist in a dynamic equilibrium (Wiśniewski *et al.*, 1968), the neurofilament protein isolated from extruded squid axoplasm is distinctly different from microtubule protein from the same source (Davison, 1970). Whether this will also be true of these proteins in mammalian systems remains to be seen. Neurofilament protein, unlike microtubule protein, does not appear to bind nucleotides. No drug that interacts specifically with these organelles is yet known. Probably because of this, no function has yet been associated with neurofilaments. The recent chemical isolation of a protein believed to be the subunit of neurofilaments (Davison, 1970) may lead to research which will clarify the function and metabolic interrelationships of these structures.

4. *Microfilaments*

A third type of fiber, the microfilament, is found along the length of the axon and in the synaptic endings. These structures are the smallest of the three being considered, possessing a diameter of about 50 Å. Unlike microtubules and neurofilaments, microfilaments occur in poorly defined tangles along the axon and often seem to end upon the axolemma itself (Wessels *et al.*, 1971). They are probably also made up of subunits of globular protein, although these have not yet been knowingly isolated. Microfilaments are strongly associated with contractility in cells (Wessels *et al.*, 1971). The drug cytochalasin B can cause the reversible disappearance of microfilaments. When the microfilaments disappear, associated contractile phenomena cease in several experimental systems. Wessels and his colleagues (1971) have reviewed the evidence which links the microfilaments, contractility, and the effects of cytochalasin B.

5. *Axolemma*

The axon membrane has been suggested as an active participant in slow axoplasmic flow, in which it may function as a peristaltic element (Weiss, 1961, 1969). This hypothesis predicts that all the components of the axon would move simultaneously. At the present time no evidence exists with which to refute the hypothesis, although the faster, more specific, transport systems must use a different mechanism.

It is possible that the axolemma is active also in fast axoplasmic transport. Again, its physical localization is ideal, stretching from the nerve cell body to the synaptic endings. Macromolecular mechanisms responsible for transduction of energy into mechanical movement could be part of the complex chemistry of the membrane. Although no direct evidence can be found to either favor or rule out this hypothesis, it is of interest that electron micrographic radioautographs of nerves through which rapidly transported proteins are migrating show an accumulation of grains near the axon membrane (Hendrickson and Cowan, 1971). Similarly, when sciatic nerves through which tritiated proteins are being transported are "beaded," freeze-substituted, and examined by radioautography using the electron microscope, grains do not appear associated with the fibrillar structures (Ochs, 1966). Although these data by no means require the participation of the axolemma, it would seem reasonable to consider the membrane at the same time we consider more fashionable structures such as the microtubules, neurofilaments, and microfilaments.

III. Effect of Drugs upon Axoplasmic Transport

The following discussion concerns all those drugs that, to the knowledge of the author, have been examined for an effect upon axoplasmic transport. The effects of one class of compounds, the antibiotics and general metabolic poisons, will not be discussed in detail due to their well-known action in other systems. Compounds of this class have been studied in transporting systems by several authors (Barondes, 1968; McEwen and Grfsatein, 1968; Sjöstrand and Karlsson, 1969; Cahill, 1970; Ochs and Ranish, 1970; Ochs, 1971; Ochs and Hollingsworth, 1971; Ochs and Smith, 1971a,b). In general, these studies agree well. Puromycin, and related antibiotics which inhibit the synthesis of protein in mammalian ribosomal systems, can prevent the synthesis of protein destined to be transported. These data suggest that transported proteins are synthesized by the same mechanisms used for other cellular proteins. This suggestion is supported by the inhibitory action of actinomycin D (Cahill, 1970), a compound known to interfere with the deoxyribonucleic acid (DNA)-dependent synthesis of ribonucleic acid (RNA).

Ochs and his colleagues have examined the effects of a number of inhibitors of respiration upon transport. The fast movement of protein through the sensory fibers in isolated sections of the cat sciatic nerve is strongly inhibited by anoxia, cyanide ion, dinitrophenol, or iodoacetate. Inhibition produced by iodoacetate can be overcome by adding lactate or pyruvate. These data support the hypothesis that glycolysis and mitochondrial oxidative pathways supply the energy for transport. Significantly, the inhibition produced by these agents appears as a decrease in the rate of transport, and not as a decrease in the amount of material transported in each length of nerve. It is possible that all those drugs that produce a decreased rate of flow may act through a primary effect upon the supply of energy.

The following sections discussed the remaining drugs which have been tested upon axoplasmic transport.

A. Tranquilizers

The movement through the sympathetic fibers of storage granules containing catecholamines has been studied by Dahlström and her collaborators (Dahlström, 1967a; Dahlström and Waldeck, 1968; Dahlström *et al.*, 1969; Dahlström and Häggendal, 1970) and by researchers at Monash University (Geffen and Rush, 1968; Livett *et al.*, 1968a,b, 1969; Geffen *et al.*, 1970). The effects of several drugs upon these systems have been examined (Dahlström and Häggendal, 1966, 1967; Kapeller and Mayor, 1967; Dahlström, 1967b, 1969, 1970). These workers have ligated the sciatic nerve, after which the accumulation of catecholamines above the ligation can be observed by means of fluorescence histochemical techniques (Hillarp *et al.*, 1966). In this experimental system, the material accumulated is believed to be norepinephrine. If two ligations are made simultaneously in one sciatic nerve, fluorescent material accumulates on the proximal side of both ligations, providing more evidence that transport is carried out by means of energy supplied locally in the nerve. Quantitative studies upon transport in the sympathetic system, both in the sciatic nerve and in the celiac plexus, have shown that certain proteins, such as dopamine β-hydroxylase and chromogranin A (both of which are associated with the storage granules) are transported at rates corresponding to the transport rates of the granules themselves (Laduron, 1968; Laduron and Belpaire, Geffen *et al.*, 1969, 1970).

The effect of reserpine upon the transport of amine storage granules has been examined by Dahlström (Dahlström, 1967a,b, 1970). If reserpine is administered systemically to an animal prior to ligation of the sciatic nerve, no fluorescence accumulates above the ligation. Furthermore, reserpine can be administered at times after a ligation has been placed, with equal efficiency in preventing the accumulation of catecholamines. The effect of reserpine can be abolished by treatment of the animal with nialamide, an inhibitor of monoamine oxidase. These results suggest that reserpine causes release of catecholamines from the storage granules, after which monoamine oxidase can destroy the released amines. Similar results have been obtained by Kapeller and Mayor (1967).

It would appear that the opening of storage granules caused by reserpine is irreversible in nature. This conclusion is based upon observations of the recovery of fluorescence after reserpine treatment. The accumulation of catecholamine-containing granules occurs at times which correspond to transport of new granules from the cell body. Furthermore, fluorescence reappears at ligations placed closer to the cell body at times earlier than it appears at ligations placed farther away. Finally, the recovery of fluorescence at the more distal of two ligatures on the same nerve can be studied. As mentioned above, treatment with reserpine will abolish the fluorescence due to catecholamines at both of the two ligations. Although recovery occurs in the usual times at the proximal ligation, no accumulation of fluorescence is seen at the distal defect. This finding suggests that the ligation placed nearer to the cell body can prevent the movement of material from the perikaryon to the more distal ligation. Taken together, the data provide strong evidence that reserpine causes an irreversible alteration of the storage granule.

Tetrabenazine was also examined for an effect upon the storage granules (Dahlström, 1967b). This compound is a short-acting tranquilizer which possesses pharmacological properties very similar to those shown by reserpine (cf. Pletscher *et al.*, 1962). Dahlström (1967b) has shown that this drug can cause disappearance of fluorescence which has accumulated at ligations placed on the sciatic nerve, in exact parallel with the effects of reserpine. Recovery of fluorescence after treatment with tetrabenazine is quite different, however, from that seen after reserpine. After depletion with tetrabenazine, recovery of fluorescence occurs simultaneously at a distal ligation on one nerve and a more proximal ligation on a second nerve. This result suggests that tetrabenazine does not inactivate the storage granule, but that the granule can pick up catecholamines *in situ* after treatment. The conclusion is strengthened by experiments involving two ligations on a single sciatic nerve. In this case, tetrabenazine causes depletion of the catecholamines that accumulate at both ligatures. In contrast to the results obtained with reserpine, however, fluorescence is now recovered simultaneously at both ligations, confirming the hypothesis that the once-depleted granules can be refilled without transport of new material.

The discussion thus far concerns the action of reserpine and tetrabenazine upon transported material. The effects of these agents upon transport itself should also be considered. A number of lines of evidence suggest that reserpine has little or no direct effect upon the transport process Experiments which involve the piling up of transported material at ligations must rely upon the transport mechanism to produce the accumulation. Although the transport system need not be operating perfectly, it must certainly be functioning to some extent. Since amine storage granules continue to accumulate in animals treated with reserpine or tetrabenazine, one must conclude that these drugs do not abolish axoplasmic flow. This conclusion is supported by experiments involving the movement of radioactively labeled proteins by slow axoplasmic transport through the motor fibers of the sciatic nerve. Injection of reserpine into the ventral horn of cats had little or no effect upon the transport of material labeled with simultaneously injected phosphate-^{32}P (Ochs *et al.*, 1962). Similarly, reserpine seems to have no effect upon fast transport through the optic nerves of rats. Intraocular injections of 0.55 mg of reserpine have no effect upon transport in this system, although synthesis of protein is slightly depressed (Paulson and McClure, unpublished data). The neurotransmitters at the synaptic endings of these two experimental systems, however, may not be sensitive to depletion by reserpine. If reserpine has a direct effect upon transport, it is more likely to be seen in adrenergic systems. It would seem fruitful to examine reserpine and other tranquilizers in various experimental systems to explore the possibility that these agents interfere with transport.

B. Drugs Affecting Fibrillar Structures

Microtubules have been implicated in a number of cell processes, one of which is intracellular transport of metabolites (Porter, 1966; Tilney and Gibbons, 1968; Newcomb, 1969). Several authors (cf. Schmitt and Samson, 1968) have suggested that microtubules may be involved in axoplasmic transport. A number of drugs, such as colchicine and vinblastine, can halt mitosis by interacting with the microtubules of the mitotic spindle (Borisy and Taylor, 1967; Malawista *et al.*, 1968). These facts lead to the prediction that antimitotic agents should be effective inhibitors of axoplasmic flow, a hypothesis suggested earlier by Schmitt (1968).

1. *Colchicine*

Of the available antimitotic compounds, colchicine has been most extensively studied. This drug is a known neuropathogen (Wiśniewski and Terry, 1967; Sjöstrand *et al.*, 1970). Colchicine blocks transport when injected into the sciatic nerve, using as a measure of activity either the accumulation of acetylcholinesterase (Kreutzberg, 1969) or amine storage granules (Dahlström, 1969). Although both these studies reported that rather large doses were necessary (about 1 mg), Karlsson and Sjöstrand (1968) have reported that intraocular injections of 50 or 100 μg of colchicine will prevent both slow and fast transport of radioactively labeled material from the eyes of rabbits. Similar doses are effective in interfering with transport through the vagus nerve (Sjöstrand *et al.*, 1970). In this case, fast transport of protein was completely blocked, whereas the slower transport of acetylcholinesterase was blocked only partially. Injection of even smaller amounts of material (1–10 μg) into the sciatic nerves of chickens caused paralysis of the legs after 72 hours and strongly inhibited both slow and fast axoplasmic flow (James *et al.*, 1970). The effect of colchicine upon at least one invertebrate system has also been studied. Fernandez has described a flow of material from the ventral ganglia through the axons of the ventral cord of the crayfish (Fernandez and Davison, 1969; Fernandez *et al.*, 1970). Injections of colchicine into nearby ganglia could halt this transport (Fernandez *et al.*, 1970; Fernandez and Samson, 1970).

2. *Vinblastine*

Other antimitotic agents can also affect transport. Vinblastine is an efficient inhibitor of mitosis (Frei *et al.*, 1964; Malawista *et al.*, 1968). This agent can also exhibit many other effects, such as interaction with bacterial ribosomes (Kingsbury and Volez, 1969). Injections of vinblastine can produce degenerative changes in nervous tissue (Wiśniewski *et al.*, 1968; Schochet *et al.*, 1968; Shelanski and Wiśniewski, 1969) and can provoke the intracellular proliferation of crystals in L cells or in leukocytes (Bensch and Malawista, 1969) and nerve cells (Bensch and Malawista, 1968). These crystals are believed to be molecular aggregates of preformed monomeric microtubule protein—a conclusion strengthened by the *in vitro* induction by vinblastine of crystalline aggregates of microtubule protein (Bensch *et al.*, 1969; Marantz *et al.*, 1969). Dahlström (1970) has reported that vinblastine can block transport of amine storage granules through the sympathetic fibers of the cat sciatic nerve if the drug is either injected into the nerve or applied topically to the ganglia of the lumbar plexus. Furthermore, injection of vinblastine into the sciatic nerve not only causes an accumulation of catecholamines proximal to the defect but prevents the usual accumulation at a ligation placed distal to the site of the injection. Fernandez and Samson (1970) have reported that vinblastine blocks axoplasmic transport in the ventral cord of the crayfish. Both these groups report that vinblastine is a more effective agent than is colchicine.

3. *Other Antimitotic Agents*

In none of the above studies were dose–response curves determined. Although Dahlström reports the effects of three doses of colchicine (Dahlström, 1969), most workers have considered only a single level of drug. Cahill and co-workers (Cahill, 1970; Cahill *et al.*, 1971; Cahill and McClure, unpublished data) have used the transport of material through the optic nerve of the rat to develop a quantitative method with which the effect of drugs can be assessed. Dose–response curves for a number of antimitotic agents have been measured (Fig. 1). Colchicine yielded a typical sigmoid curve. Transport was depressed to 50% of control values at doses of about 0.3 mg, in reasonable agreement with the results of Dahlström (1969), Kreutzberg (1969), and Karlsson and Sjöstrand (1969). Vinblastine was also effective, in agreement with earlier reports. In addition to these agents, other antimitotic compounds were tested. Vincristine, a structural analog of vinblastine, is effective as an antimitotic agent (Frei *et al.*, 1964) and is

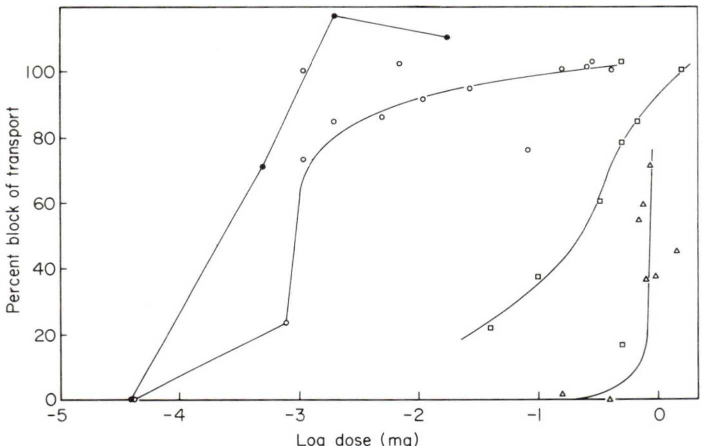

FIG. 1. Dose–response curves displaying the effects of antimitotic agents upon fast axoplasmic transport in the optic system of the rat. Drugs used: vincristine (●); vinblastine (○); colchicine (□); and griseofulvin (△). [Data from Cahill (1970) and Cahill *et al.* (1971).]

also effective in blocking transport. Colcemid, the *N*-deacetyl-*N*-methyl analog of colchicine, also blocks. The antifungal agent, griseofulvin, shown effective as an antimitotic compound by Paget and Walpole (1958, 1960) and by Malawista *et al.* (1968), was found effective against transport only at the highest doses which could be attained. Several drugs which are structurally related to antimitotic compounds but which are not themselves effective in preventing mitosis, were similarly ineffective when assayed against transport. For example, colchicoside, which is about 100 times less toxic than colchicine, did not block transport at the highest doses which could be attained (0.6 mg). It is clear that a number of antimitotic agents effectively inhibit axoplasmic transport.

The preceding results provide strong qualitative evidence for a relationship between mitosis and axoplasmic flow. In view of the known involvement of microtubules in the structure of the mitotic spindle, it is very tempting to conclude that microtubules themselves provide a link between these two processes. Quantitative comparisons, however, make this conclusion less clear-cut. The available data allow a series of antitransport agents to be ranked, in order of decreasing efficacy: vincristine > vinblastine ≫ Colcemid $\gtrsim$ colchicine > griseofulvin. These data can be compared with the relative effects of the same drugs evaluated as antimitotic agents by Tannock (1965). Dose–response curves were evaluated in the rate for vinblastine, vincristine, Colcemid, and colchicine by examining the accumulation of mitotic figures in cells of either the intestinal mucosa or a mammary tumor. The drugs were also compared on the basis of either (*1*) the dose required to achieve metaphase block, (*2*) the minimal effective dose, or (*3*) the time required for the tumor to double in size when host animals were treated with equal doses of the drugs. The four drugs were nearly equal in efficiency when judged by any of these criteria. In even the most extreme cases, the most active drug was no more than 5 times as potent as the least active. The ordering of the drugs varied when different measures of efficacy were considered. If the measure of greatest relevance to the effect of these drugs on transport in healthy tissue is considered (doses required to obtain metaphase block in the intestinal mucosa), the drugs rank as follows (numbers in parentheses refer to efficacy relative to colchicine): vincristine (2.5) > vinblastine (1.0) = colchicine (1.0) > Colcemid (0.5). These data agree poorly with those observed by Cahill (1970): vincristine (1000) > vinblastine (200) ≫ Colcemid (5) > colchicine (1). Although Tannock did not study griseofulvin, Paget and Walpole (1958, 1960) had to employ extremely high levels (10–20 mg/animal) in order to observe inhibition of mitosis in the rat.

The greatest point of contrast in the antitransport and antimitotic activities of these agents is seen when comparing vinblastine and colchicine. Vinblastine is about 1000 times more effective than colchicine in blocking transport (Fig. 1) but is of approximately equal potency as an inhibitor of mitosis (Tannock, 1965). A similar discrepancy results when the antimitotic activities of these compounds are evaluated using dividing oocytes of *Pectinaria*, the ice-cream cone worm. In this system, Malawista *et al.* (1968) find again that vinblastine is about as active as Colcemid. Both colchicine and vincristine are less active than their structurally related partners. Again, no marked differences in the activities of any of these drugs were seen. Of greater importance were results obtained with griseofulvin, which equals or surpasses vinblastine in effectiveness. Griseofulvin is a very poor antitransport agent (Cahill, 1970; Cahill *et al.*, 1971). It is, of course, possible that these discrepancies lie in different rates of uptake by different cells, different metabolic patterns in different experimental systems, or other differences. It is quite possible that the microtubules of invertebrates differ from those of vertebrates (Behnke and Forer, 1967; Olmsted *et al.*, 1971) and may respond to drugs in a different manner. Nonetheless, the lack of agreement in the quantitative relationships suggests that the involvement of microtubules in transport, although strongly supported on a qualitative level, must be viewed with caution pending further experimental data. It seems quite possible that other structures may be involved in addition to the microtubules.

4. *Cytochalasin B*

One other agent that affects fibrillar structures has been studied. Cytochalasin B affects neither microtubules nor neurofilaments, but does interfere fairly specifically with those physiological functions associated with microfilaments (Wessels *et al.*, 1971). Using the ventral nerve cord of the crayfish, Fernandez and Samson (personal communication) have shown that cytochalasin B can block both the slow (1 mm/day) flow and a faster (10 mm/day) flow. These important results suggest that subcellular fibers other than microtubules may be involved in axoplasmic transport. Studies with this interesting drug should be extended to other systems, particularly mammals.

5. *Discussion*

a. Drugs. Based upon the effects of the drugs discussed above, a number of tentative conclusions can be drawn and some suggestions for further research put forth.

Slow axoplasmic flow in a number of experimental systems is blocked by colchicine and vinblastine. In the only system thus far studied, cytochalasin B can also block the slow phase of axoplasmic flow. These results, if interpreted in terms of the commonly accepted action of the drugs, suggest that slow transport involves both microtubules and microfilaments. The interrelationships between these two organelles and transport remain to be elucidated. As a first step, the microfilament protein could be isolated and examined for possible interaction with purified microtubule protein.

The faster flow rates probably also involve the microtubules. Participation of other fibrous structures is quite likely but more difficult to justify. For example, consider the effect of cytochalasin. In the crayfish, this agent blocks a transport system that exhibits a flow rate of about 10 mm/day. This rate is clearly too low to be considered the counterpart of the 400 mm/day flow seen in mammals. Even if allowance is made for differences in temperature, the rate can be corrected upward to only 40–60 mm/day (20°–37°C; Q_{10} of 2.0 to 2.5). In fact, the rate of 40 to 60 mm/day is in excellent agreement with that seen in the so-called intermediate flow of mammals (Section II,B,3). Since this flow, in the crayfish, is blocked by either colchicine, vinblastine, or cytochalasin B, it seems likely that both microtubules and microfilaments are involved here also. There is, however, one difference between the functions subserved by microfilaments in the slow and intermediate flows. When intermediate flow is stopped by colchicine or vinblastine, the "plug" of radioactively labeled moving material remains sharply defined in the nerve, and does not broaden with time due to diffusion (Fernandez and Samson, 1970). Apparently, the material being transported stays firmly attached to the transporting mechanism. A similar sharp localization is observed when slow flow is blocked with colchicine, vinblastine, or cytochalasin B. In contrast, when cytochalasin B is used to block intermediate flow, the material whose movement has been interrupted does not remain localized but diffuses along the nerve (Fernandez and Samson, personal communication). These results suggest that microfilaments are not only involved in the movement at intermediate rates but also serve to constrain the transported material. Apparently they are not required for this function in the slow flow, suggesting that differences exist in the manner in which material transported in the two flows is bound. In order to clarify these relationships in higher animals, the effects of colchicine and cytochalasin B upon intermediate flow should be examined.

The organelles associated with the fast flow (400 mm/day) are not as well-defined. The fact that colchicine, vinblastine, and their analogs can effectively block the fast flow suggests that microtubules are involved in this phase of transport. The involvement of other filamentous structures is unclear. At the present time, the effect of cytochalasin B upon this system is unknown. As data pertaining to this point become available, the possible activity of the microfilaments will become more clear.

The preceding discussion rests heavily upon data obtained using the crayfish. It may well be, however, that results obtained when invertebrates are used to study axoplasmic transport may not be readily extrapolated to mammals. For example, treatment of crayfish with either colchicine or low temperatures (2°–3°C) produces no deficiency in the behavioral repertoire of the animals for periods as long as 20–45 days (Fernandez *et al.*, 1970; Davison, 1970). Under these conditions, axoplasmic transport is effectively prevented. These results suggest that crayfish are resistant to long-term treatments which are highly deleterious to mammals (Wiśniewski and Terry, 1967; Wiśniewski *et al.*, 1968; James *et al.*, 1970). Similar long-term support in crayfish of severed axons, which would have degenerated in mammals, has been reported by Hoy *et al.* (1967). In these respects, invertebrate axons apparently differ significantly from their mammalian counterparts. If so, results obtained when using invertebrates to study axoplasmic transport should be extrapolated to mammals only with caution.

b. Direct Observations with the Electron Microscope. If microtubules are involved in transport, agents that block transport by interfering with these structures might provide morphological defects observable with the electron microscope. In at least three studies such defects have not been observed. Colchicine can block slow axoplasmic flow through the axons of the crayfish nerve cord, yet examination of these axons under the electron microscope reveals microtubules of normal size and shape, in the same number as seen in controls (Fernandez *et al.*, 1970). Low temperatures can also disrupt the structure of microtubules (Tilney and Gibbons, 1968). Crayfish maintained at 2°–3°C do not transport axonal protein, but have normal numbers of apparently intact microtubules (Fernandez *et al.*, 1970; Davison, 1970). Finally, rats in which fast axoplasmic transport through the optic nerve has been blocked by intraocular injections of vinblastine show no defects in the axonal microtubules of the optic fibers (Cahill, 1970; Pumplin and Cahill, unpublished data). Although these results suggest that antimitotic agents may not act upon microtubules, this interpretation is too limited. It is quite possible that binding of drugs to the microtubules can produce changes which would be sufficient to block transport, but too small for direct visualization with the electron microscope. As a larger-scale example, a pilot flying at high altitudes would have difficulty detecting the point in a railroad at which the track was damaged enough to derail a train.

c. Neurofilaments and Transport. Even less than the preceding statements can be said about the possible involvement of the neurofilaments in any of the phases of transport. Lacking drugs that interact specifically with these structures, direct studies of inhibition are not possible. To date, no direct evidence links neurofilaments with transport. Nonetheless, these organelles are often considered as candidates. Lasek (1970b) has proposed a mechanism of transport which involves the neurofilaments. There are several lines of evidence, all highly circumstantial, which implicate neurofilaments in the transport process. (*1*) Their anatomy is favorable—the neurofilaments run in an unbranching fashion from the cell body linearly through long stretches of axon, and could well serve as a guiding influence for transport. (*2*) In large myelinated cells, which would need to transport proportionately more material than smaller ones, neurofilaments are more numerous (with respect to axonal cross-sectional area) than they are in small nonmyelinated cells (Porter, 1968). (*3*) As cells grow older from birth, the numbers of microtubules decrease and those of neurofilaments increase (Peters and Vaughn, 1967). During this same time the rate of slow axoplasmic transport decreases, whereas that of fast transport increases (Hendrickson and Cowan, 1971). This correlation would suggest that neurofilaments may be associated with fast transport. (*4*) Finally, neurofilaments appear to share a reciprocal metabolism fate with microtubules: in a number of cases, when one of these structures increases in number the other decreases. These results suggest that neurofilaments and microtubules may be related in function, even if they have dissimilar chemical properties. The question of neurofilaments is discussed in more detail by Davison (1970).

A final understanding of the complicated interrelationships between the various rates of axoplasmic transport and either microtubules, neurofilaments, or microfilaments, as well as the interaction between the fibrillar elements themselves, must await further experimental data. Although the evidence presently available implicates microtubules and microfilaments, the data neither compel one to accept these structures, nor force one to exclude others. Although current thinking is largely centered upon these organelles, we must not lose sight of the fact that other as yet unspecified and, perhaps, now unknown, subcellular structures may be important. In this case, as is often true, we are severely hampered by the lack of more compounds with which to arrest transport.

C. Methoxylated Phenylalkylamines

The block of axoplasmic transport by colchicine has prompted experimentation with other agents. The structures of known derivatives of colchicine were examined (Paulson and McClure, unpublished data) in an attempt to define other compounds which might block transport. The simplest structures which might be effective would appear to be trimethoxyphenylalkylamines and closely related compounds. Accordingly, 3,4,5-trimethoxyphenethylamine (mescaline) was examined for a possible effect as an inhibitor of axoplasmic transport. By using as an experimental system the transport of protein labeled by intraocular injection of tritiated amino acids, Paulson and McClure (unpublished data) have shown that mescaline blocks transport quite well, being slightly less efficient than colchicine itself. Two structurally related compounds were also tested. Both 3,4,5-trimethoxyamphetamine (TMA) and 2,4,5-trimethoxyamphetamine (TMA-2) are also effective inhibitors. Dose–response curves for the effect of each of these compounds indicate that TMA-2 > TMA > colchicine > mescaline. Although high doses of mescaline can inhibit the synthesis of proteins and could, thus, lead to an artifactual lowering of "transport" simply by depressing the incorporation of the precursor, these data were corrected for the minor depression in protein synthesis which occurred. That interference with the synthesis of protein is not responsible for the observed effect is further shown by the methoxylated amphetamines, which had no effect upon protein synthesis at levels completely blocking transport.

Mescaline and the two methoxylated amphetamines are known hallucinogenic agents. The possibility that these compounds exert their hallucinogenic action through an effect upon the transport of essential materials to the nerve ending, thereby altering neuronal integration of information, is an attractive hypothesis. The suggestion is strengthened by the fact that these three drugs have hallucinogenic effects which are ranked in the same order as those observed for their antitransport activities. Much further work must be carried out to clarify this relationship. Although the significance of these findings is not yet clear, this class of drugs provides an interesting new addition to the known antitransport agents.

D. Anesthetics

1. *General Anesthetics*

Allison and Nunn (1968) have suggested that anesthetic agents act through depolymerization of microtubules. This hypothesis was based upon the observations that high pressures and low temperatures, which are known to destabilize microtubules (Tilney and Gibbons, 1968), would elicit narcosis. In addition, colchicine treatment of some animals will produce narcosis. Finally, treatment with D_2O, an agent that stabilizes microtubules, can effectively antagonize narcosis produced by anesthetics.

In support of the hypothesis, Allison and Nunn subjected *Actinosphaerium* to treatment with halothane and observed a retraction of the axopods, which contain microtubules believed to be supportive elements. Axopods reappeared a few minutes after removal of the anesthetic. This hypothesis can be discussed in the light of several experimental findings.

a. Halothane. Fink and co-workers have conducted careful experiments designed to evaluate the effect of halothane upon transport in mammals. *In vivo* experiments were carried out by observing fast axoplasmic flow through the optic nerve and tract of rabbits under normal anesthetic levels of halothane (Fink and Kennedy, 1971a). No effect was seen, although high concentration of the anesthetic yielded a small but statistically insignificant decrease in the rate of transport (Fink and Kennedy, 1971b; Kennedy and Fink, 1971; Kennedy *et al.*, 1971). To extend their experiments to higher pressures of halothane, *in vitro* studies were conducted (Kennedy and Fink, 1971; Kennedy *et al.*, 1971). Tritiated leucine was introduced into the calamus scriptorius area of rabbits, producing a wave of radioactive protein which traveled through the vagus nerve. Sections of nerve were dissected out and maintained on nutrient solution in an atmosphere of O_2, CO_2, and varying levels of halothane. Fast transport was not affected at halothane levels up to 4%. Higher levels of halothane progressively slowed transport, with an eventual block of movement at 10.4%. The effect was reversible at levels up to 7.8% but was not reversible at 10.4%. Since in the rabbit an anesthetic dose of halothane is about 1%, and a lethal dose of halothane lies at or below 3.2%, the authors conclude that physiological levels of halothane have no effect upon fast axoplasmic transport.

The effect of halothane upon the structures of microtubules was also examined. At 7.8% halothane, when transport was slowed to about 40% of control values, the vagus nerve showed normal microtubules. Even nerves in which transport was blocked by treatment with 10.4% halothane showed normal microtubules in many axons. Hinkley and Green (1971) have also examined the effect of halothane upon the number of microtubules in the rabbit vagus nerve. These workers report that 3 and 10 mM levels of halothane (about 8 and 26 atm%, respectively) increase the density of microtubules. Halothane at these concentrations effectively blocks propagation of action potentials. Hinkley and Green conclude that microtubules are not closely related to propagation of action potentials and that the effects of halothane upon microtubules may be secondary to another activity of the anesthetic. It seems that there is little evidence to support the suggestion that the direct action of general anesthetics is upon microtubules.

b. Other General Anesthetics. Some scattered observations have been made concerning the effects of other anesthetic agents. Ochs *et al.* (1962) studied the effect of pentobarbital upon transport. The anesthetic was injected into the ventral horn of cats in a sample of phosphate-^{32}P which served to label the slow flow. The pentobarbital had little or no effect.

Kerkut *et al.* (1967) have also examined the action of pentobarbital, using an *in vitro* preparation from the snail. They find that treatment with pentobarbital for a short time (3 minutes) can delay the rapid appearance of radioactive glutamate in a perfusate of the nerve endings. Glutamate is believed to be a neurotransmitter in this system. It is not clear that the primary effect of the anesthetic is upon transport, however. It seems quite possible that pentobarbital inhibits propagation of the action potentials required to elicit release of glutamate. A more direct measurement of the transport process is required.

The effect of pentobarbital can also be assessed using animals which have been anesthetized with this agent. In our laboratory data have been gathered on cats in which the sensory fibers of the sciatic nerve were labeled by injecting L-leucine-^{3}H into the dorsal root ganglia (Anderson *et al.*, 1970; Anderson and McClure, unpublished data). Of the animals considered in this regard, about ten were inadvertently given either abnormally high doses of anesthetic or were maintained in surgical anesthesia longer than the usual period of 1 to 2 hours. All the animals so treated exhibited very poor transport. In all cases, rates of transport were less (averaging about 250 mm/day; controls were 400 mm/day) and the amount of material transported was reduced. The levels of anesthetic varied from animal to animal. In no case, however, was a lethal dose given. All the animals were well recovered from the anesthetic when the necessary nerves were harvested. Although these data by no means represent a carefully controlled study, they suggest that deep but nonfatal levels of some general anesthetics can affect transport.

Considering all these data, it is likely that normal surgical anesthesia has little or no effect upon transport. High doses, not necessarily lethal, may cause small decreases in both the amount of material transported and in the rate of transport. Lethal doses clearly depress both these parameters, but not necessarily in a direct manner. It seems quite possible that high doses may alter many aspects of metabolism, resulting in a secondary effect upon the transport system.

2. *Local Anesthetics*

Evidence has been produced which suggests that local anesthetics, such as lidocaine, can affect both the structure of microtubules and the rate of axoplasmic flow. Fink *et al.* (1971) have studied the effect of lidocaine upon transport of radioactive proteins through the rabbit vagus nerve using the *in vitro* technique already described in Section III,D,1,*a*. Lidocaine added to the culture medium at concentrations of 0.1 to 0.3% slowed transport in a reversible manner. Concentrations of 0.6% completely blocked transport, in a manner which was reversible for only short periods of time. Electron micrographs of nerves treated with 0.6% lidocaine showed no microtubules, in contrast to controls in which microtubules appeared normal. Kerkut *et al.* (1967) have reported an effect of lidocaine upon *in vitro* transport from the central nervous system of a snail through connecting nerves to the attached muscles. In this preparation, radioactive glutamate placed in the compartment containing the central nervous system will appear in a perfusate of the muscle when the nerve is stimulated. Treatment of the connecting nerve with lidocaine (10^{-4} gm/ml) for 3 minutes at the beginning of the experiment delayed the appearance of radioactive material in the perfusate by about 30 minutes. Although these data have been interpreted to mean that lidocaine can block transport, the effect of the drug in this system is difficult to evaluate. Rather than interfering with transport itself, it is possible that lidocaine is interfering with propagation of action potentials which are necessary to release the transported material.

In contrast to these reported effects, several experimenters have found that local anesthetics were unable to affect transport. Topical applications of lidocaine (Karlsson and Sjöstrand, 1968; McClure *et al.*, unpublished data) and of Ophthaine (Hendrickson and Cowan, 1971) have been used by several groups in connection with the intraocular injections necessary to study transport through the optic nerve. None of these workers have reported any effect of the drugs. Similarly, injection of lidocaine into the eyes of rats did not depress transport of labeled protein through the optic pathway (Siegel and McClure, unpublished data).

Ochs has reported experiments dealing with the effect of procaine upon both slow and fast flow in cats. Studies concerning slow transport were carried out by injecting procaine and phosphate-^{32}P into the ventral horn of the cat. At later times the appearance of radioactive material in the nerve was assessed. Using doses of procaine which should have abolished electrical activity near the site of injection, no effect upon transport was seen. The effect of the drug upon fast flow was examined by initiating transport of a pulse of radioactively labeled protein in the cat sciatic nerve, after which a section of the nerve was incubated in nutrient medium containing 1% procaine. Again, no effect upon transport was observed (Ochs and Hollingsworth, 1971).

These results are difficult to interpret. The studies using intact animals may have failed to find an effect due either to improper placement of the anesthetic or to failure to achieve high enough concentrations of the drug. Although neither consideration appears likely, they cannot be experimentally refuted. Studies employing *in vitro* preparations, however, should overcome these objections. The *in vitro* data showing a block by lidocaine of transport through the rabbit vagus nerve stand in contrast to the lack of an effect of procaine upon transport through the cat sciatic nerve. The drugs used and the systems employed are, of course, different. Although the obvious differences in the experiment may be responsible for the conflicting results, this seems unlikely. It is possible that the heavily myelinated sciatic nerve is better protected from local anesthetics, even though these levels of either procaine or lidocaine would block the electrical activity of the nerve. More experimental work will be necessary to resolve this question. In view of the great medical utility of these agents, further study seems amply justified.

E. Miscellaneous Compounds

There exist a number of experiments in which the effects of miscellaneous drugs have been studied.

1. *Aluminum Ions*

Treatment of experimental animals with aluminum ions gives rise to an experimentally induced neuropathy in which tangles of fibrillar material appear in axons (Klatzo *et al.*, 1965; Terry and Peña, 1965; Wiśniewski *et al.*, 1965, 1966). If axoplasmic flow is dependent upon the morphological integrity of intra-axonal fibers, animals treated with Al^{III} should show deficiencies of transport. Although rats treated in an acute manner with simultaneous intraocular injections of Al^{III} and L-leucine-^{3}H failed to transport radioactively labeled proteins through the axon (Cahill, 1970) this effect has since been shown to be due to inhibition of the incorporation of radioactive leucine into protein (Tanouye and McClure, unpublished data). When appropriate corrections are made, no effect of acute treatment with Al^{III} can be seen. Nonetheless, studies with animals treated chronically with this ion should be carried out. Such studies are particularly relevant in view of the medical importance of diseases in which defects in fibrous structures are seen in axons. Examples of such diseases include Alzheimer's disease (Terry *et al.*, 1964), deficiency of vitamin E (Lampert *et al.*, 1964), the Guam parkinsonism dementia (Hirano *et al.*, 1968), and postencephalitic parkinsonism. Whereas the pathological filaments seen in aluminum-induced states are not identical to those seen in the reported natural neuropathies, the effect upon transport may be similar. If so, the aluminum-induced system may prove to be a valuable model for diseases which involve a deficiency in axoplasmic transport.

2. *Neuropathic Agents*

Several other compounds known as neuropathogens have been studied. Chronic administration of acrylamide causes a small diminution in slow axoplasmic flow through the sciatic nerve of the cat (Pleasure *et al.*, 1969). This agent has a very small effect upon fast axoplasmic flow through the optic pathway of acute rats (Cahill, 1970). Tri-*o*-cresyl phosphate, a known neuropathogen (Earl and Thompson, 1952; Bischoff, 1967), caused no decrease in slow transport when administered chronically in the cat (Pleasure *et al.*, 1969). Rats treated in an acute manner with this agent similarly showed no significant decrease of transport through the optic nerve (Cahill, 1970). Tri-*p*-cresyl phosphate is also without effect upon transport in the latter system. Further study of the acrylamide-induced neuropathy might prove rewarding.

Diisopropyl fluorophosphate (DFP) has been reported to cause paralysis in the legs of chickens (Austin and Davies, 1954). In studies designed to assess the effect of DFP on transport, James and Austin (1970) report the drug has effect neither upon slow nor upon fast transport through the motor fibers of the chicken sciatic nerve.

Alkyl metals, such as tetramethyllead, triethyltin, and dimethylmercury, are active neuropathic agents. In a single series of experiments using the largest usable doses (about 4 mg), Cahill and McClure (unpublished data) found no effect of tetramethyllead upon the transport through the rat optic nerves of protein labeled with L-leucine-^{3}H injected into the eye. It would be interesting to study animals which were chronically treated with these agents.

Tetrodotoxin prevents excitation of the axonal membrane by selectively interfering with the entry of sodium ions (Narahashi *et al.*, 1964; Nakamura *et al.*, 1965). Ochs and Hollingsworth (1971) have used an *in vitro* assay employing the sensory fibers of the cat sciatic nerve to examine the effect of tetrodotoxin upon fast axoplasmic flow. At concentrations (10^{-2} mg/ml) which prevented the propagation of action potentials, transport was not affected. These data support further the conclusion that transport is not closely associated with conduction of action potentials.

γ-Aminobutyric acid has been injected into the ventral horn of cats simultaneously with phosphate-^{32}P. No effect of the drug was seen upon the subsequent slow transport of radioactive material through the sciatic nerve (Ochs *et al.*, 1962).

IV. Conclusions

Axoplasmic transport is a neural activity of ever-increasing interest to the biochemist and physiologist. Several rates of flow are seen, apparently, in every nerve; at each rate different molecules are carried, with different functions. To understand the functions of the transported molecules and the manner in which they interact with the axon and synapse, we shall probably have to employ agents that disrupt transport. Several classes of such drugs are now available: inhibitors of karyokinesis, such as colchicine; antimetabolites, such as dinitrophenol; and important but poorly studied compounds, such as the neuropathogens. New types of compounds, such as the methoxylated phenalkylamines, are becoming available. Agents about which much is now known suggest that transported proteins are synthesized upon ribosomes using messenger RNA which is, in turn, coded from DNA. Transport requires the use of metabolic energy, probably derived from carbohydrates through respiration. The act of transport probably involves intra-axonal filamentous structures, of which the microtubules and microfilaments are most strongly implicated. These data provide a promising beginning. As we expand our studies to include the many new compounds which can affect transport, a great deal of further insight into this complex and important subcellular transport system should be gained. If we examine not only the transport systems, but also the molecules being transported, we should be able to add substantially to our knowledge of intra- and intercellular communication.

References

Allen, R. D., and Kamiya, N., eds. (1964). "Primitive Motile Systems in Cell Biology." Academic Press, New York.

Allison, A. C., and Nunn, J. F. (1968). *Lancet* **ii,** 1326.

Anderson, L. E., Schlichter, D. J., and McClure, W. O. (1970). *Amer. Chem. Soc., 160th Meet., Chicago, Ill.* Abstr. No. 190.

Austin, L., and Davies, D. R. (1954). *Brit. J. Pharmacol. Chemother.* **9,** 145.

Barondes, S. H. (1967). *Neurosci. Res. Program, Bull.* **5,** 307.

Barondes, S. H. (1968). *J. Neurochem.* **15,** 343.

Barondes, S. H. (1969). *In* "Handbook of Neurochemistry" (A. Lajtha, ed.), Vol. II, pp. 435–446. Plenum, New York.

Behnke, O., and Forer, A. (1967). *J. Cell Sci.* **2,** 169.

Bensch, K. G., and Malawista, S. E. (1968). *Nature* (*London*) **218,** 1176.

Bensch, K. G., and Malawista, S. E. (1969). *J. Cell Biol.* **40,** 95.

Bensch, K. G., Marantz, R., Wiśniewski, H., and Shelanski, M. (1969). *Science* **165,** 495.

Bischoff, A. (1967). *Acta Neuropathol.* **9,** 158.
Borisy, G., and Taylor, E. W. (1967). *J. Cell Biol.* **34,** 525.
Bray, J. J., and Austin, L. (1969). *Brain Res.* **12,** 230.
Bray, J. J., Kon, C. M., and Breckenridge, B. McL. (1971). *Brain Res.* **26,** 385.
Bryan, J., and Wilson, L. (1971). *Proc. Nat. Acad. Sci. U.S.* **68,** 1762.
Burdwood, W. O. (1965). *J. Cell Biol.* **27,** 115A.
Cahill, A. L. (1970). Thesis, Univ. of Illinois, Urbana, Illinois.
Cahill, A. L., Paulson, J. C., and McClure, W. O. (1971). *Soc. Neurosci., 1st Annu. Meet., Washington, D.C.* Abstr. p. 144.
Dahlström, A. (1967a). *Acta Physiol. Scand.* **69,** 158.
Dahlström, A. (1967b). *Acta Physiol. Scand.* **69,** 167.
Dahlström, A. (1969). *Acta Physiol. Scand.* **76,** 33A.
Dahlström, A. (1970). *In* "Bayer Symposium II" (H.-J., Schümann, and G. Kroneberg, eds.), pp. 20–36. Springer-Verlag, Berlin and New York.
Dahlström, A., and Häggendal, J. (1966). *Acta Physiol. Scand.* **67,** 278.
Dahlström, A., and Häggendal, J. (1967). *Acta Physiol. Scand.* **69,** 153.
Dahlström, A., and Häggendal, J. (1970). *Advan. Biochem. Psychopharmacol.* **2,** 65.
Dahlström, A., and Jonason, J. (1968). *Eur. J. Pharmacol.* **4,** 377.
Dahlström, A., and Waldeck, B. (1968). *J. Pharm. Pharmacol.* **20,** 673.
Dahlström, A., Jonason, J., and Norberg, K.-A. (1969). *Eur. J. Pharmacol.* **6,** 248.
Davison, P. F. (1970). *Advan. Biochem. Psychopharmacol.* **2,** 289.
Droz, B. (1967). *J. Microsc.* (*Paris*) **6,** 201.
Droz, B., and Leblond, C. P. (1963). *J. Comp. Neurol.* **121,** 335.
Earl, C. J., and Thompson, R. H. S. (1952). *Brit. J. Pharmacol. Chemother.* **7,** 685.
Emmelin, N., Nordenfelt, I., and Perec, C. (1966). *Experientia* **22,** 725.
Fernandez, H. L., and Davison, P. F. (1969). *Proc. Nat. Acad. Sci. U.S.* **64,** 512.
Fernandez, H. L., and Samson, F. E., Jr. (1970). *Trans. Amer. Soc. Neurochem.* **1,** 44.
Fernandez, H. L., Hunneus, F. C., and Davison, P. F. (1970). *J. Neurobiol.* **1,** 395.
Fink, B. R., and Kennedy, R. D. (1971a). *Fed. Proc. Fed. Amer. Soc. Exp. Biol.* **30,** 215.
Fink, B. R., and Kennedy, R. D. (1971b). *Anesthesiology* **36,** 13.
Fink, B. R., Kennedy, R. D., and Hendrickson, A. E. (1971). *Annu. Meet., Amer. Soc. Anesthesiol., Atlanta, Ga.* Abstr. p. 91.
Frei, E., III, Whang, J., Scoggins, R. B., vanScott, E. J., Rall, D. P., and Ben, M. (1964). *Cancer Res.* **24,** 1918.
Frizell, M., Hasselgren, P. O., and Sjöstrand, J. (1970). *Exp. Brain Res.* **10,** 526.
Geffen, L. B., and Rush, R. A. (1968). *J. Neurochem.* **15,** 925.
Geffen, L. B., Livett, B. G., and Rush, R. A. (1969). *J. Physiol.* (*London*) **204,** 593.
Geffen, L. B., Livett, B. G., and Rush, R. A. (1970). *Circ. Res.* **26/27,** *Suppl.* **II,** 11.
Gerard, R. W. (1932). *Physiol. Rev.* **12,** 469.
Grafstein, B. (1969). *Advan. Biochem. Psychopharmacol.* **1,** 11.
Grafstein, B., and Murray, M. (1969). *Exp. Neurol.* **25,** 494.
Gutmann, E., Vodicka, E., and Zelená, J. (1955). *Chekh. Fiziol.* **4,** 200.
Held, I., and Young, I. J. (1969). *Exp. Brain Res.* **8,** 150.
Hendrickson, A. (1969). *Science* **165,** 194.
Hendrickson, A. E., and Cowan, W. M. (1971). *Exp. Neurol.* **30,** 403.
Hillarp, N.-Å., Fuxe, K., and Dahlström, A. (1966). *In* "Mechanism of Release of Biogenic Amines" (U. S. von Euler, S. Rosell, and B. Unnës, eds.), pp. 31–56. Pergamon, Oxford.
Hinkley, R. E., and Green, L. S. (1971). *J. Neurobiol.* **2,** 97.

Hirano, A., Dembitzer, H. M., and Kuland, L. T. (1968). *J. Neuropathol. Exp. Neurol.* **27,** 167.
Hoy, R. R., Bittner, G. D., and Kennedy, D. (1967). *Science* **156,** 251.
James, K. A. C., and Austin, L. (1970). *Brain Res.* **18,** 192.
James, K. A. C., Bray, J. J., Morgan, I. G., and Austin, L. (1970). *Biochem. J.* **117,** 766.
Johnson, J. L. (1970). *Brain Res.* **18,** 427.
Kapeller, K., and Mayor, D. (1967). *Proc. Roy. Soc., Ser. B* **167,** 282.
Karlsson, J.-O., and Sjöstrand, J. (1968). *Brain Res.* **11,** 431.
Karlsson, J.-O., and Sjöstrand, J. (1969). *Brain Res.* **13,** 617.
Karlsson, J.-O., and Sjöstrand, J. (1971a). *J. Neurobiol.* **2,** 135.
Karlsson, J.-O., and Sjöstrand, J. (1971b). *J. Neurochem.* **18,** 749.
Kennedy, R. D., and Fink, B. R. (1971). *Fed. Proc. Fed. Amer. Soc. Exp. Biol.* **30,** 441.
Kennedy, R. D., Myers, M. R., and Fink, B. R. (1971). *Annu. Meet., Amer. Soc. Anesthesiol., Atlanta, Ga.* Abstr. p. 129.
Kerkut, G. A., Shapiro, A., and Walker, R. J. (1967). *Comp. Biochem. Physiol.* **23,** 729.
Kidwai, A. M., and Ochs, S. (1969). *J. Neurochem.* **16,** 1105.
Kingsbury, E. W., and Voelz, H. (1969). *Science* **166,** 768.
Klatzo, I., Wiśniewski, H., and Streicher, E. (1965). *J. Neuropathol. Exp. Neurol.* **24,** 187.
Koenig, H. (1958). *Trans. Amer. Neurol. Ass.* **83,** 162.
Kreutzberg, G. W. (1969). *Proc. Nat. Acad. Sci. U.S.* **62,** 722.
Laduron, P. (1968). *Arch. Int. Pharmacodyn. Ther.* **171,** 233.
Laduron, P., and Belpaire, F. (1968). *Life Sci.* **7,** 1.
Lampert, P., Blumberg, J. H., and Puntschew, A. (1964). *J. Neuropathol. Exp. Neurol.* **23,** 60.
Lasek, R. J. (1967). *Nature (London)* **216,** 1212.
Lasek, R. J. (1968a). *Exp. Neurol.* **21,** 41.
Lasek, R. J. (1968b). *Brain Res.* **7,** 360.
Lasek, R. J. (1968b). *Brain Res.* **7,** 360.
Lasek, R. J. (1970a). *Brain Res.* **20,** 121.
Lasek, R. J. (1970b). *Int. Rev. Neurobiol.* **13,** 289.
Levi-Montalcini, R., and Angeletti, P. U. (1968). *Physiol. Rev.* **48,** 534.
Livett, B. G., Geffen, L. B., and Austin, L. (1968a). *Nature (London)* **217,** 278.
Livett, B. G., Geffen, L. B., and Austin, L. (1968b). *J. Neurochem.* **15,** 931.
Livett, B. G., Geffen, L. B., and Rush, R. A. (1969). *Biochem. Pharmacol.* **18,** 923.
Lubińska, L. (1964). *Progr. Brain Res.* **13,** 1.
Lubińska, L., Niemierko, S., and Oberfeld, B. (1961). *Nature (London)* **189,** 122.
Luco, J. V., and Eyzaguirre, C. (1955). *J. Neurophysiol.* **18,** 65.
Lux, H. D., Schubert, P., Kreutzberg, G. W., and Globus, A. (1970). *Exp. Brain Res.* **10,** 197.
McEwen, B. S., and Grafstein, B. (1968). *J. Cell Biol.* **38,** 494.
Malawista, S. E., Sato, H., and Bensch, K. G. (1968). *Science* **160,** 770.
Marantz, R., Ventilla, M., and Shelanski, M. (1969). *Science* **165,** 498.
Mayor, D., and Kapeller, K. (1967). *J. Roy. Microsc. Soc.* **87,** 277.
Miani, N. (1962). *Nature (London)* **193,** 887.
Miani, N. (1963). *J. Neurochem.* **10,** 859.
Miani, N. (1964). *Progr. Brain Res.* **13,** 115.
Nakamura, Y., Nakajima, S., and Grundfest, H. (1965). *J. Gen. Physiol.* **48,** 985.
Narahashi, T., Moore, J. W., and Scott, W. R. (1964). *J. Gen. Physiol.* **47,** 965.

Newcomb, E. H. (1969). *Annu. Rev. Plant Physiol.* **20**, 53.
Norström, A., and Sjöstrand, J. (1971). *J. Neurochem.* **18**, 29.
Ochs, S. (1966). *In* "Macromolecules and Behavior" (J. Gaito, ed.), pp. 20–39. Appleton, New York.
Ochs, S. (1971). *Proc. Nat. Acad. Sci. U.S.* **68**, 1279.
Ochs, S. and Burger, E. (1958). *Amer. J. Physiol.* **194**, 499.
Ochs, S., and Hollingsworth, D. (1971). *J. Neurochem.* **18**, 107.
Ochs, S., and Johnson, J. (1969). *J. Neurochem.* **16**, 845.
Ochs, S., and Ranish, N. (1969). *J. Neurobiol.* **1**, 247.
Ochs, S., and Ranish, N. (1970). *Science* **167**, 878.
Ochs, S., and Smith, C. B. (1971a). *Fed. Proc. Fed. Amer. Soc. Exp. Biol.* **30**, 665.
Ochs, S., and Smith, C. B. (1971b). *J. Neurochem.* **18**, 833.
Ochs, S., Dalyrymple, D., and Richards, G. (1962). *Exp. Neurol.* **5**, 349.
Ochs, S., Johnson, J., and Ng, M.-H. (1967). *J. Neurochem.* **14**, 317.
Ochs, S., Sabri, M. I., and Johnson, J. (1969). *Science* **163**, 686.
Olmsted, J. B., Witman, G. B., Carlson, K., and Rosenbaum, J. L. (1971). *Proc. Nat. Acad. Sci. U.S.* **68**, 2273.
Paget, G. E., and Walpole, A. L. (1958). *Nature* (*London*) **182**, 1320.
Paget, G. E., and Walpole, A. L. (1960). *AMA Arch. Dermatol.* **81**, 750.
Parker, G. H. (1932). *Amer. Natur.* **67**, 147.
Peters, A., and Vaughn, J. E. (1967). *J. Cell Biol.* **32**, 113.
Peters, A., Palay, S. L., and Webster, H. deF. (1970). "The Fine Structure of the Nervous System." Harper, New York.
Pleasure, D. E., Mishler, K. C., and Engel, W. K. (1969). *Science* **166**, 524.
Pletscher, A., Brossi, A., and Gey, K. F. (1962). *Int. Rev. Neurobiol.* **4**, 275.
Porter, K. R. (1966). *Principles Biomol. Organ., Ciba Found. Symp.*, **1965** pp. 308–356
Porter, K. R. (1968). *In* "Neuronal Fibrous Proteins" (F. O. Schmitt and F. E. Samson Jr., eds.), p. 154. MIT Press, Boston, Massachusetts.
Renaud, F. L., Rowe, A. J., and Gibbons, I. R. (1968). *J. Cell Biol.* **36**, 79.
Routtenberg, A., Sladek, J., and Bondareff, W. (1968). *Science* **161**, 222.
Samuels, A. J., Boyorsky, L. L., Gerard, R. W., Liber, B., and Brust, B. (1951). *Amer. J. Physiol.* **164**, 1.
Schmitt, F. O. (1968). *Proc. Nat. Acad. Sci. U.S.* **60**, 1092.
Schmitt, F. O., and Samson, F. E., Jr. (1968). *Neurosci. Res. Program, Bull.* **5**, **117**.
Schochet, S. S., Jr., Lampert, P. W., and Earle, K. M. (1968). *J. Neuropathol. Exp. Neurol.* **27**, 645.
Shelanski, M. L., and Taylor, E. W. (1967). *J. Cell Biol.* **34**, 549.
Shelanski, M. L., and Taylor, E. W. (1968). *J. Cell Biol.* **38**, 304.
Shelanski, M. L., and Wiśniewski, H. (1969). *Arch. Neurol.* (*Chicago*) **20**, 199.
Sjöstrand, J. (1969). *Exp. Brain Res.* **8**, 105.
Sjöstrand, J., and Karlsson, J.-O. (1969). *J. Neurochem.* **16**, 833.
Sjöstrand, J., Frizell, M., and Hasselgren, P.-O. (1970). *J. Neurochem.* **17**, 1563.
Slater, C. R. (1966). *Nature* (*London*) **209**, 305.
Stephens, R. E. (1968). *J. Mol. Biol.* **32**, 277.
Stephens, R. E. (1970). *Science* **168**, 845.
Tannock, I. F. (1965). *Exp. Cell Res.* **47**, 345.
Taylor, A. C., and Weiss, P. (1965). *Proc. Nat. Acad. Sci. U.S.* **54**, 1521.
Taylor, E. W. (1965). *J. Cell Biol.* **25**, 145.
Terry, R. D., and Peña, C. (1965). *J. Neuropathol. Exp. Neurol.* **24**, 200.

Terry, R. D., Gonatas, N. K., and Weiss, M. (1964). *Amer. J. Pathol.* **44,** 269.
Tilney, L. G., and Gibbons, J. R. (1968). *Protoplasma* **65,** 165.
Weisenberg, R. C., Borisy, G. C., and Taylor, E. W. (1968). *Biochemistry* **7,** 4466.
Weiss, P. (1961). *In* "Regional Neurochemistry" (S. S. Kety and J. Elkes, eds.), pp. 220–242. Pergamon, Oxford.
Weiss, P. (1969). *In* "Cellular Dynamics of the Neuron" (S. H. Barondes, ed.), Symp. Int. Soc. Cell Biol., Vol. 8, pp. 3–34. Academic Press, New York.
Weiss, P., and Hiscoe, H. (1948). *J. Exp. Zool.* **107,** 315.
Weiss, P., and Holland, Y. (1967). *Proc. Nat. Acad. Sci. U.S.* **57,** 258.
Weiss, P., Wang, H., Taylor, A. C., and Edds, M. V. (1945). *Amer. J. Physiol.* **143,** 521.
Wessels, N. K., Spooner, B. S., Ash, J. F., Bradley, M. O., Luduena, M. A., Taylor, E. L., Wrenn, J. T., and Yamada, K. M. (1971). *Science* **171,** 135.
Wiśniewski, H., and Terry, R. D. (1967). *Lab. Invest.* **17,** 577.
Wiśniewski, H., Terry, R. D., Peña, C., Streicher, E., and Klatzo, I. (1965). *J. Neuropathol. Exp. Neurol.* **24,** 139.
Wiśniewski, H., Karczewski, W., and Wiśniewska, K. (1966). *Acta Neuropathol.* **6,** 211.
Wiśniewski, H., Shelanski, M. L., and Terry, R. D. (1968). *J. Cell Biol.* **38,** 224.
Yamada, K. M., Spooner, B. S., and Wessels, N. K. (1970). *Proc. Nat. Acad. Sci. U.S.* **66,** 1206.

The Metabolism of the Tetrahydrocannabinols

LOUIS LEMBERGER

Lilly Laboratory for Clinical Research
Marion County General Hospital, and
Departments of Pharmacology and Medicine
Indiana University School of Medicine
Indianapolis, Indiana

I. Introduction

Cannabis sativa, the hemp plant from which marihuana and hashish are derived, is one of the most widely used source of drugs known to man. The use of this plant for medicinal purposes was first described in 2737 B.C. by the Chinese Emperor Shen Nung, and extracts of *Cannabis* were recognized in the *United States Pharmacopoeia* until as late as 1937. Its nonmedical use is well known. With the recognition of the increasingly widespread use of *Cannabis* preparations, much controversial debate has been generated in political and social circles. Possible harmful effects of the drug and the

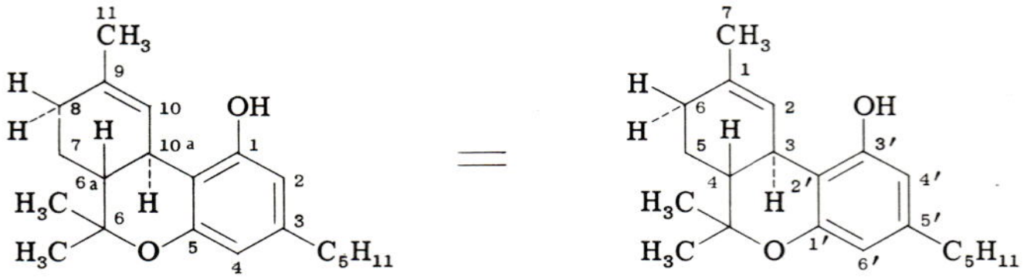

Δ^9-THC Benzopyran or formal numbering system = Δ^1-THC Monoterpenoid numbering system

FIG. 1. Nomenclature for tetrahydrocannabinol.

possibility of its legalization and acceptance as a recreational substance, such as alcohol, coffee, tea, and cigarettes, are both being discussed. *Cannabis sativa* is most widely used in the United States in the form of either marihuana, the dried flowering tops of plants, or hashish, a resin derived from the flowering tops of the Cannabis plant.

Cannabis sativa exists in various forms (Doorenbos *et al.*, 1971). The plant is usually diecious, i.e., male and female plants grow separately with both plants producing flowers. In the past, it was thought that only the female plant produced pharmacologically active constituents and, therefore, only the female plant was officially recognized as a source of *Cannabis* preparations for medicinal purposes. Recent studies have demonstrated that the flowering tops of both male and female plants contain approximately similar quantities of tetrahydrocannabinols (THCs) (Ohlsson *et al.*, 1971; Fetterman *et al.*, 1971) and that extracts from both sexes are pharmacologically equipotent (Valle *et al.*, 1968). The plant, an annual, is capable of attaining heights in excess of 15 ft and can grow under the most adverse conditions. The characteristic leaf is palmately compound and contains an odd number (usually five or seven) of coarsely serrated leaflets. *Cannabis* contains a multitude of chemical constituents, with the cannabinoids* receiving the most attention. More than twenty cannabinoids have been isolated and their chemical structures elucidated (Shani and Mechoulam, 1970; Mechoulam, 1970). Some confusion exists as to the chemical nomenclature of the tetrahydrocannabinols, since two numbering systems have been extensively used by various workers (Fig. 1). The formal or dibenzopyran numbering system treats the cannabinoids as substituted dibenzopyrans, whereas the monoterpenoid numbering system considers them as substituted terpenes. Consequently, one of the THCs can be

* Mechoulam (1970) uses the term cannabinoids to include the C_{21} compounds typical of and present in *Cannabis sativa,* their carboxylic acids, analogs, and transformation products.

referred to as either Δ^9-THC or Δ^1-THC, both describing the identical chemical structure. The former numbering system will be used throughout this review.

The classic work of Adams *et al.* (1940; Adams, 1942) and Todd (1942) speculated that the active constituents of marihuana were a mixture of isomers of THCs. However, it was not until 1964 that Mechoulam and co-workers synthesized and characterized Δ^9-THC and subsequently demonstrated that it was the major pharmacologically active constituent of marihuana and hashish (Gaoni and Mechoulam, 1964; Mechoulam and Gaoni, 1967a,b; Edery *et al.*, 1970). Additional pharmacological studies in animals (Grunfeld and Edery, 1969) and man (Isbel *et al.*, 1967; Hollister *et al.*, 1968; Waskow *et al.*, 1970) have substantiated this finding. Δ^8-Tetrahydrocannabinol, an isomer of Δ^9-THC, is also biologically active; however, this compound represents only a small portion (1–10%) of the total THC content of marihuana (Hively *et al.*, 1966). The variation of THC content in plants depends primarily on genetic factors, although environmental factors, such as climate, light, and soil, also play an important role. There are two genotypes of *Cannabis sativa:* one which is low in THC and high in cannabidiol and the other, conversely, which is low in cannabidiol and high in THC. The former is used for fiber production whereas the latter, with a high THC content, is used for its euphoriant effects (Ohlsson *et al.*, 1971; Fetterman *et al.*, 1971). Within a specific genotype, there is considerable variation in the THC content of different portions of the plant. The greatest percentage of THC is present in the flowers and floral bracts (i.e., the floral part closest to the leaf) with the lowest concentration in the seeds and roots (Fetterman *et al.*, 1970).

Cannabinolic acids (Fig. 2) are the major cannabinoids in nature and can be slowly converted to the decarboxylated compounds upon storage. For example, in fresh samples of *Cannabis*, 95% of the THC present is in the form of its acid (an inactive compound); however, with aging this material forms the active Δ^9-THC (Waller, 1971).

The chemistry of the cannabinoids has been extensively reviewed by Mechoulam (1970). Investigations of the structure–activity relationship of the cannabinoids revealed the following: (*1*) the pyran ring is an essential requirement for psychotomimetic activity, e.g., cannabidiol is inactive (Adams *et al.*, 1940; Edery *et al.*, (1971); (*2*) the presence of a carboxyl group in position 4 or 6 renders the compound inactive (Mechoulam, 1970); (*3*) (+) Δ^9-THC (dextrorotatory) is inactive, whereas its optical isomer, (−)Δ^9-THC (levorotatory), is active (Mechoulam and Gaoni, 1967a); (*4*) maximal activity is seen if the double bond is in the Δ^9 or the Δ^8 position, $\Delta^{6a,10a}$-THC being relatively inactive (Edery *et al.*, 1971); (*5*) the activity

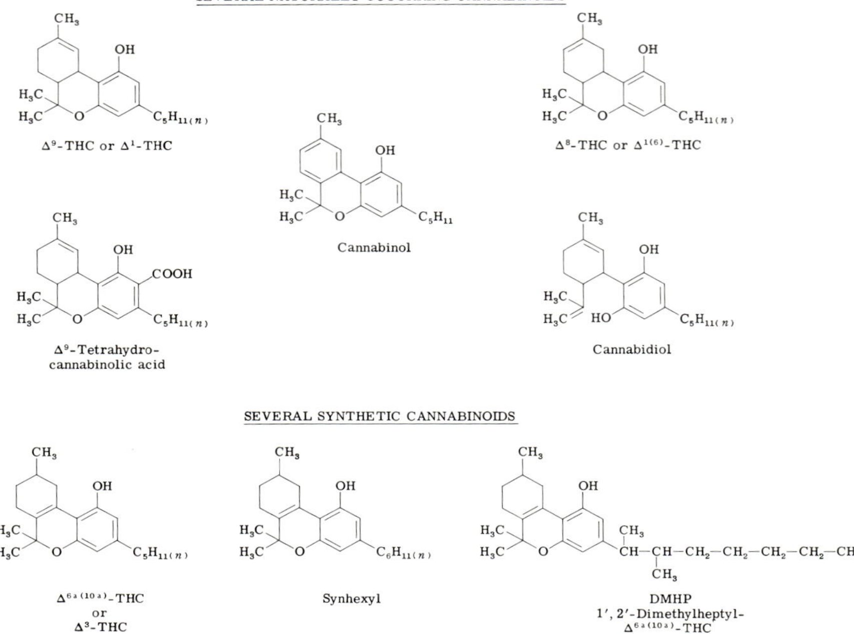

FIG. 2. Structures of some naturally occurring and synthetic cannabinoids.

of $\Delta^{6a,10a}$ compound can be increased, however, by the replacement of the pentyl side chain with a hexyl side chain to form synhexyl (Fig. 2) which is an active compound; (*6*) the substitution of a dimethylheptyl side chain for the pentyl side chain in the $\Delta^{6a,10a}$ analog of THC results in a marked increase in pharmacological activity. The resulting compound $\Delta^{6a,10a}$-dimethylheptyl THC (DMHP or EA1476) was shown to be a potent hypothermic and hypotensive agent in dogs (Boyd and Meritt, 1965; Hardman *et al.*, 1971).

In addition to those naturally occurring cannabinols containing a pentyl side chain, other cannabinol homologs have recently been identified. These include Δ^9-tetrahydrocannabivarin (the propyl side-chain homolog of Δ^9-THC) (Merkus, 1971) and Δ^9-tetrahydrocannabiorcol (the methyl homolog of Δ^9-THC) (Vree *et al.*, 1971a,b) which have been isolated from Nepalese hashish and Brazilian marihuana, respectively. Although these compounds are present in extremely small quantities, it remains to be determined whether they are biologically active.

The total synthesis of Δ^9-THC was first reported by Gaoni and Mechoulam (1964). However, this method required considerable use of column chromatography for purification and was tedious. Several years later, Fahrenholtz *et al.* (1967) synthesized Δ^9-THC by the condensation of olivetol and diethyl α-acetoglutarate; but this method was also tedious and required many inter- and intramolecular condensations before synthesis of Δ^9-THC was finally achieved. Simultaneously, however, Petrzilka and Sikemeier (1967a) described what is now the classic synthesis for Δ^9-THC. These authors demonstrated that, under acidic conditions, they could synthesize optically active Δ^8-THC by the direct condensation of (+)*cis*- or (+)*trans*-*p*-menthadiene-(2, 8)-ol-(1) and olivetol. They were then able to shift quantitatively the double bond from the Δ^8 to the Δ^9 position resulting in a simplified synthesis for Δ^9-THC (Petrzilka and Sikemeier, 1967b).

Biomedical research has been severely hampered by the lack of standardization of marihuana and by the marked variation in potency of the preparations studied. This was largely the result of the poor state of our knowledge of the chemistry of the cannabinoids and the lack of reference standards with which to measure the THC content of preparations. Prior to the recent use of synthetic Δ^9-THC and the development of methodology for determining the THC content of *Cannabis* preparations, research was unfortunately not as sophisticated as we would have expected. Researchers resorted to using marihuana, the origin of which was not known, and in many cases clinical studies were carried out with "alleged" marihuana which had been confiscated by local law enforcement agencies. Thus, the results of many studies concerning the pharmacological effects of marihuana which appear in the literature through the late 1960s must be treated cautiously. The recognition by the National Institutes of Mental Health (NIMH) of the state of affairs up to this time has succeeded in beneficially affecting marihuana research. The NIMH developed a program for large-scale synthesis of Δ^9-THC and the cultivation of a standardized, chemically assayed *Cannabis sativa*. These materials were then made available to qualified, interested researchers.

Since no sensitive means of assaying the THC were available, it was impossible to do any meaningful studies concerning the absorption, distribution, and metabolism of these compounds in animals or humans. The need for radioactive Δ^9-THC was obvious, and Miras (1965) and co-workers were successful in isolating Δ^9-THC-^{14}C from *Cannabis* plants grown in an environment containing carbon dioxide-^{14}C. With the advent of the chemical synthesis of Δ^9-THC the radioactive material was soon produced. First ^{3}H-labeled Δ^9-THC was synthesized (Burstein and Mechoulam, 1968; Agurell *et al.*, 1969) and shortly thereafter, ^{14}C-radiolabeled Δ^9-THC (Timmons *et al.*, 1969; Nilsson *et al.*, 1969) became available for metabolic studies.

II. Nonenzymic Transformations of Cannabinoids

Since inhalation is the route of administration most widely used for marihuana, several laboratories have investigated the effect of combustion and smoking on the constituents of *Cannabis*. In some cases the results are equivocal since the techniques, temperatures of combustion, and other conditions varied among laboratories. These differences are, however, difficult to resolve since each group is critical of the conditions used by others stating that their study best simulates the smoking of marihuana by actual users. Von Claussen and Korte (1968) reported that during the smoking process, carboxylic acids of the cannabinoids are decarboxylated liberating the free cannabinols such as THC and cannabidiol.

Manno *et al.* (1970), using a smoking machine, analyzed the constituents of marihuana smoke and calculated the dosage of Δ^9-THC which should be delivered in a cigarette. They calculated that if a marihuana cigarette were smoked in 10 minutes and if each inhalation of smoke were retained in the alveoli and bronchial tree for 30 seconds, then about half of the original quantity of Δ^9-THC in the cigarette would be absorbed. They found less than 0.1% of cannabinoids in the butt or "roach," as it is called by experienced marihuana smokers; there was no evidence for isomerization of Δ^9-THC to Δ^8-THC.

Mikes and Waser (1971), using artificially smoked cigarettes impregnated with synthetic Δ^9-THC, also did not find any evidence for isomerization of Δ^9-THC nor for the formation of any new pyrolysis products. In their study, cigarette butts were found to contain about 22% of the originally added Δ^9-THC after completion of the smoking process. Interestingly, their data suggest that, with smoking, a small percentage of cannabidiol may be converted to Δ^9-THC by closure of the pyran ring. However, this observation has not been confirmed by other researchers in this field. Coutselinis and Miras (1970), using a similar experimental design, studied the effect of smoking on radiolabeled Δ^9-THC-^{14}C. They found that Δ^9-THC was more labile when it was the only cannabinoid present. When studied in the form of a resin or a mixture of cannabinols, less of the material was destroyed during the smoking process. This is of interest since Galanter and Wyatt (1971) noted that a cigarette of known THC content appeared to be more potent psychologically in man than a placebo cigarette containing the identical quantity of synthetic Δ^9-THC. Another possible explanation for the increased activity of crude marihuana when compared to synthetic Δ^9-THC is that some material acting as a synergistic agent is present in marihuana thereby potentiating THC. Recent evidence by Paton and Pertwee (1971) suggests that cannabidiol may play such a role. They found cannabidiol potentiated pentobarbital sleep time and showed that *in vitro* its effects were on the liver microsomal system. If cannabidiol should inhibit the metabolism of Δ^9-THC, then marihuana would have a "built-in" synergistic agent.

Truitt (1971) and co-workers have also concluded that about 50% of the total dose of THC is delivered to the smoker when the butt is completely consumed since they found that almost 21% of added Δ^9-THC remained in the butt after smoking.

Agurell and Leander (1971) recently reported that 14–29% of the cannabinoids added to cigarettes are transferred to the respiratory system. This transfer occurs with the mainstream smoke. However, this figure would be increased if the cigarettes were totally consumed, since the cannabinoids usually remaining in the butt would also be inhaled. They calculate that the experienced *Cannabis* smoker, using deep inhalations, absorbed in excess of 80% of the cannabinoids presented to the lungs in the mainstream smoke. The results of their studies demonstrated that, except for decarboxylation of the cannabinolic acids, the smoking process produced only negligible changes in the original cannabinoid fraction of marihuana presented to the smoker in the mainstream smoke.

III. *In Vitro* Metabolism of Tetrahydrocannabinols

Tetrahydrocannabinol, being a lipid, nonpolar compound, would be expected to be a substrate for the hepatic microsomal enzyme system. These enzymes are known to metabolize a variety of drugs (Axelrod, 1954a; Brodie *et al.*, 1958), steroids (Kuntzman *et al.*, 1964), and other naturally occurring compounds (Jepson *et al.*, 1962; Axelrod, 1963; Lemberger *et al.*, 1965). The hepatic microsomal enzyme system requires reduced nicotinamide adenine dinucleotide phosphate (NADPH) and molecular oxygen (Axelrod, 1954a; Brodie *et al.*, 1958). This system catalyzes a variety of reactions; many being oxidations, in which cytochrome P-450 serves as the terminal oxidase. Supporting evidence for a role of the liver in the metabolism of Δ^9-THC comes from the marked concentration of radioactivity in this organ after administration of radiolabeled Δ^9-THC to animals. These two pieces of information led to the investigation of the *in vitro* metabolism of the THCs.

As is usually the case in areas of great scientific interest, many laboratories in different parts of the world were examining the metabolic fate of the THCs in liver microsomal enzyme preparations. Within a short period of time, reports appeared in the literature describing the structural identification of one of the major *in vitro* metabolites of THC. Wall and co-workers (1970) in the United States and Nilsson *et al.* (1970) in Sweden incubated radiolabeled Δ^9-THC with the 10,000 *g* liver supernate (this fraction contains the microsomal enzymes) obtained from rats and rabbits, respectively, and isolated a polar metabolite of Δ^9-THC by solvent extraction and either thin-layer chromatography or column chromatography. Both groups identified and proved the structure of this metabolite as 11-OH-Δ^9-THC by mass spectrometry and nuclear magnetic resonance spectrometry. This metabolite represented approximately 40% of the substrate initially present. Simultaneously, Foltz *et al.* (1970) in the United States and Mechoulam, Burstein, and co-workers (Burstein *et al.*, 1970; Ben-Zvi *et al.*, 1970) in Israel and the United States described the 11-hydroxylation of Δ^8-THC and characterized its structure. All of these laboratories reported that in preliminary behavioral studies in mice or rats, the 11-OH-Δ^9-THC or its Δ^8 analog were as potent or more potent pharmacologically than the parent compounds Δ^9- or Δ^8-THC. Christensen *et al.* (1971) reported that 11-OH-Δ^9-THC had pharmacological activity approximately 2 to 15 times that of Δ^9-THC, depending upon its route of administration—the intracerebral route produced greater effects than the intravenous route.

In addition to the formation of 11-hydroxylated metabolites of Δ^9-THC, Wall *et al.* (1970); Wall (1971) isolated and identified 8,11-dihydroxy-Δ^9-THC as representing approximately 30% of the original Δ^9-THC and 8-β-hydroxy-Δ^9-THC, which was only a minor metabolite. The former is inactive (Christensen *et al.*, 1971), whereas the latter shows pharmacological activity (Wall *et al.*, 1970; Mechoulam *et al.*, 1971; Wall, 1971). Incubation of Δ^9-THC with human liver obtained at autopsy resulted in the formation of 11-hydroxy-Δ^9-THC and 8,11-dihydroxy-THC (Christensen *et al.*, 1971). By using Δ^8-THC as a substrate for the liver microsomal system, Wall (1971) confirmed the formation of 11-OH-Δ^8-THC as the major metabolite and, in addition, identified 7α,11-dihydroxy-Δ^8-THC and 7β,11-dihydroxy-Δ^8-THC as additional metabolites. In retrospect, the finding of the hydroxylation of the methyl groups (on C-11) and on C-8 of Δ^9-THC or C-7 of Δ^8-THC is not surprising since these positions are allylic to the double bond. A similar metabolic conversion is seen with the barbiturate, hexobarbital, the metabolism of which has been studied extensively with hepatic drug-metabolizing enzymes. Maynard *et al.* (1971) have recently reported the hydroxylation in the 1′ and 3′ positions of the side chain of Δ^8-THC using a dog liver 10,000 *g* supernate fraction fortified with the necessary cofactors. This, however, appears to be only a minor metabolite of Δ^8-THC, and no reports of side-chain oxidation of Δ^9-THC have as yet been published.

Recently, Nakazawa and Costa (1971), using microsomes prepared from rat lung, demonstrated that Δ^9-THC was metabolized. They suggested that the two products formed are unique to lung and are not found in liver homogenates. These compounds of which chemical structure has not yet been elucidated, appear to be more polar than Δ^9-THC but less polar than 11-OH-Δ^9-THC. The conversion of Δ^9-THC to its metabolites in lung tissue is enhanced by pretreatment of the rats with 3-methylcholanthrene (20 mg/kg for 4 days); surprisingly, these metabolites are not formed in hepatic tissue. Gilman and Conney (1963) showed that 3-methylcholanthrene could induce enzymes, localized in the microsomal fraction of lung tissue, which were capable of metabolizing drugs. However, the doses necessary for induction were approximately one-tenth as large as those used in the Δ^9-THC study. Nakazawa and Costa (1971) reported that pretreatment with 3-methylcholanthrene enhanced the behavioral effects of Δ^9-THC suggesting that these two new metabolites might be active compounds. The finding that lung tissue is capable of metabolizing Δ^9-THC is important since one of the major routes of marihuana administration in humans is by inhalation.

The metabolism of cannabinol, a pharmacologically inactive constituent of marihuana, has been studied by Widman *et al.* (1971) and Wall (1971) and co-workers. Cannabinol is hydroxylated in the C-11 (methyl group) of the aromatic ring similarly to Δ^8- and Δ^9-THC and the resultant 11-OH-cannabinol is its major metabolite. Two minor metabolites of cannabinol tentatively identified by Wall (1971) are the side-chain hydroxylated products of cannabinol and 11-OH-cannabinol, in which the hydroxyls are located on the 2′ position of the pentyl side chain.

Nilsson *et al.* (1971) studied the *in vitro* conversion of cannabidiol by a rat liver microsomal enzyme system and isolated three metabolites. These were identified as 11-hydroxycannabidiol (the major metabolite), a pentyl side-chain hydroxylated product of cannabidiol, and a cannabidiol has been tentatively identified in which the methyl group on C-6 is hydroxylated to form a primary alcohol. An alternative structure for this latter metabolite is cannabidiol with a hydroxyl group on C-8. It remains to be determined if the hydroxylated metabolites of cannabidiol are biologically active.

The *in vitro* hepatic metabolism of Δ^9-THC, Δ^8-THC, and cannabinol are summarized in Fig. 3. To date, *in vitro* metabolic studies have been carried out in livers obtained from rabbit, dog, mouse, rat, guinea pig, and human autopsy material, and all appear to make the hydroxylated compounds.

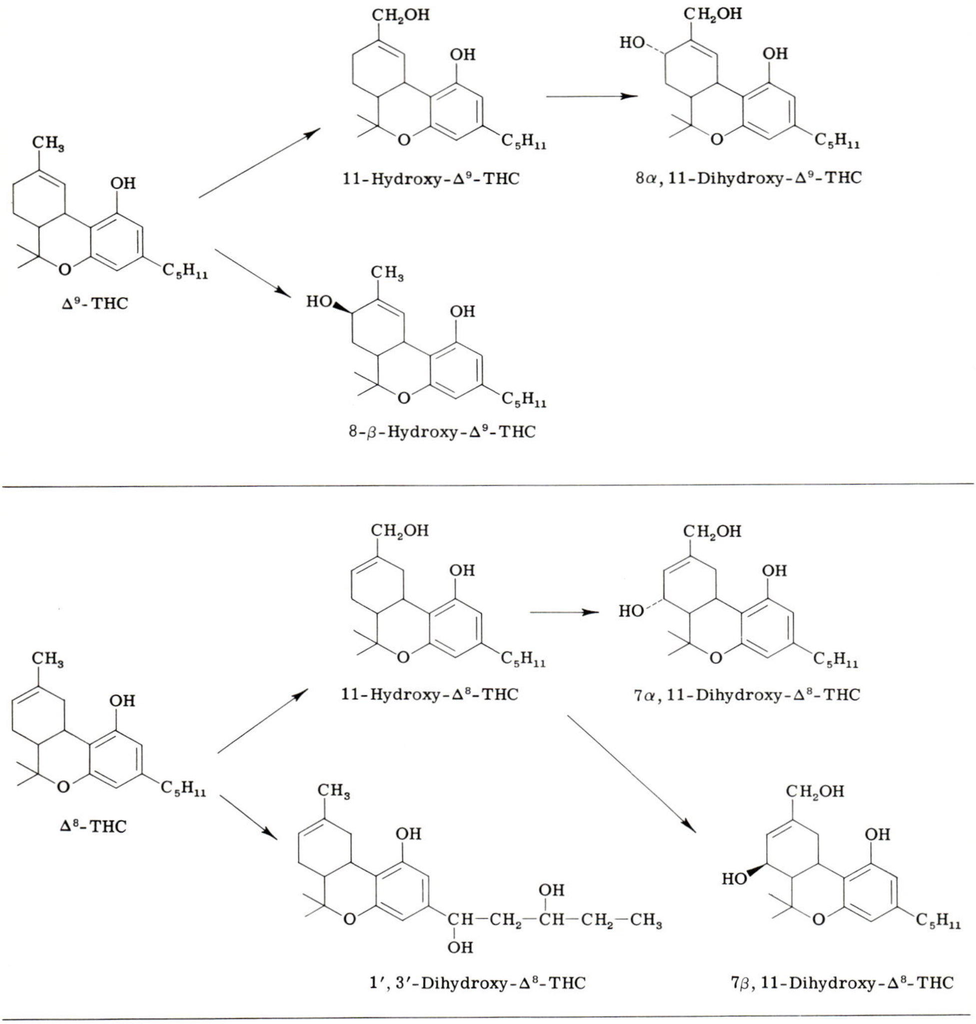

Δ^9-THC

11-Hydroxy-Δ^9-THC

8α, 11-Dihydroxy-Δ^9-THC

8-β-Hydroxy-Δ^9-THC

Δ^8-THC

11-Hydroxy-Δ^8-THC

7α, 11-Dihydroxy-Δ^8-THC

1′, 3′-Dihydroxy-Δ^8-THC

7β, 11-Dihydroxy-Δ^8-THC

FIG. 3. Metabolic pathways for Δ^9-tetrahydrocannabinol (Δ^9-THC), Δ^8-THC, and cannabinol after *in vitro* incubation with the hepatic microsomal enzyme system.

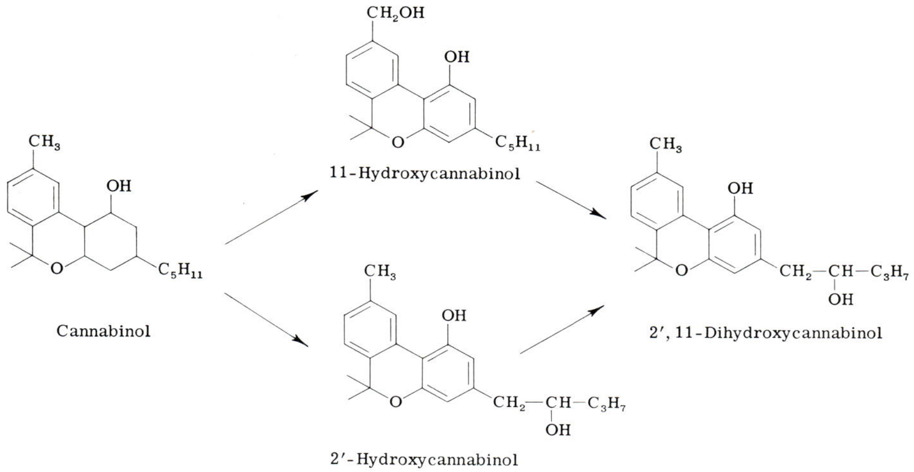

Cannabinol

11-Hydroxycannabinol

2′-Hydroxycannabinol

2′, 11-Dihydroxycannabinol

FIG. 3 (continued). See caption on facing page.

IV. *In Vivo* Studies with Δ⁹-Tetrahydrocannabinol

A. ABSORPTION

As stated earlier, the results of much of the research in the field of marihuana pharmacology must be interpreted cautiously due to a lack of pure, chemically defined materials. Furthermore, there are two considerations which are of importance regarding the present day *in vivo* research being conducted: (*1*) the vehicle in which the Δ^9-THC is prepared and (*2*) the route of administration. The vehicle problem is one which is inherent to Δ^9-THC since this is a lipophilic compound and is not soluble in any of the usual solvents used for *in vivo* studies (i.e., saline and water). Attempts have been made to synthesize soluble derivatives of Δ^9-THC (Howes, 1970), such as the ether or ester, as well as the alteration of several of the ring systems by the addition of nitrogen-containing heterocyclic rings (Pars and Razdan, 1971). Unfortunately, some of these compounds have been either inactive or have increased toxicity. Therefore, suitable solvents or additives must be used to solubilize Δ^9-THC or its analogs in aqueous solutions for oral or parenteral administration. Some of the techniques used include (*a*) first binding or suspending the Δ^9-THC in an albumin solution and diluting it with saline, (*b*) solubilizing the drug in a surfactant such as Tween 80 (polysorbate 80), Triton-X, or polyvinylpyrrolidone (PVP), and (*c*) simply dissolving the drug in a solvent such as polyethylene glycol, propylene glycol, sesame oil, dimethyl sulfoxide (DMSO), or ethanol and administering the solution directly. The last approach may affect the interpretation of pharmacological studies due to possible additive or synergistic effects of the Δ^9-THC and the vehicle used as well as variable rates of absorption.

The importance of the vehicle in which Δ^9-THC is administered has been extensively studied by Perez-Reyes *et al.* (1971). These investigators administered Δ^9-THC-^{3}H orally to human subjects. The drug was prepared in capsules containing Δ^9-THC-^{3}H (37 mg) dissolved in either sesame oil or ethanol or emulsified in 5.5% sodium glycocholate (a bile salt). Their subjects reported an intense and unpleasant psychological "high" when sodium glycocholate and sesame oil were used as the vehicles, whereas the high from Δ^9-THC dissolved in ethanol was described as moderate and very pleasant. The high reported after Δ^9-THC in sodium glycocholate had its onset 15–30 minutes after administration, whereas the onset of the high was reported to occur within 1 hour when sesame oil or ethanol was used as the vehicle. Plasma levels of total radioactivity were of considerably higher amplitude and longer duration after the sesame oil and sodium glycocholate vehicles than after the ethanol vehicle and appeared to parallel the psychologic high.

In addition to the variability and difficulty in comparing results between laboratories due to the choice of vehicle for Δ^9-THC, the choice of suitable route of administration has also been of great importance and added to some of the controversy. Most studies involving metabolism and disposition use small animals such as rats or mice and, for the sake of convenience, drugs are usually administered by the intraperitoneal or subcutaneous route. It is now clear from radioautographic studies (McIsaac *et al.*, 1971; Ho *et al.*, 1971; Kennedy and Waddell, 1971; Idänpään-Heikkilä *et al.*, 1971) that Δ^9-THC is not completely absorbed from the injection site after either intraperitoneal or subcutaneous injection. Thus it appears that for acute experiments in animals the intravenous route would give the most consistent results.

Isbell *et al.* (1967) compared the smoked route and orally administered Δ^9-THC in man. They estimated the potency of Δ^9-THC to be 2.6 to 3 times greater after smoking than after oral ingestion and suggested that more rapid absorption could be a possible explanation. Indeed, the initial plasma levels of radioactivity after Δ^9-THC-^{14}C administration are greater after smoking (Lemberger *et al.*, 1971c, 1972a).

B. Disposition

1. *Tissue Distribution*

Prior to the availability of radiolabeled Δ^9-THC, studies on the disposition of this drug in tissue and biological fluids were not feasible unless very large doses were administered since there existed no sensitive method for detecting Δ^9-THC in biological fluids after a pharmacological dose. After the oral administration of a large dose (100 mg/kg) of nonradiolabeled Δ^9-THC to rats, Forney and co-workers (King and Forney, 1967; Forney, and Kiplinger, 1971) were able to measure Δ^9-THC by gas–liquid chromatography in blood, brain, liver, lung, and spleen after 3 hours. The levels in these tissues declined after 12 hours. However, in the epididymal fat pads, Δ^9-THC became measurable at this time.

The first studies using radioactivity were those of Miras (1965) and co-workers (see Joachimoglu *et al.*, 1967). They obtained Δ^9-THC-^{14}C, of low specific activity (3.7 μCi/gm), from plants grown in an atmosphere of $^{14}CO_2$ after its isolation by chromatographic techniques. Because of the relatively low specific activity, sufficient sensitivity was not attained. Furthermore, there existed the possibility of impurities with chromatographic properties similar to Δ^9-THC. However, they were able to conclude that after 90 minutes less than 0.5% of an intraperitoneally administered dose was present in the brain and about 5% in the liver and that the rat excreted the radioactivity slowly over several days in the form of metabolites of Δ^9-THC, since no unchanged Δ^9-THC was present in the urine. Agurell *et al.* (1969, 1970) administered Δ^9-THC-^{3}H of high specific activity intravenously in the form of an emulsion to rats and rabbits. In the rat they noted that only 50% of the administered dose was eliminated during the first week and suggested that the remainder existed in the body bound to tissues. Subsequently, they studied the distribution of radioactivity in rabbits, 2 and 72 hours, after the intravenous injection of Δ^9-THC-^{3}H. At 2 hours, the highest concentration of the radioactivity was found in urine and bile, the major excretory routes. However, when tissues other than kidney were examined at 2 hours, the lung was found to contain the highest concentration of radioactivity, having about twice that of liver, the organ containing the next largest quantity. Radioactivity was also present in significant concentrations in adrenals, spleen, and ileum. In contrast, brain and spinal cord had the lowest concentration of radioactivity of any tissues examined. This is of particular interest since this drug exerts its effects predominantly on the central nervous system (CNS) and suggests that Δ^9-THC is extremely potent in its effect on neuronal tissue. At 72 hours, radioactivity present in adipose tissue had increased in concentration whereas all other tissues had considerably less radioactivity than at earlier times.

In a similar experiment in rats, Klausner and Dingell (1971) studied the tissue distribution of intravenously administered Δ^9-THC-^{14}C prepared in a solution of 30% propylene glycol and 70% rat serum. The rats were killed after 15 minutes and the diethyl ether-extractable radioactivity measured. (This procedure should extract all of the Δ^9-THC and part of the radioactivity present as metabolites.) Their findings confirmed the observations of Agurell *et al.* (1970) that lung contained the highest concentration of radioactivity and brain the least. In addition to determining total radioactivity, they measured the Δ^9-THC concentration in tissue at various times (15–120 minutes) by extraction into petroleum ether (which presumably measures only the parent drug). The highest concentration of unchanged Δ^9-THC was present in lung at 15 minutes (70.3 μg/gm), declining to less than 5% (3.3 μg/gm) of its earlier value by 2 hours. The Δ^9-THC concentration in fat at 15 minutes (2.3 μg/gm) more than doubled (5.4 μg/gm) by 2 hours. These results are consistent with the fact that Δ^9-THC is a very lipophilic compound and is redistributed from blood and other tissues into adipose tissue. It might be of some clinical relevance since in man this drug is taken repeatedly and may be deposited in fat with prolonged usage.

Ho *et al.* (1970) studied the distribution of Δ^9-THC-^{3}H in rats after its inhalation. The results obtained by this route of administration are similar to those after the intravenous route. These investigators found that radioactivity persisted in the brain for at least 7 days, presumably most of this was present in the form of metabolites, since after 1 day, only 30% was present as the unchanged Δ^9-THC.

In mice, Christensen *et al.* (1971) compared brain and liver levels of radioactivity and Δ^9-THC after the intravenous or intracerebral injection of Δ^9-THC-^{14}C and found that 10 minutes after an intravenous dose, about 1% of the radiolabel was present in the brain, of which about one-third was present in the form of THC metabolites. After intracerebral injection, the major portion of radioactivity was present as unchanged Δ^9-THC suggesting that brain tissue is unable to metabolize Δ^9-THC.

McIsaac *et al.* (1971) administered Δ^9-THC-^{3}H intravenously to squirrel monkeys and examined the regional distribution of radioactivity in the brain. The animals were sacrificed at various times and half of the brain examined for radioactivity using radioautographic techniques. The total radioactivity and unchanged Δ^9-THC were determined in the other hemisphere by solvent extraction and chromatography. In general, most of the radioactivity was localized in the gray matter, very little being in the white matter after 15 minutes. They estimated that about 80% of the radioactivity was present as unchanged Δ^9-THC at this time. Similar results were reported by Kennedy and Waddell (1971) in their radioautographic studies in the rat. In the monkeys, the radioactivity appeared to be uniformly distributed in all cortical regions, cerebellar cortex, caudate, pons, thalamus, hippocampus, and medulla, and there was considerably less radioactivity in the hypothalamus.

Layman and Milton (1971) performed similar studies in rats administering Δ^9-THC-^{3}H intraperitoneally. Brains were dissected into four major regions (cerebral cortex, hippocampus, cerebellum, and medulla and pons). They were unable to demonstrate any selective distribution in any area of the brain, all areas containing about equal concentrations of radioactivity. They found peak levels of radioactivity at 1 hour with low but measurable activity present even 1 month after the administration of the radioactive compound.

Considering the widespread usage of marihuana among young people and women of childbearing age, the importance for teratological studies as well as the distribution of Δ^9-THC in pregnant animals is obvious. Teratogenic effects appear to be associated with the injection of marihuana extracts (Persaud and Ellington, 1967, 1968; Gerber, 1969). However, no such effects were seen after relatively large doses of pure synthetic Δ^9-THC (Borgen and Davis, 1971; Pace *et al.*, 1971). Idänpään-Heikkilä *et al.* (1969) injected Δ^9-THC-^{3}H into pregnant hamsters either intraperitoneally or subcutaneously. They examined the placental and fetal tissues 15 or 30 minutes after injection and found that levels of placental radioactivity were 2–3 times that present in the fetus. In contrast, Pace *et al.* (1971), using the rat, reported that the maternal cotyledons of the placenta effectively prevented the passage of most radioactive Δ^9-THC into the fetus resulting in the accumulation of very low levels of radioactivity in the fetus. The difference in results may be explained by a species difference or by the difference in the route of administration.

2. *Plasma Levels*

The binding of Δ^9-THC-^{3}H to human plasma protein was extensively studied *in vitro* by Wahlqvist *et al.* (1970) using electrophoretic techniques. They demonstrated that 80–95% of Δ^9-THC was bound to the plasma proteins, predominantly in the lipoprotein fraction. Dingell *et al.* (1971) have obtained similar results using zonal ultracentrifugation. 11-Hydroxy-THC, one of the metabolites of Δ^9-THC, is also bound to plasma proteins

(Widman *et al.*, 1971); however, it is primarily bound to the albumin fraction.

In vivo, the blood levels of Δ^9-THC and its metabolites have been studied in many species including man. In the rabbit, Agurell *et al.* (1970) found that after intravenous administration, Δ^9-THC-^{3}H rapidly disappears from plasma, and after 30 minutes only 3–4% of the radioactivity is present as unchanged drug. The radioactivity declines in what appears to be a biphasic curve with the half-life ($t_{1/2}$) of the latter curve being about 2 hours.

In the rat, Klausner and Dingell (1971) also found a biphasic plasma decay curve; however, the $t_{1/2}$ for this species was 21 hours for the latter phase.

In man, Lemberger *et al.* (1970a, 1971a) investigated the plasma levels of intravenously administered Δ^9-THC-^{14}C. In normal volunteers who had no previous exposure to *Cannabis*, Δ^9-THC-^{14}C disappeared from plasma rapidly during the first few hours (with a $t_{1/2}$ of 30 minutes). After this initial time, the Δ^9-THC levels fell more slowly with a $t_{1/2}$ of 56 hours. Total radioactivity and ether-extractable radioactivity showed a similar biphasic plasma decay curve. When this study was repeated in chronic marihuana smokers (subjects who smoked marihuana daily for at least 1 year prior to the experiment), a biphasic plasma decay curve was also seen. However, the $t_{1/2}$ of the latter phase was only 27 hours. Since both groups of subjects appeared to be similar in all respects except for the fact that one group was composed of chronic marihuana smokers and that the difference was not due to a difference in apparent volumes of distribution between the two groups, it is suggested that a constituent of the marihuana cigarette (whether Δ^9-THC itself, another cannabinoid, or a polycyclic hydrocarbon formed during the smoking process) may induce enzymes which speed up the rate of disappearance of Δ^9-THC. In rat lung, the conversion of Δ^9-THC to its metabolites is increased by treatment with a polycyclic hydrocarbon (Nakazawa and Costa, 1971). The initially rapid decrease of Δ^9-THC-^{14}C in the plasma may in part be due to redistribution of the Δ^9-THC from the intravascular compartment into tissues and to metabolism of the Δ^9-THC-^{14}C.

In man, Δ^9-THC and its metabolites were detectable in plasma for at least 3 days. Since in most instances levels in plasma are a reflection of tissue levels, it appears that Δ^9-THC and its metabolites are also stored in human tissues. This is of considerable significance since it is known from animal studies that the highest concentration of Δ^9-THC and its metabolites are present in lung tissue and in man inhalation is the usual route of administration.

The addition of Δ^9-THC-^{14}C to a placebo marihuana cigarette and its administration to human subjects by inhalation demonstrated that Δ^9-THC disappears in a similar fashion after inhalation or intravenous administration (Lemberger *et al.*, 1971c; Galanter *et al.*, 1972). The oral administration of Δ^9-THC-^{14}C (dissolved in ethanol) to man revealed that 90–95% of the oral dose was absorbed from the gastrointestinal tract (Lemberger *et al.*, 1971d; Weiss *et al.*, 1972) and that plasma levels increased slowly, reaching a peak at 3 hours and then gradually declining (Lemberger *et al.*, 1971b,d). :The plasma levels of radioactivity after the oral, intravenous, and inhalation of Δ^9-THC-^{14}C are shown in Fig. 4. After oral administration of Δ^9-THC dissolved in ethanol, the peak psychological

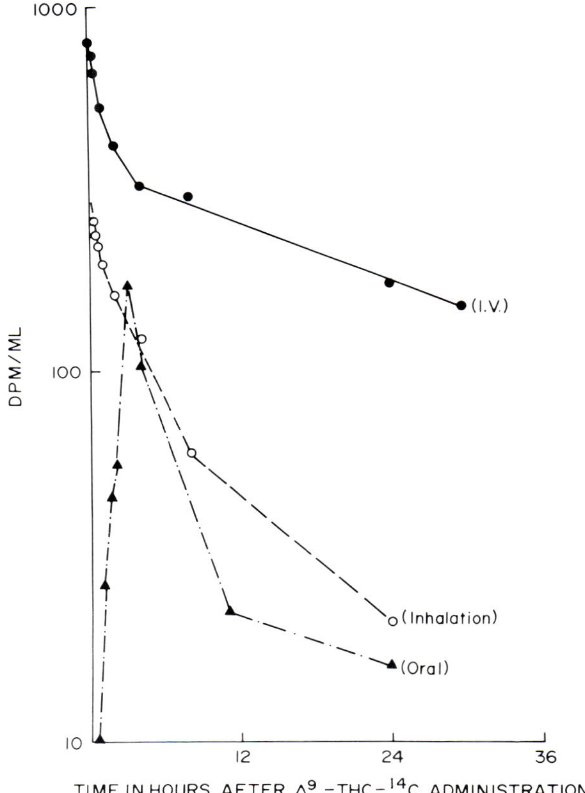

FIG. 4. Plasma levels of Δ^9-tetrahydrocannabinol-^{14}C (Δ^9-THC) and its metabolites (total plasma radioactivity) after oral and intravenous administration and after inhalation of Δ^9-THC-^{14}C.

effect occurs at about 3 hours (Hollister *et al.*, 1968) and can also be correlated with the plasma levels of radioactivity (Lemberger *et al.*, 1971c,d). Plasma levels of radioactivity after orally administered or inhaled Δ^9-THC-^{14}C correlate well with the pharmacological effects (Lemberger *et al.*, 1971b,c, 1972a, Galanter *et al.* 1972; Weiss *et al.*, 1972). Of considerable interest is the fact that the psychological effects appear to correlate with the levels of metabolites rather than the levels of unchanged Δ^9-THC (Lemberger *et al.*, 1971c, 1972a). This will be discussed below in greater detail (Section VI).

Recently, Agurell *et al.* (1971) synthesized 11-hydroxy-Δ^8-THC-^{3}H by acid-catalyzed exchange and studied its metabolic disposition in rabbits after intravenous administration. These investigators found 11-hydroxy-Δ^8-THC-^{3}H to be rapidly removed from the blood initially. However, after 10 minutes, there was a reappearance of the unchanged drug in the circulation. They reported a good correlation between the blood levels of 11-hydroxy-Δ^8-THC and its gross pharmacological effect. In the rabbit, after 11-hydroxy-THC-^{3}H administration, the radioactivity was excreted predominantly in the urine. Only a small percent of the total urinary radioactivity was in the form of the parent drug; the remainder appeared to have properties consistent with that of a carboxylic acid.

Lemberger *et al.* (1972b) administered 11-hydroxy-Δ^9-THC-^{3}H intravenously to infrequent marihuana users and demonstrated that the unchanged drug disappeared from plasma in a biphasic fashion with a $t_{1/2}$ of the later phase of 22 hours. The pharmacokinetics were similar to those seen after Δ^9-THC administration. In man 11-hydroxy-Δ^9-THC was excreted in both urine and feces in approximately the same manner as Δ^9-THC, i.e., 22% excreted in urine and 50% excreted in feces. The metabolites present in urine and feces after 11-hydroxy-Δ^9-THC administration were found to be qualitatively and quantitatively the same as those seen after Δ^9-THC administration to man.

C. Excretion

Δ^9-Tetrahydrocannabinol is extensively metabolized in all species examined thus far and its metabolites are excreted in urine and feces, the relative distribution being dependent upon the species. In the rat, about 50% of the administered dose of Δ^9-THC-^{3}H was recovered in excrements within 10 days; 7–12% is excreted in the urine, and about 40% in the feces (Agurell *et al.*, 1969; Klausner and Dingell, 1971). In the rabbit, Agurell *et al.* (1970) recovered 60% of the administered dose in 3 days; about 45% was found in urine, whereas only 15% of the radioactivity was present in feces. Mantilla-Plata and Harbison (1971) have shown that after the intraperitoneal injection of Δ^9-THC-^{14}C to pregnant mice, 90% of the dose of radioactivity was recovered in 5 days; 80% was present in the feces and 10% in the urine. Forrest *et al.* (1972) have studied the excretion of Δ^9-THC-^{3}H in both the rhesus and squirrel monkey after oral administration. In the squirrel monkey they found only 1–5% of the radioactivity excreted in urine and about 60% excreted in feces. In the rhesus monkey 22–26% of the administered radioactivity was excreted in the urine and about 46% in the feces. It thus appears that the rhesus monkey may be a good animal model for studying Δ^9-THC disposition and metabolism since this species most closely resembles man (Lemberger *et al.*, 1971a) in the manner in which metabolites of Δ^9-THC are excreted.

After the intravenous administration of Δ^9-THC-^{14}C to nonmarihuana smoking human volunteers (Lemberger *et al.*, 1971a), 67% of the administered dose was excreted in 1 week in urine and feces, 22% in the former and 45% in the latter. In chronic marihuana smokers, a larger (71%) but not significantly different percentage of the total dose was recovered in the excrement. However, there was a significantly greater increase in the urinary excretion of radioactivity when users (31%) and nonusers (22%) were compared. After the oral administration of either Δ^9-THC-^{14}C dissolved in ethanol (Lemberger *et al.*, 1971c) or Δ^9-THC-^{3}H dissolved in ethanol, sesame oil, or emulsified in sodium glycocholate (Perez-Reyes *et al.*, 1971), a similar pattern of the excretion of the metabolites was found.

In all species, the rate of excretion of radioactive metabolites of Δ^9-THC was greatest during the initial collection periods and tapered off with successive time intervals. The rate of disappearance of the drug in different species appears to correlate with the plasma half-lives; for example, the rabbit has a short half-life and rapidly metabolized and excreted Δ^9-THC, whereas man has a long half-life and excretes the drug more slowly. The excretion of Δ^9-THC in several species is illustrated in Table I.

D. Metabolism

In vivo metabolic studies confirm certain of the *in vitro* findings. 11-Hydroxylation appears to be an important route of metabolism for Δ^8-THC and Δ^9-THC *in vivo* and has been shown to occur in mice (Christensen *et al.*, 1971), rabbits (Burstein *et al.*, 1970; Ben-Zvi *et al.*, 1970), and rats (Foltz *et al.*, 1970). In man, 11-hydroxy-Δ^9-THC appears to be formed rapidly since it is present in plasma within 10 minutes after administration of Δ^9-THC (Lemberger *et al.*, 1970a). In mice, Christensen *et al.* (1971) found 11-hydroxy-Δ^9-THC present within 30 seconds after intravenous injection of Δ^9-THC. At 3 minutes, both 11-hydroxy and 8,11-dihydroxy metabolites

TABLE I

EXCRETION OF RADIOACTIVITY AFTER ADMINISTRATION OF RADIOLABELED Δ^9-TETRAHYDROCANNABINOL IN SEVERAL SPECIES

Species	Route	% Dose recovered	Time period (days)	% Radioactivity excreted: In urine	% Radioactivity excreted: In feces	Ref.
Rat	i.v.	50	10	10	40	Agurell *et al.* (1969)
Rabbit	i.v.	60	3	45	15	Agurell *et al.* (1970)
Mouse	i.p.	90	5	10	80	Mantilla-Plata and Harbison (1971)
Man Nonuser	i.v.	67	7	22	45	Lemberger *et al.* (1971a)
Chronic user	i.v.	71	7	31	40	Lemberger *et al.* (1971a)

were present in the blood. In man, 11-hydroxy-THC and 8,11-dihydroxy-THC are excreted primarily in the feces (Lemberger *et al.*, 1971d); the 11-hydroxy metabolite represents about 22% of the total radioactivity recovered in feces, whereas 8,11-dihydroxy-Δ^9-THC represents slightly less. Unidentified radioactive compounds are also present in feces having characteristics of more polar compounds and perhaps are conjugates of Δ^9-THC metabolites. In urine, only a small quantity (about 3%) of the total radioactivity recovered was present as 11-hydroxy-Δ^9-THC.

Miras and Coutselinis (1970) studied the disposition of Δ^9-THC-^{14}C in chronic hashish smokers (smoking duration of 20 to 30 years) who had indwelling biliary cannulas. After the inhalation of 100 mg of Δ^9-THC-^{14}C, they found unchanged Δ^9-THC and several polar metabolites in the bile. The presence of Δ^9-THC in the bile and its absence in feces indicate that there is an enterohepatic circulation for Δ^9-THC or that the bacterial flora further metabolize Δ^9-THC. The former hypothesis appears most feasible since this would be consistent with the findings of Klausner and Dingell (1971) using the isolated perfused liver.

After the administration of Δ^9-THC to rabbits, Agurell *et al.* (1970) found a radioactive compound excreted in urine which was acidic in nature and not subject to hydrolysis by β-glucuronidase. In man (Lemberger *et al.*,

1970a, 1971b,d) about 20 to 30% of the radioactivity in an administered dose of Δ^9-THC-^{14}C appeared in the urine, almost all in the form of metabolites since unchanged Δ^9-THC was not detected. About 90% of the urinary radioactivity had properties suggesting that there were one or more acidic metabolites present since most of the urinary radioactivity was extractable from pH 3 but not from a neutral pH. It is possible that these polar, acidic, urinary metabolites present in human urine are identical with those found by Agurell *et al.* (1970) in the rabbit. In contrast to the urine, acidic compounds were not excreted in human feces (Lemberger *et al.*, 1971b). It would appear that this metabolite (or metabolites) found in humans and rabbits is not of major importance in the rat and may be in some way related to the finding that in this species only a small percent of the administered dose is excreted via the urine.

Recently, Burstein and Rosenfeld (1971), in an elegant series of experiments, were able to isolate one of the acidic metabolites from rabbit urine. They purified it by a combination of column and thin layer chromatography, subjected the material to mass spectral analysis, and have tentatively identified the metabolite as 11-carboxy-2′-hydroxy-Δ^9-THC. Furthermore, they postulated that the other acidic metabolites might be amides or esters of the 11-carboxy compound. Cochromatography of the metabolite isolated from rabbit urine with material obtained from the urine of humans given radiolabeled Δ^9-THC suggests that these acidic metabolites are identical (Burstein and Rosenfeld, 1971).

V. Factors Affecting Δ^9-Tetrahydrocannabinol Metabolism

The knowledge that Δ^9-THC is a substrate for the hepatic microsomal enzyme system has prompted numerous laboratories to study the effects of other drugs known to affect these enzymes on the *in vitro* and *in vivo* metabolism of Δ^9-THC.

A. Stimulation

From the classic studies of Conney and Burns (1959, 1962, 1963) and Remmer (1958a,b, 1962), it is well known that pretreatment of animals or man (Burns and Conney, 1965) with a variety of drugs or chemicals of a diverse chemical nature can stimulate the metabolism of other drugs taken concomitantly. In fact, after repeated administration, a drug may stimulate its own metabolism. These compounds act to stimulate new enzyme synthesis with a resultant increase in the liver microsomal enzymes responsible for metabolizing drugs and naturally occurring compounds. This phenomenon has been termed "enzyme induction."

Several investigators have attempted to induce the metabolism of Δ^9-THC by pretreatment of animals with phenobarbital. Conney and Burns (1962) and Remmer (1962) have shown phenobarbital to be a potent enzyme inducer. Wall *et al.* (1970) and Nilsson *et al.* (1970) in their *in vitro* metabolic studies routinely employed phenobarbital pretreated animals. Livers from animals not pretreated with phenobarbital give similar results. However, there was a lesser yield of metabolites (Wall, 1971). In an *in vivo* study, phenobarbital pretreatment of mice was shown to reduce the mortality induced by Δ^9-THC, presumably by increasing the metabolism of Δ^9-THC to pharmacologically inactive compounds (Mantilla-Plata and Harbison, 1971). Burstein and Kupfer (1971) studied the metabolism of Δ^9-THC incubated with rat liver microsomes obtained from animals pretreated with the insecticide, 1,1,1-trichloro-2-bis (*p*-chlorophenyl) ethane (DDT), a known potent inducer of hepatic microsomal enzymes (Hart and Fouts, 1965). Liver microsomes obtained from rats pretreated with DDT metabolized Δ^9-THC at a faster rate than control rats and more of the hydroxylated metabolites were formed. Lung microsomes prepared from rats pretreated with 3-methylcholanthrene, another microsomal enzyme inducer, were shown to metabolize Δ^9-THC (Nakazawa and Costa, 1971) faster than lung microsomes prepared from control animals. In man, chronic *Cannabis* users appear to metabolize Δ^9-THC more rapidly than nonusers (Lemberger *et al.*, 1971a). Whether this is due to Δ^9-THC increasing its own metabolism or some other component of marihuana smoke is not known. Welch *et al.* (1969) have shown that placental tissue from women who were chronic tobacco smokers metabolized 3,4-benzopyrene *in vitro* to a greater extent than placental tissue from nonsmokers of tobacco. It remains to be determined if a common constituent of marihuana and tobacco smoke, i.e., polycyclic hydrocarbons, is responsible for the induction of Δ^9-THC and benzopyrene metabolism in humans. In animals, attempts have been made to determine whether subacute Δ^9-THC treatment induces its own metabolism. However, no direct evidence for this is yet available.

B. Inhibition

In theory, any drug that is metabolized by the liver microsomal enzyme system responsible for the metabolism of Δ^9-THC is also capable of inhibiting the metabolism of Δ^9-THC by acting as an alternative substrate. Δ^9-Tetrahydrocannabinol binds to cytochrome P-450 of hepatic microsomes producing a Type I spectral shift similar to that produced by hexobarbital

(Cohen *et al.*, 1971; Nebert and Lemberger, 1971). Cohen *et al.* (1971) demonstrated that Δ^9-THC has a good affinity for cytochrome P-450 and, therefore, should be a potent inhibitor of other Type I microsomal oxidations. In fact, Δ^9-THC inhibits the oxidation of aminopyrine and hexobarbital (Dewey *et al.*, 1970; Dingell *et al.*, 1971).

Several interactions have been noted to occur between marihuana or Δ^9-THC and other drugs administered to animals. Sleeping times after administration of hexobarbital (Garriot *et al.*, 1967) and pentobarbital (Kubena and Barry, 1970) have been reported to be prolonged if the animals were pretreated with Δ^9-THC. Since Δ^9-THC is itself a CNS depressant, one explanation for this finding is that there is an additive or synergistic effect between Δ^9-THC and the barbiturates. Another possible explanation is that Δ^9-THC potentiates the barbiturates by inhibiting their metabolism. The latter view is supported by *in vitro* studies which clearly show that Δ^9-THC can inhibit the metabolism of hexobarbital (Cohen *et al.*, 1971; Dingell *et al.*, 1971). Kubena and Barry (1970) examined the synergistic effect of Δ^9-THC on sleep time by employing barbital, a barbiturate which is supposedly not metabolized by hepatic microsomal enzymes, and indeed showed that the sleeping time produced by this drug was also prolonged by Δ^9-THC in rats. It appears likely, therefore, that both a direct CNS depressant effect and inhibition of the liver microsomes may be involved in Δ^9-THC potentiation of barbiturate sleeping times.

Paradoxically, pretreatment of rats with Δ^9-THC prior to the administration of amphetamine (Garriot *et al.*, 1967) or methamphetamine (Kubena and Barry, 1970; Phillips *et al.*, 1971b) results in a potentiation of both the amplitude and the duration of the spontaneous activity elicited by the amphetamines. This effect is related to the dose of Δ^9-THC employed. Drugs that block the metabolism of amphetamines will potentiate their pharmacological effects (Consolo *et al.*, 1967; Sulser *et al.*, 1966; Lemberger *et al.*, 1970b). In the case of inhibitors which are also CNS depressants, such as chlorpromazine, the overall pharmacological picture depends upon the dosage administered (Sulser and Dingell, 1968). The mechanism by which Δ^9-THC potentiates amphetamine is not known; however, an effect on amphetamine metabolism must be considered.

β-Diethylaminoethyl diphenylpropylacetate (SKF-525A), the classic inhibitor of the hepatic microsomal enzyme systems (Axelrod 1954a; Cooper *et al.*, 1954) is a potent inhibitor of the *in vitro* metabolism of Δ^9-THC (Dingell *et al.*, 1971). Pretreatment with this compound has been found to potentiate the toxicity and mortality due to Δ^9-THC (Mantilla-Plata and Harbison, 1971).

Sofia and Barry (1970) investigated the interaction of Δ^9-THC, barbital, and SKF 525A in an attempt to determine if Δ^9-THC was responsible for the effects seen after its administration or if it was active only after conversion to an active metabolite (i.e., 11-hydroxy-Δ^9-THC). They found the combination of SKF 525A and Δ^9-THC prolonged barbital sleeping time more than did either drug alone. The SKF 525A, by inhibiting the *in vivo* metabolism of Δ^9-THC, appeared to allow potentiation of the effect of the barbital. They concluded that Δ^9-THC must be the active compound and that an active metabolite was not responsible for the effects. The possibility of an active metabolite will be considered below (Section VI).

The interaction between a single dose of Δ^9-THC and ethanol has been examined in animals (Phillips *et al.*, 1971a; Dewey *et al.*, 1971) and in man (Manno *et al.*, 1971). The combination of these drugs resulted in a potentiation of their depressant effects. The chronic usage of ethanol is known to affect the liver microsomal enzymes which metabolize drugs (Rubin and Lieber, 1971), whereas inhibitory effects have been seen after acute alcohol administration. There is no direct evidence to support either the view that the combination of Δ^9-THC and ethanol are inhibiting each other's metabolism or the possibility that the synergism is due to an effect on the CNS.

C. Sex Difference

A sex difference is seen in rats with respect to the metabolism of drugs (Quinn *et al.*, 1958) and steroids (Kuntzman *et al.*, 1964) by the microsomal enzymes. The male rat metabolizes drugs and steroids more rapidly than the female although the administration of testosterone to female rats can abolish the difference. Burstein and Kupfer (1971) reported that microsomes obtained from male rats metabolize Δ^9-THC at a faster rate than those from females. The behavioral response of rats after the administration of marihuana extract distillate also indicated that a sex difference existed (Cohn *et al.*, 1971). The extract was more potent in the female than in the male when a series of behavioral parameters including response to handling and ability to remain suspended from a bar were determined, suggesting that metabolism might be playing some role in terminating the effects of Δ^9-THC.

VI. Pharmacological Activity—Δ^9-Tetrahydrocannabinol vs. an Active Metabolite

Prior to the elucidation of the metabolites of Δ^9-THC, it was assumed by many that Δ^9-THC was the active component of marihuana. However, based upon their findings that Δ^9-THC was much more active in animals after intraperitoneal administration than subcutaneous administration, Grunfeld and Edery (1969) suggested that a metabolite of Δ^9-THC was responsible for its effects. Indeed these findings are consistent with the hypothesis that Δ^9-THC was enzymatically converted to more active metabolites when passing through the liver. It is possible, however, that the parent compound was not absorbed well after subcutaneous administration. With the knowledge of the metabolic products of Δ^9-THC and the isolation of 11-hydroxy-Δ^9-THC and 11-hydroxy-Δ^8-THC in sufficient quantities for animal testing, it was shown that, in fact, 11-hydroxy-THCs are as potent, or more potent, than the corresponding Δ^8- and Δ^9-THCs (Foltz *et al.*, 1970; Truitt, 1970; Nilsson *et al.*, 1970; Burstein *et al.*, 1970; Ben-Zvi *et al.*, 1970; Wall *et al.*, 1970; Christensen *et al.*, 1971). In chronic *Cannabis* smokers, there is indirect evidence (Lemberger *et al.*, 1971b,c,d; Weiss *et al.*, 1972) that, after oral administration and inhalation (Lemberger *et al.*, 1971c, 1972a, Galanter *et al.*, 1972), metabolites of Δ^9-THC are responsible for its activity. The oral administration of Δ^9-THC in a pharmacological dose (20–30 mg) in conjunction with radiolabeled Δ^9-THC made possible the correlation of blood levels of Δ^9-THC with its pharmacoligcal effects. By this route, the blood levels of unchanged radioactive Δ^9-THC were relatively low in comparison to the quantity of total radioactivity (representing metabolic products of Δ^9-THC) present in the plasma at the peak psychological effect. Calculation of the plasma concentration of unchanged Δ^9-THC showed it to be of the same magnitude as that found initially after an intravenous dose of 0.5 mg of Δ^9-THC. In contrast to the pharmacological effects evidenced after the oral route, there were only minimal effects after the intravenous route even though both had similar blood levels of unchanged Δ^9-THC. This would be consistent with the hypothesis that a metabolite of Δ^9-THC is in part responsible for the biological effects. After inhalation of Δ^9-THC-^{14}C levels of unchanged Δ^9-THC are high initially, but it is the plasma levels of the metabolites which show a temporal correlation with the psychological effects (Lemberger *et al.*, 1971c; Galanter *et al.*, 1972). Additional indirect evidence for this hypothesis comes from the studies of Harris and co-workers (1971) who administered radiolabeled Δ^9-THC to pigeons intramuscularly. They observed the animals' behavior and at various times after administration of the drug determined plasma levels of total radioactivity and unchanged Δ^9-THC. They found plasma levels of unchanged Δ^9-THC reached a peak before the behavioral effects were manifested, whereas plasma levels of Δ^9-THC metabolites coincided with the peak of the behavioral effects.

Studies in animals designed to stimulate or inhibit the metabolism of Δ^9-THC have attempted to resolve this question. Sofia and Barry (1970) studied the influence of SKF 525A on the potentiating effects of Δ^9-THC on barbital sleeping time in mice and found that the drug potentiated the effect of Δ^9-THC on barbital sleeping time. They concluded that Δ^9-THC itself and not a metabolite was responsible for its effects since the conversion to a metabolite had been inhibited. However, Truitt (1971) has found that 11-hydroxy-Δ^8-THC also potentiates barbital sleeping time. In mice, SKF 525A increased the toxicity of Δ^9-THC, whereas pretreatment with phenobarbital decreased the mortality (Mantilla-Plata and Harbison, 1971). Kaymakcalan and Deneau (1971) found the analgesic effect of Δ^9-THC to be enhanced in hepatectomized rats, indicating to them that Δ^9-THC itself was the active drug, not a metabolite.

These findings can be explained or clarified if one assumes that both the parent compound (Δ^9-THC) and its metabolite (11-hydroxy-Δ^9-THC) are active compounds, whether equipotent or whether, perhaps, 11-hydroxy-Δ^9-THC is more active. A parallelism can be drawn from amphetamine metabolism where it has been shown that this drug and its metabolite, *p*-hydroxyamphetamine, are both potent sympathomimetic amines (Axelrod 1954b). If both Δ^9-THC and 11-hydroxy-Δ^9-THC are active and, as is known, 11-hydroxy-Δ^9-THC is also converted by hepatic microsomal enzymes to 8,11-dihydroxy-Δ^9-THC (an inactive metabolite), then the effect of inhibitors (i.e., SKF 525A) of the microsomal enzymes or stimulators (i.e., phenobarbital) would be exerted at both enzymic steps. Thus, all the effects interpreted as preventing the conversion of Δ^9-THC to 11-hydroxy-Δ^9-THC would also prevent the metabolism of 11-hydroxy-Δ^9-THC. Accordingly, if the second enzymic conversion was more sensitive than the first, then 11-hydroxy-Δ^9-THC might accumulate, in the case of the inhibitor studies, or be metabolized faster, in the case of the stimulator studies. This could account for the enhanced or decreased effects from inhibitors or stimulators, respectively. The recent studies of Gill and Jones (1971) appear to clarify some of the controversy regarding the results of studies using SKF 525A. These investigators administered Δ^9-THC-^{3}H of high specific activity intravenously to mice and attempted to correlate the brain levels of either Δ^9-THC and its metabolite (11-hydroxy-Δ^9-THC) with the degree of catalepsy produced. Both Δ^9-THC and 11-hydroxy-Δ^9-THC brain levels correlated with the catalepsy. Prior treatment of the mice with SKF 525A resulted in only slight inhibition of the hydroxylation of Δ^9-THC, however, it markedly inhibited the further metabolism of 11-hydroxy-Δ^9-THC. Thus, after SKF 525A pretreatment, brain levels of 11-hydroxy-Δ^9-THC were markedly increased. These results are consistent with the previously stated hypothesis that a metabolite of Δ^9-THC is responsible for the behavioral effect.

An alternative hypothesis must also be considered. Since Δ^9-THC can also be metabolized by lung tissue, the possibility exists that after the administration of drugs such as SKF 525A, which influence liver microsomal enzyme systems, or following hepatectomy, the Δ^9-THC is converted to more active metabolites in the lung.

Recent studies by Lemberger *et al.* (1972b) provide direct evidence that 11-hydroxy-Δ^9-THC may be the active form of Δ^9-THC. After intravenous administration of 11-hydroxy-Δ^9-THC (1 mg total dose), they found a marked increase in subjective symptoms, a pronounced psychologic "high," and a marked tachycardia. These effects were rapid in onset and persisted for several hours. Their findings that the metabolic fate of 11-hydroxy-Δ^9-THC was both quantitatively and qualitatively similar to that seen after the administration of Δ^9-THC suggests that after the administration of marihuana of hashish, the Δ^9-THC is rapidly converted in man to 11-hydroxy-Δ^9-THC which is responsible for the majority of the pharmacologic effects.

VII. Methods for Determining Δ^9-Tetrahydrocannabinol or Its Metabolites in Biological Fluids

The routine determination of Δ^9-THC and its metabolites in man or animals is necessary for further research endeavors and is important in the area of forensic medicine. The limited use of radioactivity has enabled investigators to establish a foundation upon which further research may be built; however, it is not practical or feasible for large-scale studies or to examine, in a large population, the effects of chronic marihuana usage. Methods for measuring blood levels of Δ^9-THC are actively being sought. These methods include the coupling of gas–liquid chromatography with mass spectrometry and the development of a radioimmunoassay. The difficulty presented by the first method is due to the extremely low levels of Δ^9-THC present in plasma (in the picogram range). In addition, since this is a lipophilic drug, it is difficult to separate it from interfering lipid substances normally present in plasma. Radioimmunoassay appears to be more practical since it should have both sensitivity and specificity.

Studies have been reported on the detection of *Cannabis* derivatives in urine. Since Δ^9-THC is almost completely metabolized in man (Lemberger *et al.*, 1970a) and animals (Agurell *et al.*, 1969), it would be unprofitable to attempt to identify this compound in urine. However, attempts to identify a metabolite should be more rewarding. In man the major urinary metabolite or metabolites of Δ^9-THC appears to be acidic in nature (Lemberger *et al.*, 1971b) and may be similar to the acid metabolite described in rabbit urine (Agurell *et al.*, 1970). The tentative identification of the chemical structure of these compounds (Burstein and Rosenfeld, 1971) should simplify the development of a rapid method for detecting *Cannabis* usage in the near future.

Christiansen and Rafaelsen (1969) administered orally 750 mg of *Cannabis* resin in the form of a tea to 10 volunteers and collected their urine. Employing thin-layer chromatography, they were able to identify cannabidiol in the urine and found several other unidentified compounds. Even with this large dose of *Cannabis* they were unable to find any unchanged Δ^9-THC. These investigators extracted the urines with petroleum ether; the polar metabolites of Δ^9-THC would not be extracted by their technique. Thus, using this method, Kanter *et al.* (1971) were unable to detect any positive reaction in urines of subjects who received pure synthetic THC.

Andersen *et al.* (1971) have developed a relatively specific method for assaying *Cannabis* in human urine. This method involves extracting urine with petroleum ether to remove substances which might give false positive reactions, followed by the extraction of the urine at pH 3.8 with diethyl ether, dehydration of the metabolites to cannabinol derivatives, and subsequent thin-layer chromatography. With this technique a positive reaction is indicated by the occurrence of two specific chromatographic spots. After oral administration of *Cannabis* resin containing 14 mg of THC to a human volunteer, they were able to find positive reactions during the first 6–7 hours. This is consistent with the findings of Lemberger *et al.* (1971a) and Perez-Reyes *et al.* (1971) that the major portion of urinary radioactivity after Δ^9-THC-^{14}C administration was excreted within the first 24 hours, primarily during the first 8 hours.

Although Δ^9-THC is not detectable in urine after *Cannabis* or Δ^9-THC administration in doses used experimentally in the laboratory, Miras and Coutselinis (1970) reported the isolation of a substance appearing to be identical with Δ^9-THC from the urine of chronic hashish smokers. They isolated a few milligrams of this substance from 50 liters of urine obtained from chronic hashish smokers who had been smoking about 3 to 7 gm of hashish daily. Despite this, Agurell *et al.* (1969) believe that attempts to devise a method for identification of *Cannabis* users, based on the excretion of unchanged cannabinols including Δ^9-THC, would be fruitless. This view is supported by studies of the metabolism and excretion in humans (Lemberger *et al.*, 1970a).

VIII. Biochemical Correlates of Clinical Findings

A. Tolerance vs. Reverse Tolerance

Tolerance can be defined as a diminishing effect of a drug which occurs after its repeated administration. The availability of large supplies of synthetic Δ^9-THC have facilitated animal investigations designed to answer the question whether or not tolerance to the effects of marihuana develops. In animals, several studies (Silva *et al.*, 1968; McMillan *et al.*, 1970; Frankenheim *et al.*, 1971) have reported the development of tolerance to some of the effects of Δ^9-THC. In these studies the doses employed were high (up to 10 mg/kg/day). In man, Δ^9-THC is active in doses as low as 6 μg/kg (Kiplinger *et al.*, 1971) and, therefore, the animal model might not be a true representation of what occurs in man. In addition, tolerance may develop for only some of the multiple effects of Δ^9-THC; other effects might be unaltered with repeated drug administration. If, in fact, tolerance develops to unwanted or toxic side effects of a drug, then the tolerance is beneficial. If, however, tolerance to beneficial pharmacological effects develops, then the tolerance is a distinct disadvantage. It is not known whether this tolerance is of a metabolic nature (i.e., the induction of enzymes produces a faster disappearance of the drug and, hence, lower blood levels as has been postulated for the barbiturates) or if it is a cellular tolerance similar to that postulated to occur with opiate derivatives (Jaffe, 1970). In contrast, Phillips *et al.* (1971a) reported an increased sensitivity to Δ^9-THC after its repeated administration to rats. They observed an increase in the severity of symptoms produced with various dosages of Δ^9-THC. Marihuana users claim that marihuana smokers do not achieve a "high" the first time they engage in the use of this drug. The first scientific study to demonstrate this was reported by Weil *et al.* (1968). They found chronic users of marihuana achieved a high after a dose of marihuana (2 gm), whereas about 90% of the naive subjects (nonusers of marihuana) did not respond to the same dose of marihuana. This effect has been referred to as "reverse" tolerance. This alleged "reverse" tolerance appears to be a complex phenomenon.

Further evidence, suggesting a difference in the response to smoking marihuana depending upon the extent of previous exposure, comes from the studies of Meyer *et al.* (1971). These investigators found that heavy marihuana smokers were more sensitive to the high and appear to require less drug than casual users. In addition, using self-evaluation, heavy users reported a greater level of high than did casual users. The heavy users also reported a shorter duration of the high than did the casual users.

Additional evidence for an alleged reverse tolerance is that the intravenous administration of Δ^9-THC (0.5 mg) to nonusers of marihuana is devoid of any pharmacological effect. In contrast, chronic users who were informed that they were receiving the same nonpharmacological dose of Δ^9-THC (0.5 mg) reported effects similar to those after smoking marihuana and these effects lasted for as long as 90 minutes (Lemberger *et al.*, 1971a). The dosage of Δ^9-THC administered to these subjects ranged between 5 to 7 μg/kg. Kiplinger *et al.* (1971a,b) studying the dose–response relationship for Δ^9-THC have shown that long-term marihuana smokers are able to obtain pharmacological effects after smoking a marihuana cigarette designed to deliver a 6.25 μg/kg dose of Δ^9-THC.

The finding that chronic users of marihuana metabolize Δ^9-THC faster than nonusers suggests that with chronic marihuana usage, hepatic microsomal enzyme systems are induced. If the metabolite of Δ^9-THC is, in fact, the active compound, then this might in part explain the alleged "reverse" tolerance since this metabolite would be formed at a faster rate in marihuana users. Other important factors to be considered in explaining reverse tolerance are an alteration in receptor sensitivity for Δ^9-THC, a familiarity through learning and, consequently, a heightened response to the effects of Δ^9-THC, and, because of its marked lipid solubility and resultant tissue storage, a possibility of cumulative effects occurring after repeated administration of Δ^9-THC. A well-controlled prospective clinical study is needed to resolve this controversy of whether tolerance or reverse tolerance develops in man.

B. Spontaneous Recurrence ("Flashback")

There have been many reports of spontaneous recurrences or flashback phenomena after the ingestion of lysergic acid diethylamide (LSD). These effects have been described as occurring as long as 6 months to 1 year after the drug's administration, and it appears unlikely that these are related to the actual presence of drug in the subjects. Keeler *et al.* (1968) reported 4 cases of spontaneous recurrence of the effects of marihuana. In 3 of 4 cases, the individuals had smoked considerably large quantities of marihuana within a short time interval and experienced symptoms similar to those produced by marihuana for up to several weeks. It is possible that with the acute administration of relatively large doses, the material accumulates in tissues and is released from its tissue stores, after some appropriate stimulus, over a short time period, in this way producing the recurrent effects. In contrast to the experience with LSD, there have been no reported incidents of flashbacks occurring from marihuana after prolonged marihuana-free intervals. Since many marihuana users also partake in the use of other drugs, there is a possibility that recurrence represents an interaction with another drug or medicine. In addition, it is well known that marihuana and hashish are adulterated with other pharmacologically active compounds (Canadian Commission, 1970; Kok *et al.*, 1971) and, therefore, one must be cautious in attributing adverse effects specifically to being caused by marihuana. Likewise, it is important to be cautious in attributing fatalities to marihuana until sufficiently sensitive methods are available to determine the absence of other toxic substances in fatal cases associated with marihuana usage.

IX. Concluding Remarks

Because of the long history of *Cannabis* usage in man, Δ^9-THC is unique in that its pharmacology has been examined in humans almost simultaneously with the animal studies. Within the past few years there has been rapid progress made in elucidating the pharmacology of this interesting group of compounds, primarily as a result of the knowledge of its basic chemistry.

From pharmacological studies of Δ^9-THC and its analogs, it appears that this group of compounds merit further investigation as possible therapeutic agents. It is interesting that the THCs appear to have actions in many important areas where new potent drugs would be welcome by the clinician, e.g. (*a*) antihypertensives, (*b*) analgesics, (*c*) anticonvulsants, (*d*) hypnotics and sedatives, (*e*) antidepressants, (*f*) tranquilizers, (*g*) antipsychotics, (*h*) chemotherapeutic agents, (*i*) for the treatment of glaucoma, and (*j*) general anesthetics.

References

Adams, R. (1942). *Harvey Lect.* **37,** 168.

Adams, R., Pease, D. C., and Clark, J. H. (1940). *J. Amer. Chem. Soc.* **62,** 2194.

Agurell, S., and Leander, K. (1971). *Acta Pharm. Suecica* **8,** 685.

Agurell, S., Nilsson, I. M., Ohlsson, A., and Sandberg, F. (1969). *Biochem. Pharmacol.* **18,** 1195.

Agurell, S., Nilsson, I. M., Ohlsson, A., and Sandberg, F. (1970). *Biochem. Pharmacol.* **19,** 1333.

Agurell, S., Nilsson, I. M., Nilsson, J. L. G., Ohlsson, A., Widman, M., and Leander, K. (1971). *Acta Pharm. Suecica* **8,** 698.

Andersen, J. M., Nielsen, E., Schou, J., Steentoft, A., and Worm, K. (1971). *Acta Pharmacol. Toxicol.* **29,** 111.

Axelrod, J. (1954a). *J. Pharmacol. Exp. Ther.* **110,** 2.

Axelrod, J. (1954b). *J. Pharmacol. Exp. Ther.* **110,** 315.

Axelrod, J. (1963). *Science* **140,** 499.

Ben-Zvi, Z., Mechoulam, R., and Burstein, S. (1970). *J. Amer. Chem. Soc.* **92,** 3468.

Borgen, L. A., and Davis, W. M. (1971). *Toxicol. Appl. Pharmacol.* **20,** 480.

Boyd, E. S., and Meritt, D. A. (1965). *J. Pharmacol. Exp. Ther.* **149,** 138.

Brodie, B. B., Gillette, J. R., and LaDu, B. N. (1958). *Annu. Rev. Biochem.* **27,** 427.

Burns, J. J., and Conney, A. H. (1965). *Proc. Roy. Soc. Med.* **58,** 955.

Burstein, S., and Kupfer, D. (1971). *Ann. N. Y. Acad. Sci.* **191,** 61–66.

Burstein, S., and Mechoulam, R. (1968). *J. Amer. Chem. Soc.* **90,** 2420.

Burstein, S., and Rosenfeld, J. (1971). *Acta Pharm. Suecica* **8,** 699.

Burstein, S. H., Menezes, F., Williamson, E., and Mechoulam, R. (1970). *Nature (London)* **225,** 87.

Canadian Commission of Inquiry into the Non-Medical Use of Drugs (1970). Interim Report, p. 74.

Christensen, H. D., Freudenthal, R. I., Gidley, J. T., Rosenfeld, R., Boegli, G., Testino, L., Brine, D. R., Pitt, C. G., and Wall, M. E. (1971). *Science* **172,** 165.

Christiansen, J., and Rafaelsen, O. J. (1969). *Psychopharmacologia* **15,** 60.

Cohen, G. M., Peterson, D. W., and Mannering, G. J. (1971). *Life Sci.* **10,** Part I, 1207.

Cohn, R., Barnes, P., Barratt, E., and Pirch, J. (1971). *Pharmacologist* **13,** 297.

Conney, A. H., and Burns, J. J. (1959). *Nature (London)* **184,** 363.

Conney, A. H., and Burns, J. J. (1962). *Advan. Pharmacol.* **1,** 31–58.

Conney, A. H., and Burns, J. J. (1963). *Advan. Enzyme Regul.* **1,** 189.

Consolo, S., Dolfini, E., Garattini, S., and Valzelli, L. (1967). *J. Pharm. Pharmacol.* **19,** 253.

Cooper, J. R., Axelrod, J., and Brodie, B. B. (1954). *J. Pharmacol. Exp. Ther.* **112,** 55.

Coutselinis, A. S., and Miras, C. J. (1970). United Nations Document ST/SOA/SER. S/24.

Dewey, W. L., Harris, L. S., Howes, J. F., Kennedy, J. S., and Anderson, R. N. (1970). *In* "Committee on Problems of Drug Dependence." Nat. Res. Counc. Publ., pp. 6818–6826. Nat. Acad. Sci., Washington, D.C.

Dewey, W. L., Harris, L. S., Dennis, B., Fisher, S., Kessaris, J., Kersons, L., and Watson, J. (1971). *Pharmacologist* **13,** 296.

Dingell, J. V., Wilcox, H. G., and Klausner, H. A. (1971). *Pharmacologist* **13,** 296.

Doorenbos, N. J., Fetterman, P. S., Maynard, B. S., Quimby, M. W., and Turner, C. E. (1971). *Ann. N.Y. Acad. Sci.* **191,** 3–12.

Edery, H., Grunefeld, Y., Ben-Zui, Z., and Mechoulam, R. (1971). *Ann. N.Y. Acad. Sci.* **191,** 40.

Fahrenholtz, K. E., Lurie, M., and Kierstead, R. W. (1967). *J. Amer. Chem. Soc.* **89,** 5934.

Fetterman, P. S., Keith, E. S., Waller, C. W., Guerrero, O., Doorenbos, N. J., and Quimby, M. W. (1971). *J. Pharm. Sci.* **60,** 1246.

Foltz, R. L., Fentiman, A. F., Leighty, E. G., Walter, J. L., Drewes, H. R., Schwartz, W. E., Page, T. F., and Truitt, E. B. (1970). *Science* **168,** 844.

Forney, R. B. and Kiplinger, G. F. (1971). *Ann. N.Y. Acad. Sci.* **191,** 74–80.

Forrest, I. S., Green, D. E., Otis, L. S., and Würsch, M. S. (1972). *Fed. Proc. Fed. Amer. Soc. Exp. Biol.* **31,** 506.

Frankenheim, J. M., McMillan, D. E., and Harris, L. S. (1971). *J. Pharmacol. Exp. Ther.* **178,** 241.

Galanter, M., and Wyatt, R. J. (1971). Unpublished observations.

Galanter, M., Wyatt, R. J., Lemberger, L., Weingartner, H., Vaughan, T. B., and Roth, W. T. (1972). *Science* (in press).

Gaoni, Y., and Mechoulam, R. (1964). *J. Amer. Chem. Soc.* **86,** 1646.

Garriot, J. C., King, L. J., Forney, R. B., and Hughes, F. W. (1967). *Life Sci.* **6,** 2119.

Gerber, W. F. (1969). *Toxicol. Appl. Pharmacol.* **14**, 276.

Gill, E. W. and Jones, G. (1971). *Acta Pharm. Suecica* **8**, 700.

Gilman, A. G., and Conney, A. H. (1963). *Biochem. Pharmacol.* **12**, 577.

Grunfeld, Y., and Edery, H. (1969). *Psychopharmacologia* **14**, 200.

Hardman, H. F., Domino, E. F., and Seevers, M. H. (1971). *Pharmacol. Rev.* **23**, 295–315.

Harris, L. S., McMillan, D. E., and Dewey, W. L. (1971). Unpublished observations.

Hart, L., and Fouts, J. (1965). *Naunyn-Schmiedebergs Arch. Pharmakol. Exp. Pathol.* **249**, 486.

Hively, R. L., Mosher, W. A., and Hoffman, F. (1966). *J. Amer. Chem. Soc.* **88**, 1832.

Ho, B. T., Fritchie, G. E., Kralik, P. M., Englert, L. F., McIsaac, W. M., and Idänpään-Heikkila, J. (1970). *J. Pharm. Pharmacol.* **22**, 538.

Ho, B. T., Fritchie, G. E., Englert, L. F., McIsaac, W. M., and Idänpään-Heikkilä, J. E. (1971). *J. Pharm. Pharmacol.* **23**, 309.

Hollister, L. E., Richards, R. K., and Gillespie, H. K. (1968). *Clin. Pharmacol. Ther.* **9**, 783.

Howes, J. F. (1970). *Pharmacologist* **12**, 258.

Idänpään-Heikkilä, J., Fritchie, G. E., Englert, L. F., Ho, B. T., and McIsaac, W. M. (1969). *New Engl. J. Med.* **281**, 330.

Idänpään-Heikkilä, J. E., McIsaac, W. M., and Ho, B. T. (1971). Unpublished observations.

Isbell, H., Gorodetzsky, C. W., Jasinski, D., Claussen, U., Spulak, F. V., and Korte, F. (1967). *Psychopharmacologia* **11**, 184.

Jaffe, J. H. (1970). *In* "The Pharmacological Basis of Therapeutics" (L. S. Goodman and A. Gilman, eds.), p. 279. Macmillan, New York.

Jepson, J. B., Zaltzman, P., and Udenfriend, S. (1962). *Biochim. Biophys. Acta* **62**, 91.

Joachimoglu, G., Kiburis, J., and Miras, C. (1967). United Nations Document ST/SOA/Ser. S/15.

Kanter, S. L., Hollister, L. E., Moore, F., and Green, D. (1971). *Clin. Chem.* **17**, 636.

Kaymakcalan, S., and Deneau, G. A. (1971). *Pharmacologist* **13**, 247.

Keeler, M. H., Reifler, C. B., and Liptzin, M. B. (1968). *Amer. J. Psychiat.* **125**, 384.

Kennedy, J. S., and Waddell, W. J. (1971). *Fed. Proc. Fed. Amer. Soc. Exp. Biol.* **30**, 279.

King, L. J., and Forney, R. B. (1967). *Fed. Proc. Fed. Amer. Soc. Exp. Biol.* **26**, 540.

Kiplinger, G. F., and Manno, J. E. (1971a). *Pharmacol. Rev.* **23**, 339–347.

Kiplinger, G. F., Manno, J., Rodda, B. E., and Forney, R. B. (1971b). *Clin. Pharmacol. Therap.* **12**, 650.

Klausner, H. A., and Dingell, J. V. (1971). *Life Sci.* **10**, 49.

Kok, J. C. F., Fromberg, E., Geerlings, P. J., Van Der Helm, H. J., Kamp, P. E., Van Der Slooten, E. P. J., and Willems, M. A. M. (1971). *Lancet* **1**, 1065.

Kubena, R. K., and Barry, H. (1970). *J. Pharmacol. Exp. Ther.* **173**, 94.

Kuntzman, R., Schneidman, K., Jacobson, M., and Conney, A. H. (1964). *J. Pharmacol. Exp. Ther.* **146**, 280.

Layman, J. M., and Milton, A. S. (1971). *Brit. J. Pharmacol.* **42**, 308.

Lemberger, L., Kuntzman, R., Conney, A. H., and Burns, J. J. (1965). *J. Pharmacol. Exp. Ther.* **150**, 292.

Lemberger, L., Silberstein, S. D., Axelrod, J., and Kopin, I. J. (1970a). *Science* **170**, 1320.

Lemberger, L., Witt, E. D., Davis, J. M., and Kopin, I. J. (1970b). *J. Pharmacol. Exp. Ther.* **174**, 428.

Lemberger, L., Tamarkin, N. R., Axelrod, J., and Kopin, I. J. (1971a). *Science* **173**, 72.

Lemberger, L., Axelrod, J., and Kopin, I. J. (1971b). *Pharmacol. Rev.* **23**, 371–380.

Lemberger, L., Axelrod, J., and Kopin, I. J. (1971c). *Acta Pharm. Suecica* **8**, 692.

Lemberger, L., Axelrod, J., and Kopin, I. J. (1971d). *Ann. N.Y. Acad. Sci.* **191**, 142–152.

Lemberger, L., Weiss, J. L., Watanabe, A. M., Galanter, I. M., Wyatt, R. J., and Cardon, P. V. (1972a) *N. Engl. J. Med.* **13**, 685.

Lemberger, L., Crabtree, R., and Rowe, H. M. (1972b) *Science* (in press).

McIsaac, W. M., Fritchie, G. E., Idänpään-Heikkilä, J. E., Ho, B. T., and Englert, L. F. (1971). *Nature (London)* **230**, 593.

McMillan, D. E., Harris, L. S., Frankenheim, J. M., and Kennedy, J. S. (1970). *Science* **169**, 501.

Manno, J. E., Kiplinger, G. F., Bennett, I. F., and Forney, R. B. (1970). *Clin. Pharmacol. Ther.* **11**, 808.

Manno, J. E., Kiplinger, G. F., Scholz, N. E., and Forney, R. B. (1971). *Clin. Pharmacol. Ther.* **12**, 202.

Mantilla-Plata, B., and Harbison, R. D. (1971). *Pharmacologist* **13**, 297.

Maynard, D. E., Gurny, O., Pitcher, R. G., and Kierstead, R. W. (1971). *Experientia* **27**, 1154.

Mechoulam, R. (1970). *Science* **168**, 1159.

Mechoulam, R., and Gaoni, Y. (1967a). *Tetrahedron Lett.* **12**, 1109.

Mechoulam, R., and Gaoni, Y. (1967b). *Fortschr. Chem. Org. Naturst.* **25**, 175.

Mechoulam, R., Shani, A., Edery, H., and Grunfeld, Y. (1970). *Science* **169**, 611.

Merkus, F. W. H. M. (1971). *Nature (London)* **232**, 579.

Meyer, R. E., Pillard, R. C., Shapiro, L. M., and Mirin, S. M. (1971). *Amer. J. Psychiat.* **128**, 198.

Mikes, F., and Waser, P. G. (1971). *Science* **172**, 1158.

Miras, C. J. (1965). *In* "Hashish: Its Chemistry and Pharmacology" (G. E. W. Wolstenholme and J. Knight, eds.), Little, Brown, Boston, Massachusetts.

Miras, C. J., and Coutselinis, A. S. (1970). United Nations Document ST/SOA/SER. S/24.

Nakazawa, K., and Costa, E. (1971). *Pharmacologist* **13**, 297.

Nebert, D., and Lemberger, L. (1971). Unpublished observations.

Nilsson, J. L. G., Nilsson, I. M., and Agurell, S. (1969). *Acta Chem. Scand.* **23**, 2209.

Nilsson, I. M., Agurell, S., Nilsson, J. L. G., Ohlsson, A., Sandberg, F., and Wahlqvist, M. (1970). *Science* **168**, 1228.

Nilsson, I. M., Agurell, S., Leander, K., Nilsson, J. L. G., and Widman, M. (1971). *Acta Pharm. Suecica* **8**, 701.

Ohlsson, A., Abou-Chaar, C. I., Agurell, S., Nilsson, I. M., Olofsson, K., and Sandberg, F. (1971). *Bull. Narcotics* **23**, 29.

Pace, H. B., Davis, W. M., and Borgen, L. A. (1971). *Ann. N.Y. Acad. Sci.* **191**, 123–130.

Pars, H. G., and Razdan, R. K. (1971). *Ann. N.Y. Acad. Sci.* **191**, 15–22.

Paton, W. D. M., and Pertwee, R. G. (1971). *Acta Pharm. Suecica* **8**, 691.

Perez-Reyes, M., Lipton, M. A., and Wall, M. E. (1971). Unpublished observations.

Persaud, I., and Ellington, A. (1967). *Lancet* **2**, 1306.

Persaud, I., and Ellington, A. (1968). *Lancet* **2**, 406–407.

Petrzilka, T., and Sikemeier, C. (1967a). *Helv. Chim. Acta* **50**, 1416.

Petrzilka, T., and Sikemeier, C. (1967b). *Helv. Chim. Acta* **50**, 2111.

Phillips, R. N., Brown, D. J., Martz, R. C., Hubbard, J. D., and Forney, R. B. (1971a). *Toxicol. Appl. Pharmacol.* **19**, 107.

Phillips, R. N., Neel, M. A., Brown, D. J., and Forney, R. B. (1971b). *Pharmacologist* **13,** 297.
Quinn, G. P., Axelrod, J., and Brodie, B. B. (1958). *Biochem. Pharmacol.* **1,** 152.
Remmer, H. (1958a). *Naturwissenschaften* **45,** 522.
Remmer, H. (1958b). *Naunyn-Schmiedebergs Arch. Pharmakol. Exp. Pathol.* **233,** 184.
Remmer, H. (1962). *Proc. 1st Int. Pharmacol. Meet., Stockholm, 1961* **6,** 235.
Rubin, E., and Lieber, C. S. (1971). *Science* **172,** 1097.
Shani, A., and Mechoulam, R. (1970). *Chem. Commun.* p. 273.
Silva, M. T. A., Carlini, E. A., von Claussen, U., and Korte, F. (1968). *Psychopharmacologia* **13,** 332.
Sofia, R. D., and Barry, H. (1970). *Eur. J. Pharmacol.* **13,** 134.
Sulser, F., and Dingell, J. V. (1968). *Biochem. Pharmacol.* **17,** 634.
Sulser, F., Owens, M. L., and Dingell, J. V. (1966). *Life Sci.* **5,** 2005.
Timmons, M. L., Pitt, C. G., and Wall, M. E. (1969). *Tetrahedron Lett.* **36,** 3129.
Todd, A. R. (1942). *Sci. J. Roy. Coll. Sci.* **12,** 37.
Truitt, E. B. (1970). *Fed. Proc. Fed. Amer. Soc. Exp. Biol.* **29,** 619.
Truitt, E. B. (1971). *Pharmacol. Rev.* **23,** 273–278.
Valle, J. R., Lapa, A. J., and Barros, G. G. (1968). *J. Pharm. Pharmacol.* **20,** 798.
von Claussen, U., and Korte, F. (1968). *Justus Liebigs Ann. Chem.* **713,** 162.
Vree, T. B., Breimer, D. D., Van Ginneken, C. A. M., Van Rossum, J. M., De Zeeuw, R. A., and Witte, H. (1971a). *Clin. Chim. Acta* **34,** 365.
Vree, T. B., Breimer, D. D., Van Ginneken, C. A. M., and Van Rossum, J. M. (1971b). *Acta Pharm. Suecica* **8,** 693.
Wahlqvist, M., Agurell, S., Granstrand, B., Nilsson, I. M., and Sandberg, F. (1970). *Biochem. Pharmacol.* **19,** 2579.
Wall, M. E. (1971). *Ann. N.Y. Acad. Sci.* **191,** 23–37.
Wall, M. E., Brine, D. R., Brine, G. A., Pitt, C. G., Freudenthal, R. I., and Christensen, H. D. (1970). *J. Amer. Chem. Soc.* **92,** 3466.
Waller, C. W. (1971). *Pharmacol. Rev.* **23,** 265–271.
Waskow, I. E., Olsson, J. E., Saltzman, C., and Kratz, M. (1970). *Arch. Gen. Psychiat.* **22,** 97.
Weil, A. T., Zinberg, N. E., and Nelson, J. M. (1968). *Science* **162,** 1234.
Weiss, J. L., Watanabe, A. M., Lemberger, L., Tamarkin, N. R., and Cardon, P. V. (1972). *Clin. Pharmacol. Ther.* (in press).
Welch, R. M., Harrison, Y. E., Gommi, B. W., Poppers, P. J., Finster, M., and Conney A. H. (1969). *Clin. Pharmacol. Ther.* **10,** 100.
Widman, M., Nilsson, I. M., Nilsson, J. L. G., Agurell, S., and Leander, K. (1971). *Life Sci.* **10,** 157.

Biological Activities of Antilymphocytic Serum

FEDERICO SPREAFICO

Istituto di Ricerche Farmacologiche
"Mario Negri"
Milano, Italy

I. Introduction

In some respects the history of ALS* is reminiscent of the fairy tale about the ugly duckling. In fact, antiserum directed against lymphoid cells was first prepared at the turn of this century, but its true discovery, with the revelation of its remarkable immunodepressive activity, dates back only to the early sixties. Metchnikoff (1898, 1899) was the first to

* See List of Abbreviations at end of this section.

notice the cytotoxic and agglutinating activity of the serum of rabbits injected with spleen and lymph node cells of rats and guinea pigs, and to foretell the use of an "antiphagocytic serum for diminishing the organism's reactivity."

The *in vitro* cytotoxic activity and involvement of complement in this process were also confirmed by a number of authors at about this same time (Besredka, 1900; Christian and Leen, 1905; Moorhead, 1905; Richtie, 1908) and especially by Pappenheimer (1917a,b). Others noted the lymphopenia-producing activity of the antiserum and its capacity to modify lymphoid tissue (Flexner, 1902; Ricketts, 1902; Bunting, 1903). Subsequently, except for an occasional paper (Chew and Lawrence, 1937; Cruickshank, 1941; Miale, 1947), ALS practically fell into oblivion. Interest was not renewed until, parrallel to the growing awareness of the role of lymphocytes in immunological responses, Inderbitzin (1956) of J. H. Humphrey's group showed that ALS could suppress tuberculin responses in guinea pigs. This finding was later confirmed by Wilhelm *et al.* (1958) and Waksman *et al.* (1961) who also obtained a modest prolongation of skin homografts in the guinea pig.

After some initial failures with homologous antisera (Woodruff, 1960; Woodruff *et al.*, 1951), the first really convincing demonstration of the immunosuppressive activity of ALS was given by Woodruff and Anderson (1963a,b), who obtained marked prolongation of skin allograft survival across a strong histocompatibility barrier in rats treated with rabbit anti-rat lymphocytic serum. Since then, more than 500 reports have been published on ALS demonstrating its potential both as a curative agent and as an important tool for gaining a better understanding of the biology of the immune response. In spite of the large volume of work performed in this area, a number of important points regarding both the biology and therapeutic applications of ALS are still to be clarified. The aim of this survey is an examination of the current knowledge about ALS. No claims are made for a complete review of the available literature in the field. Instead we have selected the most relevant papers.

List of Abbreviations

ALS:	antilymphocytic serum
ALG:	antilymphocytic globulin
ALGG:	antilymphocytic immunoglobulin G
Alabs:	specific antilymphocytic antibodies
Alnex:	antiserum against membrane-free lymphoid extracts
IgM:	immunoglobulin of the M class
IgG:	immunoglobulin of the G class

IgA:	immunoglobulin of the A class
Fab′, $F(ab')_2$:	monovalent and divalent antigen-binding fragments of antibody
Fc:	crystallizable, complement-fixing fragment of antibody
GVH:	graft-vs.-host reaction
RES:	reticuloendothelial system
MLV:	murine leukemia virus
MSV:	murine sarcoma virus
SV 40:	simian virus 40
PHA:	phytohemagglutinin
PPD:	purified protein derivative (tuberculin)
Poly I:C:	polyinosinic acid–polycytidylic acid

II. Production of Antilymphocytic Serum

As commonly used, the term ALS indicates a heterologous serum, i.e., material prepared by injecting animals with lymphoid cells obtained from a different species. Antibody reacting with lymphocytes can also be obtained by immunizing animals with cells of individuals of the same species—such antibodies are frequently found, for instance, in the serum of polytransfused patients and are directed against antigens present in the blood donor but absent in the recipient. These homologous sera have some of the *in vitro* and *in vivo* properties exhibited by heterologous sera (Sell, 1969; Bach, 1970b) but will not be considered in this survey since they are not employed for immunosuppressive purposes. Only heterologous sera will be discussed.

A number of techniques have been employed for the production of ALS. As will be shown, some of these procedures seem to give better results, but a number of problems are still open, and general agreement has not been reached as to the best method for large-scale production of sera with consistently high immunosuppressive activity and low toxicity. The effectiveness of the various procedures appear to vary from species to species; moreover, individual variability within one species in the quality of serum obtained further complicates the picture. The seriousness of the problem is compounded for antihuman ALS not only because of the rather limited number of sera tested and the many variables involved, but also because a reliable *in vitro* assay correlating with the *in vivo* immunosuppressive activity has not yet been developed. However, these problems have not precluded the production of large amounts of effective material for many animal species and for clinical use.

A. Choice and Preparation of Antigen

The main sources of lymphoid cells used in producing ALS are thoracic duct or peripheral blood lymphocytes and cell suspensions from lymph nodes, thymus, or spleen, either separately or mixed, and, more recently, long-term, *in vitro* cultured, peripheral blood lymphocytes or subcellular lymphocyte fractions have also been employed. Problems of supply and potency of the immunogens as well as efforts to make the antisera less toxic and more specific led to numerous studies of the relative value of the various lymphoid cells. In fact, not all these sources have been found to be equally satisfactory. For practical reasons, the spleen has often been employed as a source of antigen especially for antihuman sera (Iwasaki *et al.*, 1967; Doak *et al.*, 1969). However, when compared with other sources of lymphoid cells, this organ has often given sera which were both more toxic and less active *in vivo* in mice, dogs, and in man (Balner *et al.*, 1969). This result is attributable to the multiple cellular composition of the organ causing the formation of irrelevant, inactive, and toxic antibodies. Lymph nodes are frequently used in the case of laboratory animals, generally with reasonably good success. Sometimes the results are at least equivalent to those obtained with thymocytes, but one cannot always be sure of obtaining an active serum without the concomitant use of adjuvants (Wood and Vriesendorp, 1969; Monaco *et al.*, 1969). Thymocytes are considered by many investigators as the best source of antigen in the mouse, rat, and dog (Nagaya and Sieker, 1965; Russe and Crowle, 1965; Shanfield *et al.*, 1968; Dormont *et al.*, 1969; Perper *et al.*, 1970a; Sterling *et al.*, 1970) although this superiority has been questioned (Wood and Vriesendorp, 1969; Ono *et al.*, 1969b). The data so far presented are too limited for sound statistical conclusions. Antihuman thymocytic sera have also been prepared (Shorter *et al.*, 1967; Monaco *et al.*, 1967b; Taylor, 1970a; Trentin, 1970a; Cohen and Sell, 1970; Najarian and Simmons, 1971) and found to be effective. No comparative judgment is yet possible; moreover, these cells are the most difficult to obtain in quantity. Thoracic duct lymphocytes require only minimal manipulation before injection and give rise to sera which are generally quite active both in animals and in man (Woodruff and Anderson, 1963a, 1964; Starzl *et al.*, 1967a; Monaco *et al.*, 1967b; Carraz *et al.*, 1967; Traeger *et al.*, 1970; Woiwod *et al.*, 1970) and, because of the purity of the material, give fewer toxic effects. According to Traeger's experience, thoracic duct drainage of one patient waiting for a kidney homograft will give enough cells for the production of sufficient ALS to treat the same patient thereafter—the cells obtained from 6 drainages give the ALS required for the treatment of 25 patients for 1 year. Thus, this cell source seems to be poorly suited for mass production. Peripheral blood lymphocytes, although requiring more processing before a reasonably pure suspension is obtained (Woiwod, 1970), would seem to be the most readily available source of antigen for large-scale production of ALS. Approximately 150×10^9 lymphocytes might be needed for the immunization of 1 horse during 1 year (Traeger *et al.*, 1970), therefore about 800 to 1500 liters of stored blood would be necessary for the production of enough ALS to treat 25 allografted patients for 1 year according to Traeger's schedule of treatment. Recently, techniques have been proposed which allow the collection of sizable numbers of lymphocytes from the blood without reduction of the other circulating elements. More relevant is the fact that there is still no agreement on the immunosuppressive potency and toxicity of sera prepared from this source of antigen; active (Pichlmayr, 1970) as well as inactive and toxic antisera were obtained (Woiwod *et al.*, 1970). A recent report further suggests that peripheral blood lymphocytes can cause the production of much higher titers of antibodies to platelets, erythrocytes, and serum proteins than thoracic duct lymphocytes (James *et al.*, 1970)—an indication of the greater difficulty in obtaining "pure" antigen from the former source. Since it is now possible to grow peripheral blood lymphocytes indefinitely in tissue culture, in principle this method would seem to represent the best source for mass production of antigenic material in terms of purity, reproducibility, economy, and logistics. By *in vitro* culturing, very high numbers of cells can be obtained (in some centers 200-liter vats are employed) from small initial inocula, and, because of the purity of the material, the production of undesirable antibodies, such as those directed against erythrocytes, platelets, and glomerular basement membrane should be minimized. In fact, horse sera prepared with this type of antigen have been found to be immunosuppressive in man, and large doses were injected intravenously without giving anemia or thrombocytopenia (Najarian *et al.*, 1969, 1970). These sera were also shown not to contain antibodies reacting with glomerular basement membrane, an obvious advantage in the prevention of nephrotoxic nephritis which is one of the major possible complications in the clinical use of ALS.

The production of antihuman ALS could also be facilitated by the use of stored antigen since this would permit more regular and standardized procedures of immunization; lymphocytes kept at −196°C have produced active sera (Traeger *et al.*, 1969; Nossa *et al.*, 1969). Furthermore, cell viability is not a necessary prerequisite for the production of *in vivo* active sera, such sera have also been obtained employing lyophilized (Bach 1970b), heated, or boiled lymphocytes (Jooste *et al.*, 1968; Winn and Daddi, 1970), as well as with cells treated with formol (Spreafico, 1968) or other chemicals (Gozzo *et al.*, 1969).

Another approach to the problem of increasing the purity and specificity of antigenic material is to use subcellular lymphoid preparations. Subcellular fractions, prepared by a variety of techniques from mouse thymocytes, have been used to produce effective and nontoxic antisera (Levey and Medawar, 1966a; Moynihan *et al.*, 1967; Lance *et al.*, 1968, 1970; Nagaya *et al.*, 1970; Warnatz *et al.*, 1969; Zola *et al.*, 1970; Hayes *et al.*, 1970). The best results were obtained with membrane-containing fractions. An additional advantage of using antigen of this type, in which the relevant materials are probably lipoproteins, is that no decline in potency nor increase in toxicity with continued immunization were observed (Lance *et al.*, 1970). Antihuman ALS using subcellular, membrane fractions of human tonsils, thymocytes, and blood lymphocytes (Lejeune *et al.*, 1970; Traeger *et al.*, 1970b) have been prepared but in some cases were found to be toxic (Woiwod *et al.*, 1970; Zola *et al.*, 1970). Antisera to mouse thymocyte soluble extracts were found to be immunosuppressive though less than antisera to membranes of the same cells (Zola *et al.*, 1971), whereas spleen extracts did not elicit the production of *in vivo* active preparations. Antisera against extracts of human peripheral lymphocytes gave results suggestive of immunosuppressive activity and low toxicity but have not yet been critically tested. It is thus apparent that many technical problems have still to be solved in this field, but it is possible that preparations of this type may represent the antigen of choice in the future, especially if it will be possible to identify the antigen responsible for the immunosuppressive activity, to purify it without great loss during preparation, and to store it without reduction of immunogenicity.

As regards the number of cells to be injected, the experience of many investigators (Levey and Medawar, 1966b; Starzl *et al.*, 1967b; Jooste *et al.*, 1968; Barth *et al.*, 1968) seems to be that high numbers of lymphoid cells have to be injected in order to obtain active antisera for experimental or clinical use. The requirement for large numbers of cells often represents a serious handicap for the production of ALS to be used in the clinic, where thymocytes or thoracic duct cells may be desirable but difficult to obtain antigens. The number of cells injected varies markedly depending on the immunization schedule chosen and on whether adjuvants are employed; e.g., a total of 2×10^9 thymocytes are used in the frequently employed "two-pulse" immunization course proposed by Levey and Medawar (1966a,b) for rabbit antimouse ALS. No indication can be given for the cellular requirement in the production of horse antihuman ALS, because of the many different procedures employed—doses ranging from a total of 2×10^9 thoracic duct cells with Freund's adjuvant, 30×10^9 peripheral cells in adjuvant, to as many as 400×10^9 spleen cells (Pichlmayr, 1970;

Woiwod, 1970) have been used. Recently, however, data have been presented showing that in the rabbit antimouse system, highly potent antisera can be obtained with very low lymphocyte doses, in the order of 1 to 10×10^6 cells plus adjuvant per injection (Gozzo *et al.*, 1971); comparable results have also been found for rabbits immunized with human thymocytes (Darrow *et al.*, 1971). If confirmed, these findings will certainly help to solve some of the practical problems encountered in the production of large batches of standardized sera suitable for use in man.

B. Choice of Animal Species

Standardized injections of lymphocytes from one species into animals of another species do not give rise to antisera of uniform activity; on the contrary, the antisera may markedly differ in their immunosuppressive potency. Theoretically the explanation may depend not only on the immunochemical and specificity characteristics of the antisera but also on the different immunogenicity of the heterologous proteins in the recipient. This subject is far from being clarified. Sufficient information for comparing several animal species as ALS producers is not yet available, and the solution of this problem is also hampered by the lack of agreement as to the best procedure of immunization, by individual variability in response of the immunized animals, and by difficulty in evaluating the activity of the antiserum. Most of the data on the immunosuppressive activity of ALS in small laboratory animals have been obtained using sera prepared in rabbits. Evidence has been presented that in the preparation of antimouse ALS, rabbits injected with lymph node cells give much more active sera that those obtained from rats, guinea pigs, and dogs (Winn and Daddi, 1970) despite comparable titers of agglutinating and cytotoxic antibodies. Analogous findings were previously reported by Jeejeebhoy (1967a) for rabbit and dog antirat ALS, the former serum showing high *in vivo* potency, whereas the latter failed to show any immunosuppressive activity. He also described variability in graft-prolonging capacity in different pools of sera prepared by the same technique and showing similar serological activity. Pigs have been found to produce strongly immunosuppressive sera against lymphocytes of rat, dog, and chicken; sheep and goats also produced strongly immunosuppressive sera, but hemagglutinins could not be removed even by multiple absorptions; calves gave potent and nontoxic sera against mouse cells (Binns *et al.*, 1971).

As regards antilymphocytic sera to be employed in man or large animals, the horse has been the most common choice not only because of the possibility of obtaining large quantities of serum but also because of experience accumulated in using this animal for the production of antisera. Moreover, antisera from horses seem to be more active than those obtained from cows and sheep (Pichlmayr *et al.*, 1967; James, 1969). Sheep have been employed with success by some investigators (Mitchell *et al.*, 1966; Fox *et al.*, 1967) for producing antidog ALS and also antihuman ALS (Alexander, 1970), but the use of goats has met with conflicting results; negative experiences have, in fact, been reported by Perper *et al.* (1970a). Rabbit antihuman ALS has also been found to be immunosuppressive (Monaco *et al.*, 1967b; Davis *et al.*, 1971). It is certainly desirable to have ALS from a number of animal species for use in patients who develop hypersensitivity to heterologous proteins of one species—a change in the type of serum may be necessary for the treatment of rejection episodes in sensitized patients or in subjects who receive a second homograft. Moreover, Amemiya *et al.* (1970) detected a 50% incidence of preformed antibodies of low titer against horse serum among a large group of candidates for organ transplantation, probably representing naturally occurring heterospecific antibodies or a consequence of past exposure to one of the widely used animal biological products (Arbesman *et al.*, 1960). The usefulness of switching from one ALS to another would, however, be limited by the fact that, in about 25% of the subjects investigated by Amemiya (1970), cross-reactivity between horse and goat globulins was observed, whereas cross-reaction with rabbit sera occurred to a less pronounced degree. Thus a comparative study carried out in depth between antihuman sera prepared in horses and rabbits could be of value. It has been known for years that in the case of other curative sera, such as those employed in the treatment of pneumonia, rabbit sera were superior; moreover, other practical considerations (low price and economy of maintenance, the possibility of having a large pool of immunized animals, and elimination of the insufficient responders, etc.) might well tip the scale in favor of the smaller animal.

C. Method of Immunization

Methods of immunization have differed considerably among the various groups of investigators regarding doses of cells, route of injection, number and timing of injections, and the use of adjuvants. No clear conclusion can yet be drawn concerning the relative merits of the various immunization schedules for producing ALS, not even in the case of laboratory animals for which an assessment of ALS activity is easier. There seems to be a countless number of permutations in the techniques that can be used for the preparation of ALS. Since important changes in the immunosuppressive property of the antiserum may follow even simple changes in the schedule of immunization, it is apparent that there is a need for greater knowledge on the best mode of preparation of ALS if this agent is to be used clinically with reasonable confidence.

For rabbit antimouse or antirat sera, one of the most frequently adopted methods is the two-pulse procedure proposed by Levey and Medawar (1966a), consisting of two intravenous injections 14 days apart of 1×10^9 lymphoid cells; the rabbits are exsanguinated 1 week later. This method has the advantage of being rapid and easy, of giving sera which are in general (but not invariably) active *in vivo*, do not contain very high levels of hemagglutinins, and should contain low levels of antibodies against irrelevant antigens of the immunizing material. Adaptation of the two-pulse method for use in bigger animals, such as the horse, has also been attempted (Shorter *et al.*, 1967) with mixed results. Perper and his group (1970b) suggest that the most desirable method of producing ALS is a short-term immunization with an early harvesting of the serum; however, Woiwod *et al.* (1970) using human spleen cells did not obtain immunosuppressive antisera by this approach. Other more complex procedures have also been used, such as that originally proposed by Monaco and his group (Gray *et al.*, 1966) which involves first an intradermal injection of cells emulsified in Freund's adjuvant, followed, after a few weeks, by multiple booster intraperitoneal or intravenous injections, and the animal being then bled 10 days later. Methods for the production of antihuman sera have been even more varied. Only recently have efforts been made, with increased experience and availability of more refined antigenic preparations, to follow more standardized procedures. As an example the method of Najarian and associates (1970) with cultured human lymphoblasts may be cited. Horses are injected at intervals of 10 days in multiple intradermal and subcutaneous sites with doses ranging from 1 to 5×10^9 cells; the horse is bled 10 liters after the third and after each successive booster injection over a period of 6 months. The sera obtained in this way contained very low titers of hemagglutinins and thromboagglutinins and could be infused intravenously in patients without any problems. Intravenous, intramuscular, or combinations of subcutaneous and intravenous injections have been employed by others (Iwasaki *et al.*, 1967; Pichlmayr, 1970; Perper *et al.*, 1970a,b; Woiwod, 1970; Traeger *et al.*, 1970a,b).

A number of investigators have employed Freund's complete or incomplete adjuvant in the preparation of antisera to be used in rodents (Nagaya and Sieker, 1965; Gray *et al.*, 1966; Denman *et al.*, 1967; Guttmann *et al.*, 1967a; Boak *et al.*, 1967; Kinne and Simmons, 1967; Skamene, 1970; Sterling *et al.*, 1970), dogs (Monaco *et al.*, 1966c) and also antihuman ALS (Monaco *et al.*, 1967b; Carraz *et al.*, 1967; Traeger *et al.*, 1968a, 1970a;

Pichlmayr, 1970; Cohen and Sell, 1970; Woiwod, 1970). Other adjuvants have also been used, such as aluminum hydroxide (Jooste *et al.*, 1968) or killed *Corynebacterium parvum* (Butler *et al.*, 1970). Experience with rabbit antimouse ALS has shown that the use of adjuvants is ill-advised because a possible increase in activity is obtained at the expense of an increased production of toxic and irrelevant antibodies (Jooste *et al.*, 1968; Taub and Lance, 1968a; Koumans and Burke, 1969). This conclusion is, however, not shared by other investigators (Davis *et al.*, 1969; Wood and Vriesendorp, 1969; Sterling *et al.*, 1970; Skamene, 1970) who did not find that adjuvants exerted adverse effects on the quality of the sera. Differences in experimental procedures preclude significant comparisons; for instance, the discrepancy in the results on the possible toxicity of adjuvant-induced sera as observed by Wood and Vriesendorp and by Koumans and Burke who employed similar procedures for the preparation of ALS, may be attributed not only to inherent differences in sensitivity of the animal species investigated (mouse vs. guinea pig) but also to the dosage of antigen injected, which was much higher in the case of the latter group of authors. Extrapolations of immunization schedules from species to species are difficult both in theory and practice. It is obvious, therefore, that only a concerted effort in which the effect of single variables (presence or absence of adjuvants, high or low doses an antigen, etc.) in one animal species will help to clarify this complex problem. Also, as to the use of adjuvants, it may be worth mentioning that increased toxicity has not been observed in primates injected with well-absorbed antihuman ALS prepared with Freund's adjuvant (Balner, 1970a; Pichlmayr, 1970).

That the use of adjuvants produces qualitatively different antibody populations (White *et al.*, 1963) may be of importance in ALS production; for instance, James (1970) has observed that Freund's complete adjuvant stimulates in horses the formation of γ_2, complement-fixing antibodies, whereas without adjuvants or with different adjuvants, the antibodies are often of the γ_1, noncomplement-fixing type. Lymphotoxicity, which requires complement, is regarded by many as important for the *in vivo* activity of ALS. In addition, the use of purer antigenic preparations should reduce the risk of an increase in undesired contaminating antibodies in the antiserum.

A related important aspect of ALS production is represented by the so-called "decay phenomenon" to which attention was originally drawn by Levey and Medawar (1966a). These authors pointed out that sera obtained after prolonged immunization, although often containing high titers of lymphoagglutinating and cytotoxic antibodies, display lower immunosuppressive activity than earlier bleedings from the same animal. This decline has been attributed to changes in physical characteristics of the antibodies or to a progressively higher interference by antibodies directed against minor and nonrelevant antigenic constituents of the immunizing inoculum. This observation was subsequently confirmed in the rabbit antimouse system by other groups (Jeejeebhoy, 1967a; Jooste *et al.*, 1968; Sutthiwan *et al.*, 1969; Wood and Vriesendorp, 1969; Lance and Medawar, 1970b). Perper *et al.* (1969, 1970b) have shown that the immunosuppressive potency of horse antirat ALS decreased, whereas the anti-inflammatory activity increased as immunization proceeded. Anti-inflammatory potency of rat spleen-immunized horses reflected the toxicity of the serum, but this effect was not observed with thymus-induced serum. Progressive loss of immunosuppresive activity with time does not appear to be a function of antigen type but of the immunization method. On the contrary, it is possible that the increase in anti-inflammatory activity and development of toxicity are related to the immunogen (Perper *et al.*, 1970b). Whether this phenomenon is of general importance in all animal species is still unclear. Starzl, Traeger, Najarian, and their co-workers have frequently used with success antisera obtained from horses immunized for many months; and Clunie *et al.* (1968) found good immunosuppressive activity in sera drawn from horses that were stimulated for 3 years. However, examples of decay have also been observed in horse antihuman ALS (Balner, 1970a; James *et al.*, 1970), a system in which immunization lasting many months and even years has been often employed. Therefore for economic and practical considerations, less intensive courses of immunization may be desirable. The effect of employing adjuvants on the decline in immunosuppressive activity has as yet not been completely clarified. The majority of investigators seem to agree that adjuvant-induced antisera do not decay as immunization proceeds (Wood and Vriesendorp, 1969; Lance *et al.*, 1970; Skamene, 1970; Zola *et al.*, 1971), although Davis *et al.* (1969) noted a loss of potency in antisera prepared with adjuvant.

III. Characterization and Purification of Antilymphocytic Antibody

In view of the complexity and heterogeneity of many immunizing preparations and because of the presence on lymphocytes of antigens in common with other cellular elements, ALS must be regarded as a complex mixture of antibodies of different specificities. The percentage of antibodies able specifically to bind *in vitro* to lymphocytes present in rabbit antimouse ALS, prepared by the two-pulse procedure, represented approximately only 5% of the total IgG molecules (Spreafico, 1970). Through purification procedures, preparations are thus obtained which maintain the entire immunosuppressive activity with maximally reduced content of contaminating antibodies and proteins. These substances are not only irrelevant to the immunosuppressive activity but also potentially or actually toxic. The most important of the contaminating antibodies are those directed against erythrocytes and platelets; their titers can vary markedly in the different preparations, depending mainly on the purity of antigen employed and the type of immunization followed. However, it is to be noted that high titers of hemagglutinins can be found even in sera prepared with very pure antigen such as thoracic duct lymphocytes. The high levels of antierythrocyte and antiplatelet antibodies as well as anticollagen activity are responsible for the frequent toxicity of antispleen ALS in clinical use; the toxicity of some peripheral blood lymphocyte antisera has also been attributed to their antiplatelet activity (James *et al.*, 1970). *In vitro* cultured lymphoblasts, however, have given sera with quite low hemagglutinin and thrombocytopenic activity, which can be absorbed without difficulty (Najarian and Simmons, 1971). Reactivity of ALS has also been described with mast cells, granulocytes, fibroblasts (Thorsby and Lie, 1968), epithelial cells (Milgrom, 1970), and hemopoietic cells (Field and Gibbs, 1968), and a cross-reactivity with macrophages is still under discussion (Jasin *et al.*, 1969; MacLaurin and Humm, 1970; Hughes, 1970).

Many antisera directed against lymphoid tissue of rodents, dogs, and humans show reactivity, using various methods, with nonlymphoid organs such as liver, kidney, lung, stomach, gut, muscle, and nervous tissue (Lawson, 1967; Lindquist *et al.*, 1969; Skamene and Russell, 1971; Oliver and Feldman, 1971). Some of this reactivity has to be attributed to antibodies reacting with serum proteins present in the organ homogenates, but other, most probably species-specific antibodies are certainly present; in other words, on the lymphocyte membrane there are lymphocyte-specific as well as species-specific antigens which are common to other cell types. The relative importance of antispecies as opposed to antilymphocyte antibodies in immunosuppression is a point of considerable interest. Suffice it here to say that ALS deprived of its antispecies antibodies still retains strong immunosuppressive activity, but antisera prepared against other cells, such as the liver, although showing lymphotoxicity *in vitro*, are not immunosuppressive *in vivo*. Antibodies present in ALS directed against histocompatibility antigens do not appear to play a role in immunosuppression (Shigeno *et al.*, 1968) and only absorption with lymphoid tissue completely abolishes the immunosuppressive activity of ALS.

Antibodies against serum proteins are also frequently detected in ALS. In horse antihuman ALS, James and his group (1970) have observed the presence of high levels of antibodies directed against IgM and IgG, albumin, fibrinogen, transferrin, β-lipo- and glycoproteins, haptoglobins as well as, although in lower amounts, against plasminogen, α_1-glycoproteins, α_1-antitrypsin, and prealbumin. The importance of these antibodies in antiserum toxicity is not yet precisely known, although it is possible that they contribute to some of the clinically observed complications, for instance coagulation disturbances or kidney damage.

Two approaches can be followed in attempting to reduce if not eliminate the contaminating antibodies in ALS. The first is obviously represented by the use of purer antigenic preparations with rationalized immunization procedures—a subject that has already been examined; the second consists of the selective absorption and fractionation of the antiserum. Whereas ALS intended for use in experimental animals can often be employed without purification or extensive absorption, isolation of the immunoglobulins and removal of the most important contaminant antibodies are absolute requirements for antisera prepared for clinical administration. In spite of possible risks inherent in purification procedures (besides their cost in time and labor), which include bacterial contamination, protein denaturation with loss of activity, and aggregate formation, the advantages of using purified serum fractions seem clear in that injection of high quantities of nonantibody protein potentially toxic and in any case antigenic, is avoided.

Antilymphocytic immunosuppressive antibodies can be of the IgM class (Brambilla *et al.*, 1968; Spreafico, 1968; Mandel and Asofsky, 1968); however, by far the majority of these antibodies are of the IgG class in rabbit (James and Anderson, 1967; James and Medawar, 1967; Monaco *et al.*, 1966b, 1967b; James, 1969) and goat sera (Starzl *et al.*, 1970a). For horse antidog serum, the lymphopenia-producing activity (which may not be representative of the immunosuppressive activity) was found to be localized in IgG (Fateh-Moghadam *et al.*, 1967). This is of great practical importance since γG globulins are easier to purify and more stable than other immunoglobulins; moreover, Kashiwagi *et al.* (1968) have observed that the risk of becoming sensitized to horse IgG is much less than to other serum globulins. Thus, it is apparent that studies on the distribution of immunosuppressive activity among the different fractions and subfractions are of great practical and theoretical importance; the removal of inactive fractions may contribute to the reduction of complications in the clinical use of ALS. Furthermore, investigations of preparations with different chemical and biological effects could help in elucidating the mode of action of antilymphocytic serum. Also in horse antimonkey ALS, the immunosuppressive activity was exclusively present in the IgG fraction (Betel *et al.*, 1970), but other groups have reported that antilymphocytic activity in equine sera has a larger spread in the 7 S γ-globulin fraction, at least during the first months of immunization (Carraz *et al.*, 1967; Iwasaki *et al.*, 1967; Pichlmayr *et al.*, 1968b). Starzl *et al.* (1970a) found that in equine antidog sera the lymphocytotoxic activity was almost exclusively present in the IgG ("slow" γG), whereas most of the leukoagglutinating activity belonged to the IgA contained in the equine T, also known as "fast" γG, fraction. These authors have also suggested that highly purified horse IgG (ALGG) show lower immunosuppressive activity than the less refined preparations containing the T fraction, which consists mainly of IgA (Starzl *et al.*, 1969a, 1970a). These findings also indicate that different types of antibodies present in different fractions may contribute to the general immunosuppressive activity of ALS. Comparable results for horse antihuman ALS have been observed by James *et al.* (1970). Except for a transient IgM lymphoagglutinin response, the other antilymphocytic activities tested (agglutination, lysis, and blast formation) were found in the 7 S serum fraction; it was also noted that differences existed in the time of appearance of the various antilymphocytic activities, agglutinins being the first to be detected, followed by cytolytic and, finally, by transforming antibodies. In contrast with the findings of Starzl and his group, James and associates (1970) found that all the immunosuppressive activity of horse antirat antilymphocytic IgG was associated with the strongly cytotoxic slow γ components, consisting predominantly of the IgG_a and IgG_b subclasses, whereas the fast γ component, weakly cytotoxic and strongly agglutinating, was not immunosuppressive. Moreover the slow γ_2 fraction readily promoted lymphocytic opsonization, whereas the γ_2 (fast) preparation was relatively ineffective in this regard.

The equine IgG fraction is certainly complex, and the discrepancy in the results may be due not only to differences in immunization schedules but also to the inconsistencies in the methods of fractionation and analysis, as well as to variations in sensitivity to fractionation procedures of antisera among different species (Martin, 1969; Spreafico, 1970). Nevertheless, it is probable that an extension of the studies on the distribution of antilymphocytic antibodies in equine IgG subpopulation will yield results of practical interest for the production of more effective and less toxic preparations. In the aforementioned study by James *et al.* (1970), it was also shown that antibodies against platelets and serum proteins reside in the same 7 S region, but hemagglutinins were predominantly of the IgM class. Therefore reduction in toxicity of ALS cannot be completely achieved by fractionation procedures and the emphasis on using purified antigen is justified. A number of techniques have been described for obtaining bulk quantities of antilymphocytic globulin and γ-globulin, such as precipitation with salts (ammonium or sodium sulfate) or organic solvents (ethanol, ether), ion-exchange or gel filtration chromatography, forced flow electrophoresis. A detailed description and appraisal of the various methods can be found in the review by James (1969), and a flow chart for the preparation of horse antihuman ALGG is presented by Woiwod (1970); Woiwod *et al.* (1970).

In an effort to obtain preparations that contain a maximum amount of active antibodies with a minimum of contaminating substances, thus presenting higher specific activity and fewer inconveniences for clinical application, a purification procedure has been developed by an absorption–elution technique, of specifically antilymphocytic, rabbit antimouse antibodies (Spreafico, 1970). The possible therapeutic use of such preparations, substantially enriched in antilymphocytic antibodies (these eluates were 8-10 times more effective *in vivo* than the starting pure ALS IgG fraction) is certainly of interest. The procedure can be adapted to large-scale production, although a number of practical problems have to be solved.

Since it is known that human toxicity of horse globulin against bacterial antigens could be effectively reduced by pepsin treatment, James and his group (1969) have tested the activities of divalent $F(ab')_2$ and univalent Fab′ antibody fragments, i.e. antibody molecules containing, respectively, two and one antibody-combining sites but lacking the complement-binding Fc portion of the molecule. These antibody fragments, although able to combine with the lymphocytes and to agglutinate them in the case of the divalent fragment, are not cytotoxic and not immunosuppressive.

Antilymphocytic immunoglobulin purification involves absorption of the most important extraneous antibodies. First it is necessary to remove antierythrocyte activity the titer of which must be lower than 1:16–1:8 in order to avoid hemolytic reactions upon injection in man. This is not easily accomplished, since high quantities of cells are often required, for instance, in Taylor's (1970a) experience up to 40 gm of erythrocyte stroma per liter of serum were necessary. Hemagglutinin absorption is easier if done on already purified material since a great part of the IgM anti-red-cell antibodies have already been removed in the process of serum fractionation. The simultaneous purification of 7 S globulins and removal of hemagglutinins by the use of DEAE–cellulose columns into which erythrocyte stroma have been incorporated, has recently been proposed by Monaco (1970a). The injection of preformed antibodies against erythrocytes and platelets during immunization may also help in reducing the levels of these antibodies. Absorption of antiplatelet activity to reasonable levels is also often difficult and time consuming but frequently necessary because of their high levels; a method for the quantitative evaluation of antiplatelet activity in ALS has been described (Kamoun and Hamburger, 1970). Indications of this type of activity in antihuman ALS can also be given by a drop in thrombocyte count in the mouse (Woiwod *et al.*, 1970). Many researchers absorb antilymphocytic preparations with whole serum, liver, and kidney of the lymphoid antigen donor species in the intent of diminishing the potential toxicity of ALS, but a reduction in immunosuppressive activity has occasionally been observed (Iwasaki *et al.*, 1967; Jeejeebhoy, 1967a). The possibility has also been advanced that the non-antilymphocytic antibodies present in ALS might not only have a detrimental effect but also might play an active role in the complex biological activity of ALS, for instance, acting in various ways on the chain of inflammatory events activated by the antigen–antibody reaction. Anticomplement antibodies may cause a reduction in those immunological and inflammatory reactions that depend on complement components for their development. Also, as proposed by Turk (1970), a similar effect might result from antibodies reacting with serum globulins which may act as precursors or carriers of pharmacological agents involved in inflammation. Because platelets seem to be implicated in at least some types of graft rejection (Gewurz *et al.*, 1966; Rosenberg *et al.*, 1971), some antithrombocyte activity might also be of some benefit.

IV. *In Vitro* Activities of Antilymphocytic Serum

Antilymphocytic antibodies combine with lymphocytes *in vitro* as has been shown by immunofluorescence (Levey and Medawar, 1967; Russell and Monaco, 1967; Brent *et al.*, 1968) and with labeled antibodies (Woodruff *et al.*, 1967; Lance, 1969a; Skamene, 1970; Spreafico, 1970). The consequences of this combination vary according to the experimental condition.

A. Leukoagglutination

Antilymphocytic sera cause leukoagglutination; it has been reported that the titer is higher with whole leukocytes as compared to purified lymphocytes (Dormont *et al.*, 1969)—a finding that is not observed in cytotoxicity where lymphocytes are clearly more sensitive than other leukocytes (Thorsby and Lie, 1968). A high variability in agglutinating and cytotoxic activities has been observed against cells of different individuals (Putnam *et al.*, 1967), but this result has not been confirmed (Thorsby and Lie, 1968; Bach and Antoine, 1968). A number of authors have, in fact, shown that, in the mouse, rat, and man, ALS is essentially species-specific (Gray *et al.*, 1966; Lawson, 1967), although cross-reactivities with related species can be observed as well as variations of activity within the same species (Iwasaki *et al.*, 1967; Caspary *et al.*, 1971). Antilymphocytic antibody divalent fragments $F(ab')_2$ are able to combine with and agglutinate the antigen, whereas the univalent Fab′ derivative is capable of combining with but incapable of agglutinating the cells.

B. Lymphocytotoxicity

When lymphocytes are incubated with ALS in the presence of complement, cell lysis occurs as observed by various techniques, the most sensitive being the determination of ^{51}Cr release from the damaged cells. The anatomical basis for cell lysis is analogous to that observed for erythrocytes and consists of the production of holes in the cytoplasmic membrane (Clarke *et al.*, 1968; Schrek *et al.*, 1969). Divalent as well as univalent antilymphocytic antibody fragments, lacking the complement-fixing portion of the molecule, are not cytotoxic; the same is true for avian antirodent ALS since these sera are incapable of fixing mammalian complement. In the determination of the lymphotoxic titer of ALS, care should be taken to employ serum of the cell donor species as source of complement, since there is considerable interspecies variation regarding the lytic efficiency of complement. This is, however, not usually done and for horse antihuman ALS, rabbit serum is considered the most active source of complement. Lymphocytes are more sensitive to the cytotoxic action of ALS than other white cells; toxicity against polymorphs can be removed by prior absorption of the serum with red cells (Thorsby and Lie, 1968). It has been reported that there is a variation in sensitivity among lymphoid cells of different origin, antithymocyte sera being more active on thymocytes than on splenic and lymph node cells (Reif, 1963; Potworoski and Nairn, 1967; Grabar *et al.*, 1968). It is known that thymocytes possess specific antigens in addition to those in common with the general lymphoid population (Boyse *et al.*, 1968; Raff, 1969).

C. Lymphocyte Transformation

The combination of ALS with lymphocytes in culture causes the transformation of these cells into blastoid elements; the percentage of this transformation, which can be objectively quantitated by measuring the incorporation of labeled uridine or thymidine in RNA and DNA, is usually high, similar to that obtained with PHA stimulation, and is proportional, within limits, to the concentration of the antibody in the medium (Grasbeck *et al.*, 1964; Greaves *et al.*, 1967; Ling *et al.*, 1967). However, the dose–

effect relationship is not a simple one (Southworth *et al.*, 1970; Bach and Bach, 1970; James, 1970) since high concentrations of serum can exert an inhibitory effect. A limited period of contact (15 minutes) with ALS is sufficient to cause transformation, but the longer the time of contact the greater the degree of change (Holt *et al.*, 1966). Peak transformation is observed on the third to fifth day of culture, i.e., earlier than in antigen-stimulated cultures. Morphologically the blasts induced by ALS do not show differences from those obtained with other specific (antigens) or nonspecific stimulants such as PHA. Transformation does not require complement which, by inducing lysis, reduces transformation; however, for noncytotoxic but still stimulating ALS concentrations, complement seems to exert a synergistic effect (Holt *et al.*, 1966). Marked variability in transforming capacity of different antisera can be observed, but significant individual differences in the cell sensitivity have not been found (Ling *et al.*, 1967). Antilymphocytic antibody-induced transformation is not due to anti-immunoglobulin antibodies present in the antisera (Foerster *et al.*, 1969) nor to antiallotype antibodies (Knight and Ling, 1967). It also appears not to be caused by simple protein accumulation on lymphocyte membrane since rheumatoid factor does not enhance transformation (Holt *et al.*, 1966); furthermore, there is no correlation between agglutinating and stimulating activities. The antibodies responsible for this phenomenon are present in the 7 S region and can be separated from those showing cytotoxic or agglutinating activity, because fractions that have a high degree of cytotoxic and agglutinating activity are poorly transforming. On dilution, however, their lymphostimulating activity can increase (James *et al.*, 1970), and whether this is due to the presence of inhibitors, to feedback inhibition, or to other reasons is not known. In the serum of horses immunized with human lymphoid cells, transforming activity appeared later than lymphoagglutinins and lysins. Again, whether this is due to a real delay in the formation of antibodies of a special class or subclass, affinity, or specificity or whether other antilymphyocytic activities masked their existence in earlier bleeds of the serum, is not known. Univalent antilymphocytic antibody fragments do not induce lymphotransformation, whereas the divalent fragments are lymphotransforming (James, 1969).

In addition to inducing lymphostimulation, ALS interferes with the action of other specific and nonspecific lymphocyte stimulants, such as PHA, (Mosedale *et al.*, 1968), tuberculin (Greaves *et al.*, 1967; Eysvoogel *et al.*, 1969), or in mixed lymphocyte cultures (Greaves *et al.*, 1967). These interactions have recently been investigated by Moller (1970) who has shown that the simultaneous stimulation of lymphocytes with two nonspecific mitogens or with a nonspecific stimulant together with an antigen, will result in synergy when both agents are present in suboptimal concentrations, whereas antagonism will result whenever optimal amounts of the two stimuli are employed. The hypothesis has, therefore, been put forward that the cell will be transformed and synthesize DNA when a minimum critical number, the lower threshold, of membrane receptors has been triggered, but failure to transform will occur when the number of activated sites is above a critical maximum number, the higher threshold. Within these two limits it would appear that the lymphocyte responds only to the number of activated sites, disregarding the quality of these sites; in other words, it does not discriminate between specific (i.e., antigenic) and nonspecific stimuli.

D. Other *In Vitro* Activities

Another important *in vitro* activity of ALS is its inhibitory effect on immunologically active cells. *In vitro* incubation with high doses of ALS in the presence of complement reduces the number of spleen hemolytic plaque-forming cells (Allen *et al.*, 1969; Ogburn *et al.*, 1969); the experimental conditions employed are such that this suppressive activity can easily be referred to a cytotoxic effect. Coating of the lymphocyte membrane and consequent prevention of contact between membrane receptors and antigen, is probably the mechanism by which ALS inhibits the cytotoxicity displayed by activated lymphocytes on target cells (Holm and Perlman, 1969; Holm, 1969; Lundgren, 1969); a situation that may be regarded as a model for the effector mechanism of allograft rejection.

Lymphocytes from normal, nonimmunized mice and humans can form "rosettes" when incubated with sheep erythrocytes; this immunocytoadherence phenomenon presumably is the result of a "natural" antibody on the lymphocyte membrane which has specificity or cross-reactivity for the sheep red cells. In contrast to ALS resistance by rosette-forming cells of immunized animals, upon preincubation with the lymphocytes ALS can inhibit spontaneous rosette formation at very low concentrations, much lower than those showing detectable agglutination or cytotoxicity. Inhibition of rosette formation by ALS can be observed in complement-free medium; sensitivity, however, is greatly increased by the presence of complement (Bach, 1970a; Bach and Antoine, 1968; Bach *et al.*, 1969a,b). This ALS inhibition is attributed to coating of the lymphocyte surface by antibodies present in the antiserum which block the membrane receptors. Anti-immunoglobulin antibodies appear to be responsible for the rosette inhibition obtained in complement-free medium, since this inhibition is no longer observed when ALS is absorbed with the host's serum. On the other hand, inhibition in the presence of complement is not due to the anti-immunoglobulin activity of ALS, and a mechanism of nonlethal cell toxicity has been suggested (Bach, 1970a). The interest in this inhibitory activity of ALS rests on the demonstration that a good correlation exists between the graft-prolonging capacity of ALS and its rosette inhibitory activity *in vitro*. Greaves *et al.* (1969) have also shown that the incubation of lymphocytes with very low concentrations of antilymphocytic serum in the presence of complement, will lead to opsonisation of the lymphocytes as evidenced by attachment to and phagocytosis by macrophage monolayers. It has been suggested (Bach *et al.*, 1970) that this activity is mediated by cytophilic antibodies present in ALS, i.e., by antibodies having antibody specificity for lymphocytes in their Fab part of the molecule and "cytophilic" specificity for the macrophages in their Fc portion.

Electrophoretic mobility of lymphocytes is reduced by ALS (Bert *et al.*, 1970; Phondke *et al.*, 1970) presumably because of the neutralization of the ionogenic groups as a result of the interaction of surface antigen with antibody. Stimulation by ALS of adenyl cyclase in lysates of human peripheral lymphocytes has also been observed (Colobert, 1970) as well as modifications in amino acid uptake (Betuel *et al.*, 1970).

V. *In Vivo* Effects of Antilymphocytic Serum

A. Effect on Circulating Lymphocytes

The injection of ALS in animals and in man is followed by a decrease in the number of circulating lymphocytes; the fall is rapid and reaches its peak within 1 hour after intravenous injections and in approximately 6 hours using the intraperitoneal or subcutaneous routes. The degree of lymphopenia can be very marked, down to 1% of normal levels (Monaco *et al.*, 1966b), but, in general, it is not absolute. Its duration after single injections is variable from few hours to 2 to 3 weeks; with chronic schedules of treatment long-lasting lymphopenia is observed, and approximately 2 weeks are needed in the mouse before a return to normal values is seen (Gray *et al.*, 1966). A higher degree of lymphopenia is observed in animals immunologically tolerant to the heterologous antilymphocytic globulins (Denman and Frenkel, 1967) as well as in thymectomized animals in whom longer periods for a return to normal limits are also required (Monaco *et al.*, 1965b). The lymphopenic effect of ALS is proportional to the injected dose (Sacks *et al.*, 1964) which can explain the tendency of lymphocyte levels to rise on prolonged treatment since it is customary to reduce progressively the frequency of administration. On prolonged treatment, a change in the type of circulating lymphocytes can be observed (Denman *et al.*, 1968a; Taub, 1969) due to the prevalence in the blood of short-lived small lymphocytes, together with the appearance of immature-looking lymphoid elements, the level of which can occasionally reach 20% of the total lymphocytes (Taub and Lance, 1968b; Dormont *et al.*, 1969). Parallel to the fall in circulating elements, a reduction in the number of lymphocytes in the thoracic duct is found (Agnew, 1968), where many damaged elements or cells coated by the heterologous globulins can be observed. It is important to note that the reduction in the cellular output from the duct persits even when the total blood lymphocyte level has returned to normal.

Lymphopenia has to be regarded as a specific effect of ALS, and it is not simply due to stress since it is only slightly influenced by adrenalectomy, and normal nonantilymphocytic serum it is not or very poorly lymphopenic, but is caused by a direct and/or indirect cytocidal activity of ALS. The phenomenon appears to be complement-dependent as indicated by the fact that the antilymphocytic antibody fragments $F(ab')_2$ are not lymphopenic (Anderson *et al.*, 1967). Associated with the fall in circulating lymphocytes are a prompt and marked, although transient, reduction in blood complement levels (Guttmann *et al.*, 1967b) and a rise in the urinary excretion of uric acid as seen in patients undergoing ALS therapy (Monaco *et al.*, 1967b). The antibodies responsible for this effect are at least in part different from those inducing agglutination and cytotoxicity since there is no strict correlation between these activities (Jeejeebhoy, 1967a,b; Jeejeebhoy and Vela-Martinez, 1968). A direct relationship between the degree of lymphopenic and immunosuppressive activities was observed by Lawson (1967) and by Kinne and Simmons (1967) but has not been confirmed by the majority of investigators (Jeejeebhoy and Vela-Martinez, 1968; Shanfield *et al.*, 1968; Dormont *et al.*, 1969; Taub and Lance, 1968a). A coincident return to normal values of circulating lymphocytes with the reappearance of immunological reactivity after the suspension of ALS administration has been described (Lawson, 1967), but this finding has not been confirmed by others (Abaza *et al.*, 1966; Rule and Judd, 1968). Changes regarding other blood elements can also be observed after injection of ALS. A transient fall in the number of polymorphs has been found in animals and man (Pichlmayr *et al.*, 1967; Lawrence *et al.*, 1968), occasionally followed by granulocytosis with myeloid hyperplasia during prolonged treatments (Lawson, 1967; Russell and Monaco, 1967; Starzl *et al.*, 1967b; De Mesteer *et al.*, 1968). Thrombocytopenia as a consequence of contaminating antibodies has been recorded (Balner and Dersjant,

1967; Starzl *et al.*, 1967a; Calne *et al.*, 1968; Kashiwagi *et al.*, 1968; Woodruff *et al.*, 1969; Najarian and Simmons, 1971), especially with antisera to human spleen. This represented a major problem in early human ALS therapy, occasionally causing severe hemorrhagic syndromes; however, with the use of more refined antisera, as already discussed, such profound drops in platelet numbers are no longer observed, although a reduction is still often seen, possibly due to the sharing of antigens between lymphocytes and platelets. Anemia of moderate degree has also been noticed in animals receiving unabsorbed antisera (Balner and Dersjant, 1967; Lance, 1968a; Shanfield *et al.*, 1968), and reports of its occurrence in humans have also been recorded.

B. Effect on Lymphoid Organs*

The early descriptions of histological modifications of lymphoid organs by ALS are somewhat confusing, the contradictory results being attributable to the differences in the experimental conditions concerning the type of treatment, animal species, and quality of the antiserum and to the lack of distinction between specific and nonspecific effects of ALS. General agreement has now been reached that ALS induces quite selective morphological alterations in lymphoid organs. (Turk and Willoughby, 1967, 1969; Taub and Lance, 1968a; Baroni *et al.*, 1969; Everett *et al.*, 1970; Turk, 1970). The most prominent change is represented by a marked depletion of small lymphocytes from the paracortical areas of the lymph nodes and from periarteriolar cuffs of the spleen. In these areas early signs of cell death can be seen as well as macrophages engulfing lymphocytes, and eventually reticulohistiocytes with marked phagocytic activity replace the lymphocytes. Pronounced phagocytosis of small lymphocytes by macrophages in the cortical lymph sinuses as well as at the corticomedullary junction, especially in relation to the postcapillary zones, is also found in the nodes. In contrast, germinal centers and medullary areas in the lymph nodes and follicular areas in the spleen are as a rule, unaffected by ALS as well as the proliferation of plasma cells in the medullary cords and in the corticomedullary zone. The last element of the characteristic triad of ALS-induced histological modifications is represented by the fact that thymus histology is not significantly altered. Sera containing high titers of toxic antibodies may induce extensive and generalized depletion of lymphocytes in lymph nodes, spleen, and thymus, but these lesions should be considered nonspecific and extraneous to the immunosuppressive activity of ALS.

* See, also, the article by G. R. F. Krueger, "Morphology of Chemical Immunosuppression" in this volume.

The above-mentioned selective histological changes can be detected in the lymph nodes within a few days after a single, active dose of antiserum, whereas those in the spleen usually require a more prolonged treatment to become observable; lymphocyte depletion is more profound if ALS is given to thymectomized animals (Monaco *et al.*, 1965a). Transformation of some lymphocytes of the long-lived variety into blasts can also be noted in these organs (Tyler *et al.*, 1969; Everett *et al.*, 1970), a finding also observed, although to a lesser extent, in animals treated with normal heterologous immunoglobulins. After chronic ALS administration, lymphoid depletion can be obscured by hyperplasia and hypertrophy of germinal centers, medullary and follicular zones (Taub and Lance, 1968a), originally considered by some authors to be the most distinctive changes induced by ALS (Levey and Medawar, 1966a,c; Pichlmayr *et al.*, 1967; Iwasaki *et al.*, 1967). This change has to be considered as a nonspecific feature representing the morphological equivalent of the immune response of the host against the heterologous proteins constituting ALS, in fact these changes are not observed if ALS is injected in animals previously rendered tolerant to the foreign immunoglobulins.

According to the majority of investigators, the thymus is not modified histologically by ALS. A modest reduction in the number of small lymphocytes has been observed by some (Gray *et al.*, 1966; Nagaya and Sieker, 1965, 1967; Denman and Frenkel, 1968a,b), but the specificity of this finding is questionable. The great sensitivity of thymus to the action of endotoxins is known (Landy *et al.*, 1965).

Lymphopoiesis in the lymphoid organs is not decreased by ALS; on the contrary, an increase of possible compensatory origin, in the production of cells, mainly of short-lived lymphocytes, is observed (Denman and Frenkel, 1968a,b; Denman *et al.*, 1968a; Leuchars *et al.*, 1968; Taub, 1969, 1970). As regards other lymphoid organs, Peyer's patches are also depleted in lymphocytes after ALS administration (Gray *et al.*, 1966), whereas the changes in bone marrow are more complex. A moderate and transitory drop in total cell number of bone marrow is observed together with a considerable reduction in the number of lymphoid elements (De Mesteer *et al.*, 1968; Baroni *et al.*, 1969) and erythroblastopenia (Rodriguez-Paradisi *et al.*, 1971), regardless whether or not ALS was contaminated by hemagglutinins. In the study by Rodriguez-Paradisi, myelocytes and neutrophilic and eosinophilic granulocytes increased in the marrow, but Harris *et al.* (1969) found that these cells decreased. Erythroblastosis in the spleen is a frequent finding on prolonged treatment of mice with ALS (Taub and Lance, 1968a); stem cells, megakaryocytes, and myeloid elements also increase in the spleen (Ledney, 1967; De Mesteer *et al.*,

1968; Rodriguez-Paradisi *et al.*, 1971), perhaps to compensate the lympho-erythroblastomegakaryocytopenia of the bone marrow.

The implications of the histological changes in lymphoid organs caused by ALS on understanding the mode of ALS action are discussed in Section VII.

No significant modifications have been observed in nonlymphoid organs (except in the kidneys) of animals submitted to ALS treatment, although critical studies have not yet been performed. Signs of myocardial and hepatic necrosis have in a few instances been detected (Iwasaki *et al.*, 1967; Pichlmayr *et al.*, 1967; Lawson *et al.*, 1967) but were considered as expressions of terminal infections and not directly caused by ALS, or as a result of cross-reacting antibodies. Hydropic degeneration of the pancreas, submucosal edema of the large intestine, and interstitial myocarditis with mononuclear infiltration were occasionally observed by Cohen *et al.* (1970) in mice of some strains submitted to long treatments with ALS prepared with adjuvants; no pulmonary lesions were described. Continuous life-long treatment of mice with ALS did not significantly influence development, weight gain, the reproductive capacity (Nehlsen, 1971). Changes in the kidney may frequently follow therapeutic treatments with ALS, directly attributable to the use of heterologous globulins and to cross-reacting antibodies. The lesions which consist of glomerular membrane thickening, increased mesangial matrix, adhesions between tufts and capsules, epithelial crescents with subendothelial and subepithelial deposits of immunoglobulins, can progress to obliteration of capillary lumen, fibrotic and fibrinoid alterations, hyalinization, and complete loss of structure of the glomerulus (Lindquist *et al.*, 1969; Cohen *et al.*, 1970). These changes are further discussed in Sections VIII and IX.

C. Immunosuppressive Activity of Antilymphocytic Serum

This is by far the most important of the biological activities of ALS: it can be affirmed that this agent by inhibiting an extensive array of immune phenomena, is certainly the most powerful, least toxic, and the only real specific immunosuppressant now available.

1. *Effect on Allograft Survival*

Although attempts to prolong skin allograft survival by using ALS had previously been made (Waksman *et al.*, 1961), the first really significant results showing the remarkable immunosuppressive activity of ALS were obtained by Woodruff and Anderson (1963a,b, 1964) who were able to prolong the survival of first-set skin allografts in rats across a strong histocompatibility barrier. These findings have since been confirmed by many investigators and extended to other animal species such as mice, rabbits, pigs, and monkeys (Gray *et al.*, 1964; Monaco *et al.*, 1965a,b; Jeejeebhoy, 1965a,b, 1967a,b; Nagaya and Sieker, 1965; Levey and Medawar, 1966a,b,c; Brent *et al.*, 1967; Grogan and Hardy, 1967; Govallo and Kosmiadi, 1968; Lucke *et al.*, 1968). Skin allograft survival is in fact the most common assay of the immunosuppressive activity of antisera employed for experimental purposes. Of special interest in this connection is that antihuman ALS will prolong skin graft survival exchanged between subhuman primates (Balner *et al.*, 1968a,b), a finding which forms the basis of a test for the measurement of the immunosuppressive activity of antisera to be used in the clinic.

For comparative purposes, the effect of 600 R whole-body irradiation in prolonging mouse skin allograft can be easily matched by 0.25 ml of a potent ALS, and only procarbazine can be, under some conditions, as effective as ALS (Stewart and Cohen, 1969).

The immunosuppressive effect is most evident when antiserum is started prior to grafting and can be further increased if the injections are continued after transplantation; the superior results obtained with pretreatment have clearly been shown also in the transplantation of other organs (Huntley *et al.*, 1966; Starzl *et al.*, 1967a; Clunie *et al.*, 1968; Monaco and Franco, 1969). However, ALS treatment is effective also when initiated after grafting; as an example, Levey and Medawar (1966b,c), giving only two injections of 0.5 ml of ALS on the second and fifth days after grafting, obtained more than 100 days survival of mouse skin transplanted across the H-2 histocompatibility barrier, whereas the mean survival time in controls was 10 days. Ono *et al.* (1969b) have observed that an immunosuppressive effect could be found even when ALS was started 5 days after heart transplantation in rabbits. Skin homograft acceptance can be rendered indefinite as long as treatment is continued and during this period the grafted skin appears healthy and does not show histological signs of rejection. However, the duration of the immune unresponsiveness obtained even with prolonged courses of ALS is not usually indefinite and slowly wanes after discontinuation of treatment until rejection occurs. Generally speaking, the activity of ALS is preventing or delaying allograft rejection can be regarded as dose-dependent; the higher the dosage, the longer the survival. Under the experimental conditions used, it does not appear that there exists a threshold above which no further effect is observed and a hyperbolic dose–response curve is obtained (Spreafico, 1971). As expected, therefore, more pronounced effects are obtained (Lance, 1968a) when the same total dose is given in repeated subdivided doses rather than in larger amounts at longer intervals; this is presumably attributable to the fact that the target cells for ALS action are susceptible only during part of their existence, namely while they are in the periphery and not when in lymphoid organs (see Section VII).

Antilymphocytic serum is capable of reversing established rejection processes and of producing considerable prolongation also of second-set skin allografts (Levey and Medawar, 1966a; Monaco *et al.*, 1966a) as well as of heterografts as shown in mice with human, rat, rabbit, or guinea pig skin grafts (Russell and Monaco, 1967; Lance and Medawar, 1968). Whereas survival of Wistar rat skin to A strain mice is about 7 days, treatment of the mice for 7 days before and after they received the graft, extended the survival to more than 30 days. Such results distinguish ALS from all other immunosuppressive agents so far studied when employed in nontoxic dosages; in addition, they clearly show that ALS can overcome antigenic differences greater than those expected in clinical homotransplantation. Antilymphocytic serum can also prevent the development of sensitization induced by allografts: if the transplanted skin is removed by the fourth day, a second graft from the same donor is then rejected with a primary type of reactivity, whereas an accelerated, second-set rejection is observed in untreated controls (Monaco and Franco, 1969). Immunological memory can also be erased with high doses of ALS as shown by the reversion to a state of virgin reactivity of antiserum-treated animals in which sensitization had been induced by a previous skin graft (Levey and Medawar, 1966a,b; Lance, 1968b). The immunosuppressive activity of ALS is observed irrespective of the route of injection, and it seems that the effect is practically the same by the subcutaneous, intramuscular, intraperitoneal, or intravenous routes; the only report indicating a greater survival of skin allografts in rats with intravenous injections (Dalton *et al.*, 1970), has not been confirmed (Shorter and Elveback, 1970b; Collste *et al.*, 1971).

After the demonstration that ALS delayed skin allograft rejection, its activity was tested in whole-organ transplantation where its immunosuppressive activity was also amply confirmed. Most of the reports have been devoted to ALS effects on renal allotransplants in the rat and on renal and liver grafts in dogs (Abaza *et al.*, 1966; Abbott *et al.*, 1966; Huntley *et al.*, 1966; Mitchell *et al.*, 1966; Monaco *et al.*, 1966c; Atai and Kelly, 1967; Fox *et al.*, 1967; Guttmann *et al.*, 1967a, 1968, 1969; Iwasaki *et al.*, 1967; Lawson *et al.*, 1967; Mikeloff *et al.*, 1967; Pichlmayr *et al.*, 1968a,b; Shanfield *et al.*, 1968; Shorter *et al.*, 1968; Starzl *et al.*, 1967a,b). The results obtained have been quite favorable—in all but one of the reports (Herman and Schloerb, 1967), ALS has been found to prolong the survival of the grafted organ. The extent of survival varied considerably in the different studies, and comparisons are impossible to make, not only because of the differences in type of treatment and potency of the antiserum employed but also because of technical, genetical, and other complicating factors. A detailed discussion of the results obtained is beyond the scope of this presentation and the reader is referred to the original reports for more precise information. As examples, the survival of renal transplants exchanged between untreated beagle dogs is approximately 10 days, whereas survivals longer than 1 year were obtained in animals receiving ALS (Starzl *et al.*, 1967a). Renal function after transplantation across strong histoincompatibility barrier in rats has been prolonged for 1 year with no histological or functional evidence of rejection (Guttmann *et al.*, 1969).

In contrast with the findings that neither divalent nor univalent antilymphocytic antibody fragments were able to prolong skin allografts (Anderson *et al.*, 1967; Riethmüller *et al.*, 1968), it was reported by Guttmann *et al.* (1967b) that large amounts of divalent fragments could prolong renal allografts in the rat. This report could not be subsequently confirmed and, in any case, the degree of immunosuppression observed by Guttmann was much lower than that obtainable with much smaller doses of intact antibody. Guttmann and his group (1967b) observed that rat kidney allografts could also be prolonged by ALS treatment of the donor animal, supposedly through a mechanism of masking by cross-reacting immunoglobulins of the foreign antigens and, thus, preventing both the afferent and efferent phases of the immune response. In Section VII, there is a discussion of this potential mechanism of immunosuppression by ALS.

The number of organs of various species whose survival upon transplantation to histoincompatible recipients has been shown to be prolonged by ALS treatment is very large, ranging from the heart in mice (Judd *et al.*, 1969; Judd and Trentin, 1971), rats (Ono *et al.*, 1969a; Van Bekkum *et al.*, 1969), and dogs (Cachera *et al.*, 1968; Halpern *et al.*, 1969), intestine and lung in dogs (Otte and Grosjean, 1967; Iwahashi *et al.*, 1970; Hardy *et al.*, 1970a), ovarian grafts in rats and mice (Yussman, 1969; Barnes, 1969), corneal homografts in rabbits (Lernor, 1970), goat heart transplanted to calves (Donawick *et al.*, 1971) to baboon kidneys transplanted to macaques (Dubernard *et al.*, 1971).

2. *Effect on Other Cell-Mediated Phenomena*

In addition to the ability to prevent or delay the onset of the immunological reactions leading to the rejection of homografts and to arrest reactions already in progress, ALS is also capable of inhibiting other cell-mediated immune responses. An important example of these phenomena is the GVH reaction which results when immunocompetent cells capable of reacting against the host are injected into recipients incapable of rejecting them.

In general, recipients used in GVH reactions fall in three main categories: newborn animals whose immunocompetence has not yet fully matured; adult animals whose reactivity has been abrogated by irradiation or drugs, and normal adult F_1 hybrids inoculated with cells derived from one of the parental strains. The immunosuppressive effect of ALS has been shown in various experimental systems which lead to a GVH reaction such as the injection of parental strain lymphoid cells in F_1 hybrids (Boak *et al.*, 1967, 1968; Levey and Medawar, 1967; Monaco *et al.*, 1967b; Van der Werf *et al.*, 1968; Van Bekkum *et al.*, 1967; Field and Gibbs, 1968) or the transfer of allogeneic lymphoid to neonatal or lethally irradiated animals (Brent *et al.*, 1967; Ledney and Van Bekkum, 1968; Ledney, 1969; Floersheim and Ruszkiewicz, 1969). It would appear that the GVH reaction can be suppressed by dosages of ALS lower than those needed for prolongation of mouse skin allografts (Mandel and Asofsky, 1968; Tridente and Van Bekkum, 1969). A GVH reaction can be suppressed by treating the lymphoid cell donor with ALS (Lance, 1968a; Ledney and Van Bekkum, 1969) from 24 hours up to 30 to 45 days before cell transfer (Mandel and Asofsky, 1968; Brent *et al.*, 1968). Appropriate timing is an important factor in showing the full immunosuppressive potency of ALS in this condition, since inactivation of the cells seems to occur at different rates in different regions of the donor lymphoid system. *In vitro* incubation with ALS even for very limited periods (5 minutes) in the absence of complement has also been shown to abolish the capacity of lymphoid cells to mount a GVH reaction upon injection (Brent *et al.*, 1967; Field and Gibbs, 1968), although poorer results are obtained as compared with *in vivo* treatments of the cell donor (Ledney and Van Bekkum, 1968). Brent *et al.* (1968) have also shown that by exposing to trypsin the ALS-treated lymphocytes, the cells can be restored to their immune reactivity.

Graft-vs.-host reaction can further be prevented by treating with ALS the lymphoid cell recipient as shown both in mice (Boak *et al.*, 1968; Ledney and Van Bekkum, 1968; Suvatte *et al.*, 1968) and in irradiated monkeys injected with allogeneic bone marrow cells (Balner and Dersjant, 1967; Van Bekkum *et al.*, 1967; Balner *et al.*, 1968b). In these animals, ALS treatment of the recipient animal has been the only way of controlling the secondary disease since neither *in vitro* treatment of the allogeneic cells nor the treatment of the donor were able to reduce GVH significantly. In addition, the use of ALS because of its greater specificity, has made possible results not achievable with chemical immunosuppressants which also act on the hemopoietic elements. In many cases of bone marrow transplantation performed under ALS protection, it could be shown that a state of chimerism or tolerance had been induced (Mandel and Asofsky, 1968; Brent *et al.*, 1968; Suvatte *et al.*, 1968; Seller and Polani, 1969). The importance of these findings, and those of Floersheim and Ruszkiewicz (1969) who, under ALS treatment, were able to graft allogeneic bone marrow in mice previously rendered aplastic with cytotoxics, for the possible clinical application of bone marrow transplantation is evident, and encouraging results have been obtained in the few clinical experiments performed (Mathé *et al.*, 1970).

Antilymphocytic serum is capable of interfering also with localized GVH reactions, such as that observed after injection of heterologous lymphoid cells under the kidney capsule of rats; this ability, as discussed later, has been proposed as an assay for measuring the immunosuppressive activity of the serum. It contrasts with the observations of Jooste *et al.* (1968) that no strict correlation exists between the GVH-depressing and skin graft-prolonging activities of antimouse ALS, Najarian and Simmons (1971) have reported that this test has value for the evaluation of antihuman antisera.

Levey and Medawar (1966a, 1967) demonstrated that anti-guinea-pig ALS could completely abolish all components of the normal and sensitized lymphocyte transfer reactions, which are resistant to other conventional immunosuppressants; this result can be obtained by treating with ALS either the donor or the recipient of the lymphoid cells. Delayed hypersensitivity reactions to a variety of stimuli have been shown to be inhibited by ALS. Following the early reports of Inderbitzin (1956), Wilhelm *et al.* (1958), and Waksman *et al.* (1961), several other investigators have confirmed that, in various animal species including man, ALS can abolish both the induction and the expression of delayed hypersentivity in immune animals to antigens such as tuberculin, ovalbumin, diphteria toxoid, dinitrochlorobenzene, and oxazolone (Nagaya and Sieker, 1965; Russe and Crowle, 1965; Willoughby *et al.*, 1965; Turk and Willoughby, 1967; Balner *et al.*, 1968a; Brunstetter and Claman, 1968; Heise and Weiser, 1970; Nelson, 1970).

As evidenced by Turk (1970; Turk and Willoughby, 1969) the activity of ALS in suppressing the peripheral manifestations of immune reactivity of sensitized animals, is complex. In fact, ALS may contain several antibodies each capable of interfering through different mechanism with the inflammatory manifestations of immune reactions. Antibodies reacting with complement can inhibit both cell-mediated and nonspecific inflammation, whereas others appear to have more specific effects on the expression of cell-mediated responses by interfering with the ability of normal cells of the host to respond to mediators released after the interaction between antigen and sensitized cells. Of importance is also the fact (Turk and Polak, 1969) that ALS can suppress tissue lesions caused by antigen–antibody and complement complexes as examplified by the Arthus reaction. It is now believed (Porter, 1967) that the lesions of rejections in patients already under immunosuppression with chemicals are also due to the formation of immune complexes between humoral antibody and target antigen rather than to exclusively cell-mediated immune reactions. It is well known that complement is involved in the production of these lesions (Cochrane and Dixon, 1969); the reduction of complement levels which can be very marked after antiserum injection, could thus explain the suppressive effect of ALS on the Arthus reaction and account for the reduction of polymorphs in these lesions, complement components being chemotactic for these elements. However, since a reduction of Arthus reaction can also be obtained with Alnex which causes only a slight decrease of complement, interference by ALS with other mediators is probably also operative. Since Alnex contains antibodies reacting with α and β globulins, it has been suggested (Turk, 1970) that these serum proteins may represent precursors or carriers of pharmacological mediators involved in the production of this type of lesion.

3. *Antilymphocytic Serum and Tolerance Induction*

The ultimate goal in clinical transplantation is the induction of a state of specific unresponsiveness of the recipient to the donor antigens. Since in animals tolerance is more easily induced if the antigenic disparity between donor and recipient is limited, the progress being made in histocompatibility typing will facilitate the establishment of tolerance in organ recipients provided that suitable methods become available. Tolerance to tissue allografts can be obtained in animals by the introduction of antigen in periods of either natural or artificial reduced immune reactivity of the host. Antilymphocytic serum, because of its potent immunosuppressive activity, is highly effective in aiding the induction of such a state of immunological tolerance, as first shown by Monaco and his group (1966a) who were able to obtain tolerance to H-2 incompatible skin grafts by the inoculation of high doses of donor lymphoid cells in ALS-treated, thymectomized mice. Adult thymectomized ALS-treated mice of the A strain, injected with 300×10^6 $(A \times C3H)F_1$ hybrid lymphoid cells, showed survivals of C3H skin grafts for more than 100 days, whereas ALS-treated and ALS-thymectomized animals not injected with cells, rejected the homograft in 25 and 60 days, respectively. In a series of careful experiments, Lance and Medawar (1969) observed that tolerance even to xenografts could be obtained in nonthymectomized animals after the administration of ALS in the first week after skin grafting and subsequent inoculation of as few as 25×10^6 F_1 hybrid spleen cells. Tolerance, although transient, has also been obtained in monkeys by the same combination of treatment (Lance and Medawar, 1970a). To obtain tolerance, treatment with ALS must be adequate—in general, the dose required for tolerance induction is the same necessary to abolish immune memory (Lance and Medawar, 1970b). The timing of antigen injection relative to ALS treatment is also crucial, in the sense that antigen must be injected shortly after ALS administration in order to observe a potentiation of allograft survival. However, if antigen is injected before or during ALS treatment, sensitization instead of tolerance can be obtained as evidenced by an accelerated rejection of the skin graft of which the survival is the index of the induced tolerant state. The dosage of antigenic cells injected is also important, the probability of tolerance induction being proportional to the number of cells injected. With inocula of over 100×10^6 cells, tolerance is consistently obtained and in some strain combinations, homograft survival may last throughout the lifetime of the recipient. Also, a very low number of cells have induced graft prolongation (Monaco, 1970b) pointing to the possibility that perhaps in this system there exist both high- and low-antigen dose zones for tolerance induction as was observed with other antigens by Mitchison (1964, 1968).

Tolerance obtained in this way extends also to humoral antibody production against the foreign tissue antigens and is accompanied by, although necessarily dependent on, a state of chimerism of the recipient with the presence of cells derived from the tolerance-inducing inoculum. The best results have been obtained with the use of living lymphoid or myeloid cells injected intravenously. Although tolerance could be regularly achieved by the introduction of antigen in ALS-treated animals, the duration of the specific unresponsive state and of cellular chimerism was not indefinite, which was probably related to a failure in maintaining antigen in the recipient above a minimal concentration for indefinite periods. Tolerànce could, in fact, be extended by repeated injections of the foreign cells and by the use of cytotoxic drugs or small doses of irradiation prior the administration of antigen (Lance and Medawar, 1970b) or by the association of thymectomy to ALS treatment (Monaco, 1970b). By the two latter means, allogeneic mouse skin graft survivals of more than 1 year have been obtained and survival of more than 100 days of rat skin in mice was observed by the combination of ALS, thymectomy, and injection of lymphoid or myeloid cells from donors pretreated with antirat lymphocyte serum (Lance and Medawar, 1969).

In view of possible clinical exploitation of these results and to avoid GVH reactions mounted by the injected allogeneic cells in the immunosuppressed host, it has been advocated to use cells obtained from donors pretreated with ALS or lymphoid populations made selectively deficient in immunologically competent cells by the methods pioneered by Dicke and colleagues (1969). The best choice would obviously be to use cell-free antigenic preparations. The value of this approach is still unclear, and no significant prolongation of graft survival has been observed by Lance and Medawar (1969) who gave single or repeated injections of spleen extracts in conjunction with ALS. Abbott *et al.* (1969) found substantial prolongation of graft survival only in thymectomized animals given a prolonged treatment with cell-free antigen starting 1 day before grafting. On the other hand, Brent and Kilshaw (1970) have shown that cell-free antigen injection immediately prior to skin graft was ineffective, whereas strongly incompatible skin graft survival was prolonged for more than 120 days by giving an appropriate dose of cell-free antigen 15–25 days before skin transplantation and injecting ALS on the second, fourth, and sixth day after grafting. The promise held by these results for inducing specific unresponsiveness in human organ recipients is obvious, although further research on more refined preparations of different organs (liver extracts, for instance, appear to be nonimmunogenic) and on the most active schedules of treatment need to be performed before the value of this approach is established.

The facilitation of tolerance induction by ALS has also been demonstrated with soluble antigens (Lance, 1970c). Pretreatment with ALS resulted in the failure of a normally immunizing dose of bovine serum albumin to sensitize mice and led to subsequent inability to respond to this antigen when normal responsiveness to unrelated antigens could be demonstrated. Analogous results with strong immunogens, such as *Salmonella* flagellin, have been obtained by Shellam (1969).

4. *Effects on Humoral Antibody Production*

Antilymphocytic serum interferes also with humoral antibody response. Whereas the immunosuppressive effect of ALS on cell-mediated responses is fairly general in most species irrespective of the type of experimental condition, the same does not seem to be true for humoral antibody production where a number of factors, especially type and doses of antigen, animal strain, and species, seem to play major roles in determining the final result.

An immunosuppressive effect of ALS has been shown on the antibody response to sheep erythrocytes in mice (Jeejeebhoy, 1965b; Monaco *et al.*, 1966a; Berenbaum, 1967; Barth *et al.*, 1968; Brambilla *et al.*, 1968), rats (Currey and Ziff, 1966; James and Anderson, 1967; Jeejeebhoy, 1965a, 1967b), and dogs (Pichlmayr *et al.*, 1967), bacterial antigens in mice and dogs (Gray *et al.*, 1964; Pichlmayr, 1967; Muschel *et al.*, 1968), and to soluble protein antigens, such as bovine serum albumin, in mice and rats (Russe and Crowle, 1965; Levey and Medawar, 1966c; James and Anderson, 1967; James *et al.*, 1968; James, 1970). Several reports have shown that ALS is active only if given prior to or together with the antigen injection; for instance, the response to sheep red cells in mice can be reduced to less than 1% of control level by a single injection of ALS given up to 4 days before antigen injection, whereas only 50% inhibition is obtained by giving the antiserum on the same day as antigen, an insignificant reduction is obtained by injecting the antiserum 24 hours after the antigenic stimulus, and no reduction in antibody response is observed if ALS is injected only 4 hours after bovine albumin (James, 1969). Thus it appears that ALS acts on antigen-sensitive cells and has little influence on the proliferative and productive phases of antibody production. In analogy to their inefficacy in prolonging homograft survival, antilymphocytic antibody fragments do not induce a reduction of the primary response to sheep erythrocytes or bovine albumin (James, 1970).

The genetic constitution of the animal seems to have an important influence on the immunosuppressive effect; for instance, Sprague-Dawley rats are not inhibited by ALS in contrast to Wistar rats (James, 1970) and mice of CBA and A strains are much more sensitive to ALS that C3H mice (James and Milne, 1971). James has suggested that ALS might be relatively inefficient in animals responding poorly to antigenic challenge, and markedly active in high responders.

The type of antigen employed is also important. Antigens are, in fact, often classed as "thymus-dependent," such as sheep erythrocytes and bovine albumin, and "thymus-independent," such as ferritin, hemocyanin, pneumococcal polysaccharides, and the T4 phage. In the mouse the immune response to the former group is absent in neonatally thymectomized animals, whereas it is normal for the second group of antigens. It appears that ALS interferes more readily with the humoral antibody response to thymus-dependent antigens; for instance, Baum *et al.* (1969) have shown that ALS pretreatment of mice results in the virtual absence of immune response to sheep erythrocytes, but the antibody titers to hemocyanin far from being reduced are actually raised. Enhanced antibody response to Type III pneumococcal polysaccharide after ALS treatment has also been found by Baker *et al.* (1970a,b) in Balb/c mice. A possible explanation for this seemingly paradoxical result may be the disruption of subtle control mechanisms due to the elimination by ALS of a population of cells (supposedly thymus-derived lymphocytes) which play a regulatory role in the complex cellular interplay in antibody production. Actually the injection of thymus cells into an ALS-treated recipient diminished the enhancement of the response seen with pneumococcal polysaccharide. However, the selective activity of ALS in interfering only with the response to thymus-dependent antigens is still disputed (James and Milne, 1971; Kerbel and Eidinger, 1971), and more extensive studies under defined conditions are required before a conclusion is reached. The contrasting results could possibly be attributed to basic differences in immune responsiveness of the various animal strains and to differences in doses of antigens and antiserum employed; it is known that the ability of ALS to suppress humoral antibody response (Lance, 1970c) as well as the thymus dependency of the response are both dose-dependent (Sinclair and Elliot, 1968; Taylor and Wortis, 1968).

Doses of ALS that are capable of suppressing the primary response fail to have a pronounced effect on the secondary humoral response—a significant reduction of the response is seen only in thymectomized animals treated with ALS. Only a moderate degree of depression of the secondary response has been observed in mice stimulated with sheep erythrocytes, bovine albumin, tetanus toxoid, bovine γ-globulin, and *Listeria monocytogenes* (Denman *et al.*, 1967; Levey and Medawar, 1967; James and Anderson, 1967; James and Jubb, 1967; Barth *et al.*, 1968; Riethmuller *et al.*, 1968; Mackaness and Hill, 1969), and some workers reported that there was no effect (Gray *et al.*, 1964; Monaco *et al.*, 1966b; Liebermann *et al.*, 1967). Lance (1968b) has shown that a course of ALS effective in wiping out immune memory to a second-set skin homograft was unable to return a sensitized animal to virgin reactivity as regards bovine serum albumin. Similarly, cell transfer experiments have shown that treatment with ALS of sensitized donors does not impair the ability of transferred cells to confer secondary immune responsiveness (Lance, 1968b, 1970b); only an *in vitro* treatment of the sensitized cells is capable of destroying this capacity (James *et al.*, 1969) which is probably explained by a failure of these antibody-coated cells to "home" in the lymphoid organs of the recipients. In studies of this type, antibody fragments were unable to inactivate sensitized lymphoid cells (Harris and Harris, 1966).

The finding of the relative inefficacy of ALS to inhibit the sensitization elicited by the intravenous administration of low doses of allogeneic lymphoid cells and yet being clearly active in the homograft response, led

Levey and Medawar (1967) to propose that ALS was in some way a specific immunosuppressant more active on cell-mediated immune responses than on humoral antibody production. Of special relevance to this contention are the results of experiments designed to evaluate simultaneously both cell-mediated and humoral antibody production. Lance and Batchelor (1968) found that high titers of graft-induced anti-H_2 hemagglutinins were present in mice bearing intact skin homografts. Similar results were obtained in rats by James and Anderson (1968): circulating antibodies against sheep erythrocytes were detectable before skin allograft rejection. Stewart and Bell (1970) observed in rabbits prolongation of allograft survival with concomitant normal antibody production to bovine albumin. Other examples of selective suppression of cellular reactivity with unimpaired humoral antibody production have been observed in various viral infections as discussed later in Section V, G. Moreover, as already pointed out, whereas, even in very limited doses, ALS can prolong homograft survival, abolish immunological memory, and easily depress the secondary homograft response, in humoral antibody production limited doses of ALS are ineffective (Berenbaum, 1967): the secondary antibody response, as discussed above, is resistant to the action of ALS and immune memory is unaffected (Lance and Batchelor, 1968). Whereas, in the humoral response, immunosuppression for a given dose of ALS can be overcome by increasing the dose of antigen (Lance, 1970c), this is not observed in cell-mediated immunity (Lance and Medawar, 1969). Although indirect, other findings also support the contention of this discriminatory activity of ALS. A wasting syndrome observed in neonatally thymectomized animals, a condition which functionally resembles in many aspects the situation given by ALS treatment, has not been seen in mice chronically treated with ALS (Lance, 1968a). Since there is substantial evidence by now that infection plays a crucial role in the etiology of this syndrome (McIntyre *et al.*, 1964), it may be concluded (Levey, 1970) that ALS-treated animals are not more susceptible to bacteria of the normal environment because their humoral response, presumably in most cases of a secondary type, is essentially unimpaired.

5. *Effect of Antilymphocytic Serum on Antibody Formation against Itself*

Despite its immunosuppressive efficacy, ALS does not inhibit antibody formation against itself, a fact which has important therapeutical consequences since both local and generalized allergic reactions can and have actually been observed in man, as is discussed in Section VIII.

In contrast to some early observations (Gray *et al.*, 1966; Iwasaki *et al.*,

1967), it is now clear that ALS, even when given in the form of highly purified IgG, is strongly immunogenic (Clark *et al.*, 1967; Lance and Dresser, 1967; Howard *et al.*, 1968), much more so than normal serum IgG (Guttmann *et al.*, 1967a; Brambilla *et al.*, 1968). The high immunogenicity of antilymphocytic IgG compared to its normal serum counterpart has also been confirmed by using specific antilymphocytic antibodies—2.5 μg doses being sufficient to induce a sizable immune response in mice in less than 10 days (Brambilla *et al.*, 1968; Spreafico, 1968). In humans, accelerated plasma clearance due to antibody formation against the foreign globulins was observed within 2 weeks after a single injection of as little as 2 mg of equine antihuman ALG (Butler *et al.*, 1971a). Probably the high immunogenicity of ALG is to be attributed to the fact that the percentage of immunoglobulin molecules in ALG which have specificity for cell membrane antigens, rapidly become attached to the lymphocyte and are subsequently phagocytized along with the cells to which they are bound—a factor that might be crucial in inducing immunization as compared to nonadhering IgG molecules. In other words, the intrinsic specificity of antilymphocytic antibody probably facilitates the processing of these heterologous proteins as antigens.

Howard *et al.* (1968) have indeed shown that one-hundredth of a dose of ALGG, although ineffective in inducing anti-γ-globulin antibody production if injected as a solution, was active if given adsorbed onto lymphocytes. Similar results showing different immunogenicity of proteins in a cell-bound form as compared to a free state had previously been obtained in other systems (Torrigiani and Roitt, 1965; Wilkinson and White, 1966).

In addition to anaphylactic hazards, a further consequence of antibody production against ALS is that its immunosuppressive effectiveness may also be reduced. Antibodies may impair the absorption of the antiserum when given intramuscularly and facilitate the rapid degradation of those molecules that manage to reach the circulation, thus preventing the interaction of antilymphocytic antibody and its target cell. In immune patients, horse ALGG may be removed completely from the circulation within minutes of injection. Some investigators (Currey and Ziff, 1968; Raju and Grogan, 1969) have failed to observe a reduction in ALS graft-prolonging activity in animals previously immunized with normal IgG, but others have shown that the immunosuppressive potency is reduced in the presence of antibodies reacting with heterologous globulins (Lance, 1968a; Judd *et al.*, 1969; Wood, 1970; Anderson and Dalton, 1971), and this reaction has also been observed in man (Butler *et al.*, 1971a). A logical approach to eliminate both possible complications and decreased effectiveness would be the induction of a state of immunological tolerance to the foreign immunoglobulins prior to treatment. Experiments in rodents have in fact demonstrated that under such conditions ALS activity can be markedly enhanced (Denman and Frenkel, 1967; Raju and Grogan, 1969; Hardy *et al.*, 1970a, Wood, 1970); as discussed later, the application of this approach to clinical therapy in man is still at an experimental phase but indications of its value have already been reported.

6. *Effect on Experimental Autoimmune Diseases*

The ability of ALS to influence the course of allergic encephalomyelitis in guinea pigs, as noted by Waksman *et al.* (1961), represents one of the first experimental observations of the immunosuppressive activity of this agent. Since then a number of other diseases of altered immunity has been shown to be modified by ALS, and this subject has been recently reviewed by Denman (1969). Autoimmune diseases with prevalent cellular immune responses have proved to be more amenable to interference by ALS, as in the case of allergic encephalomyelitis in which ALS not only has a preventive but also a curative effect on the paralytic symptoms (Leibowitz *et al.*, 1968). The development of allergic thyroiditis can also be prevented if ALS is started before immunization (Kalden *et al.*, 1969a,b; Field, 1969; Land *et al.*, 1969; Mac Sween *et al.*, 1970). Another model of experimental autoimmune disease is adjuvant arthritis in rat, considered as the result of a delayed hypersensitivity response to a disseminated antigen present in *Mycobacterium tuberculosis* which is one of the constituents of Freund's adjuvant (Pearson and Wood, 1964). Ziff and his group have shown that ALS can prevent its onset and also was very effective when injected at the time of appearance of the symptoms (Currey and Ziff, 1966, 1968; Jasin and Ziff, 1970; Possanza and Stewart, 1971).

The capacity of ALS to suppress GVH has already been discussed; it should be mentioned that the so-called homologous disease, which develops after chronic GVH reactions, has been considered to be, in some aspects, representative of human connective tissue diseases (Statsny *et al.*, 1965). However, diseases in which circulating antibodies are of prime importance, are less sensitive to the action of ALS—the hemolytic anemia of NZB mice can be prevented only if ALS treatment is started before the usual onset of the disease (Denman *et al.*, 1967, 1968b). Other pathological features observed in these animals—immune complex glomerulonephritis, macroglobulinemia, and lymphoid infiltrates in the kidney—are also resistant to the ALS therapy (Denman *et al.*, 1971). Not only did antiserum fail to prevent the appearance of autoimmune renal disease in B/W mice, but onset of the disease was accelerated (Denman *et al.*, 1966) and increased mortality occurred when treatment with ALS was applied on an already established nephropathy (Strom *et al.*, 1968). This result is not due to a possible aggravating role on the kidney of antigen–antibody complexes arising from an immune response to the heterologous proteins since earlier death occurred also in animals tolerant to the foreign proteins (Jasin and Ziff, 1970). A possible explanation can be found in the suggested viral origin of renal disease and (Strom *et al.*, 1968) noting that ALS enhances viral multiplication. Similar ALS failures have been observed in the treatment of the nephritis observable in animals neonatally injected with the lymphocytic choriomeningitis virus (Hirsch *et al.*, 1968; Volkert and Lundstedt, 1968) which is due to the deposition in the kidney of antigen–antibody complexes, and in nephrotoxic serum nephritis (Fisher and Fisher, 1970); experimental amyloidosis in mice has been favorably influenced by ALS (Ranlov, 1967). The use of this agent in the therapy of human autoimmune disease is discussed in Section VIII.

In conclusion, the available evidence indicates that, as in other types of immune reactivity, ALS is especially effective on the induction of autoimmune disorders, whereas already established forms appear to be less sensitive particularly those diseases in which circulating antibodies are important. However, since autoimmune diseases are believed to be caused by inflammatory processes directly or indirectly related to immune mechanisms, the complex anti-inflammatory capacity of ALS may still be of benefit also for the latter conditions.

7. *Potentiation of Antilymphocytic Serum Immunosuppressive Effect*

Any means of reducing the dose of the currently used chemicals or of ALS itself have important clinical implications in obtaining better immunosuppression and reduced toxicity. As yet, experience is rather limited regarding the best schedules and combinations of treatments to reach this objective.

It has been shown that corticosteroids can enhance the immunosuppressive activity of ALS. Homograft survival was 3 times longer in mice with combined treatment as compared to those receiving ALS alone (Levey and Medawar, 1966b; Simmons *et al.*, 1968), but this synergism with corticosteroids has not invariably been observed (Jeejeebhoy *et al.*, 1968).

Pretreatment with hydrocortisone caused only slight prolongation of allograft survival (Floersheim, 1969) and may even interfere with the subsequent antiserum activity (Hoehn and Simmons, 1967). A clear synergism has been reported with 6-mercaptopurine (Jeejeebhoy *et al.*, 1968), azathioprine (Starzl *et al.*, 1967b) although not in mice (Floersheim, 1969), thioguanine, methotrexate, cyclophosphamide, methylhydrazine derivatives, cytosine arabinoside, and synthetic progestins (Gunnarson *et al.*, 1969; Floersheim, 1969; Perper *et al.*, 1970a; Turcotte *et al.*, 1971). In most cases graft survival potentiation, either of an additive or truly synergistic type, is observed irrespective whether the chemical is given before or after ALS; steroids and antimetabolites give possibly the best results if used postoperatively after an initial priming course of ALS. This procedure would permit using short course of this agent and thus limit the incidence of complications. However, the value of pretreating the host with cytotoxic agents also merits careful scrutiny. Potentiation of immunosuppression is also obtained by associating ALS with thoracic duct drainage (Woodruff and Anderson, 1964), and the same effect is also obtained with preoperative irradiation. Contrasting effects were observed when irradiation is given after the antiserum—Levey and Medawar (1966b) found a curtailment of ALS activity, whereas no reduction was observed by Floersheim (1969). Thymectomy remarkably increases the immunosuppressive activity of ALS (Monaco *et al.*, 1969; Monaco, 1970b) as evidenced by marked prolongations of allograft survival and slower rates of rejection of both primary and secondary allo- and xenografts, facilitation in the induction of immune tolerance, and more profound inhibition of antibody production. Nonimmunosuppressive doses of ALS are active in previously thymectomized animals, and by this approach also peripheral lymphopenia is prolonged, lymphoid tissue depletion is increased, and the return of immunocompetence after discontinuation of the treatment is delayed.

D. Effect of Antilymphocytic Serum on Inflammatory Reactions

Antilymphocytic serum, similarly to other cytotoxic immunosuppressive agents, is capable of acting against inflammatory processes directly or indirectly caused by immune mechanisms as well as on nonspecific acute inflammatory reactions. Anti-inflammatory activity of ALS has been revealed in a number of experimental acute inflammatory reactions induced by physical, bacterial, or chemical injury (Currey and Ziff, 1966; Morris and Burke, 1967; Turk *et al.*, 1968; Turk and Willoughby, 1969), but the antiserum failed to affect chronic inflammatory processes such as granuloma formation caused by the implantation of cotton pellets. According to Turk *et al.* (1968), the anti-inflammatory activity seems more effective on acute vascular changes such as vasodilatation and altered vascular permeability, and these investigators also reported that ALS does not appear to antagonize histamine, serotonin, or bradykinin but possibly acts on other still unclarified vasoactive mediators. A possible choice would be complement. It is known that a marked drop in complement levels follows ALS injection, partly due to direct anticomplement antibodies and partly due to its temporary consumption after the combination of ALS with lymphocytes. The role of complement as a mediator in acute inflammation has been reviewed by Osler (1961), and Turk *et al.* (1968) have shown that the anti-inflammatory effects of ALS can to some extent be reproduced in guinea pigs by treatment with anticomplement serum. Antibodies capable of reacting with polymorphs or ALS-induced changes in adrenal steroid hormone levels do not appear to be the only factors responsible since this effect is obtained also with antisera absorbed with granulocytes as well as in adrenalectomized animals. Increased plasma levels of corticosterone can be observed in mice and rats (Spreafico *et al.*, 1972) after injection of ALS; although a single injection caused only a slight elevation, hormone levels can be trebled after a limited course of antiserum and reach normal values in about 3 days after discontinuation of the treatment. The hormone rise can be blocked by dexamethasone pretreatment and is specific in the sense that it is not observed after normal serum or with lymphocyte-absorbed ALS injections and it is not accompanied by changes in the body or adrenal weights. Antibodies cross-reacting *in vitro* with adrenal homogenates have been reported by Lawson (1967), but preliminary findings in this laboratory seem to indicate that the increase in corticosterone level may not be mediated only through a direct action on the adrenals, but may also involve the hypophysis. Separation of the anti-inflammatory from the immunosuppressive activity has been reported by Perper *et al.* (1969), who noted that, in contrast to the early appearance and subsequent frequent decline of graft-prolonging activity, the anti-inflammatory potency of the serum is initially low and increases with the progression of immunization—an obvious indication that the antibodies responsible for these two activities are of different specificity. Billingham *et al.* (1970) have found anti-inflammatory activity both in the IgG fraction and in a second, not further characterized fraction; these authors suggest that the second component may represent an anti-inflammatory protein which can be detected in the serum and exudates of many animal species during acute inflammation (Billingham *et al.*, 1969).

Activity against nonspecific inflammation should be differentiated from ALS effects on the inflammatory consequences of immune reactions. The interaction of sensitized lymphocyte and specific antigen leads to the release of several nonantibody factors which, although still not completely characterized in their nature and true biological role, are increasingly believed to represent the molecules through which lymphocytes act in the expression and possibly also in the regulation of the immune response. The soluble factors generated by the antigen–lymphocyte interaction, which may be important in this context, are the inflammatory factor described by Dumonde *et al.* (1969) and Bennet and Bloom (1968), the cytotoxic protein found originally by Kolb and Granger (1968), the migration inhibition factor (David, 1966), and macrophage chemotatic (Ward, 1968) and agglutinating factors (Lolecka *et al.*, 1970) which may lead to an accumulation of macrophages at inflammatory sites. In addition, a lymph node permeability factor has been described by Willoughby *et al.* (1963) in membrane-free extracts of lymphoid cells—a mediator believed to be released only during specific immune reactions and not in nonspecific inflammations. Since ALS may contain antibodies reacting with many lymphocyte contituents, it is possible that the anti-inflammatory activity of the antiserum is mediated by inactivation of these substances. In fact, ALS has been shown to interfere with the *in vitro* release of the migration inhibitory factor (Ranløv and Hardt, 1970; Pekarek *et al.*, 1971).

E. Antilymphocytic Serum and Infections

Antilymphocytic serum has been observed to influence the evolution of infections induced by several types of causative agents. In some cases the effect is most probably due to the reduction of the host's immune responsiveness, whereas, in others, altered production of certain types of antibodies or impairment of nonspecific cellular resistance processes in macrophages of the type discussed by Mackaness and Blanden (1967), may play a greater role.

A larger number of results are available as regards ALS effects on viral infections. The first indications of increased susceptibility to viruses were reported by Abaza *et al.* (1966) for distemper virus in dogs submitted to prolonged treatment with ALS, and these findings were subsequently confirmed in monkeys by Balner and Dersjant (1967). The effect of ALS on infections have at the present time been investigated for a large number of viruses: vaccinia, influenza, murine hepatitis, yellow fever, lymphocytic choriomeningitis, Langat, and herpes simplex (Hirsch and Murphy, 1968b; Hirsch, 1970a; Nahmias *et al.*, 1969; Zisman *et al.*, 1970; Jandasek, 1970). As expected, in view of the importance of cell-mediated immunity in resistance to viruses (Allison, 1967), the infection is aggravated in proportion to the participation in the response of cell-mediated immunity as with oncogenic viruses, but, where delayed-type reactivity is unimportant as with influenza virus, ALS has practically no effect (Hirsch and Murphy, 1968b). Furthermore in situations where the host's immune response is responsible for the lesions, ALS improves the course of the disease, as for Langat virus (Rook and Webb, 1970) and in lymphocytic choriomeningitis (Gledhill, 1967; Volkert and Lundstedt, 1968) where the symptoms and mortality are prevented and a persistent viral carrier state is induced which leads to subsequent development of immune complex nephritis. Hirsch (1970a) has emphasized that the route of infection is also important as regards the subsequent effect of ALS. Mortality from several viral agents injected intracerebrally is not increased by ALS treatment, whereas an increase in mortality is noted after peripheral inoculations—a further indication of the nonprotective role of cellular responses in viral infections of the nervous system (Weigand and Hotchin, 1961). Treatment with ALS can also activate latent infections tolerated by normal animals as was observed for murine hepatitis virus by Allison (1970) and for distemper virus in immunized dogs by Woodruff (1967).

It is noteworthy that these *in vivo* findings are paralleled by markedly enhanced replication of viruses in cultured ALS-induced lymphoblasts (Edelman and Wheelock, 1968; Poste, 1970). Increased virus growth, which is proportional to the number of blasts present in the culture, is not limited to ALS-induced blasts but is observed also in lymphoblasts induced by other specific or nonspecific stimulants. The augmented nucleic acid and protein synthesis accompanying lymphostimulation, could increase cellular capacity for viral growth; the increase in the amount, and the reduction in stability, of lysosomal enzymes observable in these cells could also facilitate viral uncoating and thus replication.

The possible effects of ALS on other aspects of the host's defense against viruses are still largely unknown—an interferon-like factor has been detected in lymphocytes by Green *et al.* (1969) which may be antagonized by ALS. Of greater importance could be changes in interferon activity induced by ALS. Barth *et al.* (1969) were the only group to detect a drop in interferon levels after ALS treatment in poly I:C-stimulated mice; the fall was, however, limited and transient, and has not been observed by Hirsch and Murphy (1968a) and Hirsch *et al.* (1970). Falcoff (1970) has even reported the induction of interferon production by ALS in human lymphocytes. The discrepancies in the results probably depend on the differences in experimental conditions and nature of stimulants used; in any case, it seems clear that the pathogenetic significance of modifications in interferon levels must be questioned and that the effects of ALS upon viral infections, whether cytopathic or oncogenic, are mediated mainly via a depression of cellular immune responsiveness.

As regards bacterial infections, it has been shown (Gaugas, 1968; Gaugas and Rees, 1968; Allison, 1970) that ALS greatly increases bacterial dissemination and reduces survival of mice infected with *Mycobacterium tuberculosis*. Similar results have been observed with *Mycobacterium leprae murium* and *Mycobacterium leprae*, where thymectomy and ALS produce lesions containing few lymphocytes and many infected macrophages resembling the lesions of lepromatous leprosy in man. The cellular infiltration caused by subcutaneous injection of staphylococci were reduced by ALS but no effect on the course of the infection could be seen (Morris and Burke, 1967). Furthermore, ALS treatment potentiates growth and mortality by *Mycoplasma* (Allison, 1970), *Candida albicans* (Smolin and Okimoto, 1968), reduces destruction of *Nippostrongylus brasiliensis* (Kassai *et al.*, 1968), and reduces the size of granulomata caused by *Schistosoma mansoni* (Domingo and Warren, 1968). Antithymocyte serum abolishes the innate resistance of rats to rodent malaria without arresting antibody production (Spira *et al.*, 1970), which is an indication that cell-mediated immunity is substantially involved in resistance to plasmodia in animals, and, also emphasizes the potential of ALS in helping to analyze the role of the different types of immune response in protection and development of infectious processes.

F. Effect on Reticuloendothelial Function

Effects of ALS injection on the activity of the RES are complex and not yet completely ascertained. Differences in the treatment used, quality of the antisera, type of testing colloid employed have contributed to the contrasting findings.

It appears that the initial effect of ALS is to cause RES blockade as regards a variety of colloids such as carbon, aggregated albumin, and gelatinized lipid emulsion (Grogan, 1969; Pisano *et al.*, 1969; Gill and Gotjamanos, 1969; Kinnaert *et al.*, 1969). The blockade, the degree of which is dose-dependent, is of rapid onset being observable 15 minutes after intravenous injection of ALS or 1 hour after intraperitoneal administration, but it is of relatively short duration since as early as at 24 or at 48 hours a state of normal or increased RES activity reappears, as also noted by Marshall and Knight (1969) for the phagocytosis of *Salmonella thyphimurium* organisms. Not all testing substances seem to behave similarly in the early periods after ALS injection; in fact for colloidal carbon the response seems to be biphasic, blockade being preceeded by a 4-hour period of increased phagocytosis (Sheagren *et al.*, 1970). This effect has not been observed for aggregated albumin where depression occurs immediately. After multiple injections of ALS, enhancement of particle removal is more prominent than depression (Sheagren *et al.*, 1970; Grogan, 1970); the hyperphagocytosis is, in any case, of short duration and wanes in a few days despite continuation of ALS treatment.

As regards the mechanisms responsible for modified RES activity, a number of factors may play a role in inducing blockade. A massive and rapid accumulation of lymphocytes within the macrophages of the liver, spleen, and lymph nodes follows ALS injections, therefore opsonized lymphocytes could compete with the test colloids for the macrophages and/or for heat-labile serum factors (opsonins, complement), as indicated by the fact that the injection of normal serum can reverse the blocking effect of ALS. In addition, because of ALS cross-reactivity with macrophages, direct damage to these cells could occur and has, indeed, been reported (Di Luzio and Pisano, 1970); however, since RES activity returns to normal or even increases as early as 1 day after ALS injection, it would appear that if this direct toxic effect is really present, it is promptly repaired. Changed in the blood flow of the liver have also been suggested (Sheagren *et al.*, 1970). Still uncertain are the reasons for the increased phagocytosis in animals submitted to prolonged ALS treatment since hepato- and splenomegaly are not consistent findings in these animals. It has been shown that increased adrenal activity can be associated with an enhanced RES activity (Di Carlo *et al.*, 1963), and, since multiple injections of ALS induce an increase in circulating levels of corticosterone (Spreafico *et al.*, 1972), hormonal changes may, therefore, play a role in this phenomenon, but direct evidence is needed before a conclusion can be reached.

G. Antilymphocytic Serum and Tumors

The existence of a direct relationship between the host's immunological capability and its susceptibility to tumor induction and proliferation has been so well ascertained that it needs no further emphasis (Smith, 1968; Klein and Oettgen, 1969). Thus it is not surprising that when the immune responsiveness is depressed by whatever means, an increased tumor frequency and reduced latent period is observed.

Since the first results by Allison and Law (1968a) on the enhancing effect of ALS on Moloney virus tumor induction in mice, the number of reports on ALS and tumor induction has multiplied. It has by now been shown that ALS determines a marked increase in the frequency of virus-induced neoplasms by agents such as MLV, MSV, polyoma, Rauscher, SV-40, and adenovirus 12 (Allison *et al.*, 1967; Allison and Law, 1968b; Hirsch and Murphy, 1968a,b; Law *et al.*, 1968; Tevethia *et al.*, 1968; Vandeputte, 1968; Varet *et al.*, 1968; Al-Falluji *et al.*, 1969; Hook *et al.*, 1969; Gaugas *et al.*, 1969; Vredevoe and Hays, 1969; Vandeputte, 1970; Allison, 1970; Law, 1970a,b).

In general, the facilitating activity of ALS on the induction of viral neoplasms is higher than that obtained with thymectomy or with the use of chemical immunosuppressants and its degree is proportional to the importance of the cell-mediated component of the immune response. As an indication of this high ALS activity, it may be recalled that adult Balb/c mice, normally resistant to the leukemogenic effect of Moloney virus, can be rendered leukemic at high frequencies and with a short latency period after only two injections of 0.1 ml of ALS (Law, 1970a). Antilymphocytic serum is capable not only of preventing the establishment of antitumor immunity but also of erasing it when already present (Cerilli and Treat, 1969; Rabbat and Jeejeebhoy, 1970). As already discussed, in the case of oncogenic viruses production of circulating antibodies appears to be less easily interfered with by ALS as compared to cell-mediated immune responses. Tevethia *et al.* (1968) were able to show, using the SV-40 virus system, that ALS readily suppressed the induction of transplantation immunity without inhibition of antiviral antibody formation. Similar results were obtained by Law (1970a) for oncogenic DNA viruses, but a reduction of antiviral antibodies was seen in the case of MLV. The facilitating activity of ALS on the appearance and growth of tumors does not appear to be restricted solely to virus-induced neoplasms but has also been documented, although with less impressive results, for other types of primary malignancies, such as those induced by chemical carcinogens, which can develop, after ALS treatment, with higher frequency, more rapidly and reach larger sizes. Facilitating effects of ALS were, in fact, observed in mice for methylcholanthrene sarcomas (Balner and Dersjant, 1969; Cerilli and Treat, 1969; Rabbat and Jeejeebhoy, 1970) but not confirmed by Wagner and Haughton (1971), in mice and hamsters for dimethylbenzanthracene carcinomas (Grant and Roe, 1969; Woods, 1969), and in mice for urethan-induced lung adenomas (Trainin and Linsker-Israeli, 1970).

Antilymphocytic serum also can increase the frequency of take and growth of several other tumors of different origin in syngeneic, allogeneic, and xenogeneic systems, as found in mice transplanted with Walker carcinoma (Anigstein *et al.*, 1966, 1967; Kubista *et al.*, 1967), Ehrlich carcinoma (Franchi and Van Bekkum, 1969), sarcoma 180 (Deodhar *et al.*, 1968), myelomas (Mandel and De Cosse, 1969), and sarcomas induced by methylcholanthrene (Bremberg *et al.*, 1967; Fisher *et al.*, 1969) or by benzpyrene (Hellmann *et al.*, 1968). Furthermore, human tumor cells can proliferate in animals pretreated with ALS (Monaco *et al.*, 1967a; Phillips and Gazet, 1967, 1968, 1969, 1970; Stanbridge and Perkins, 1969).

Cancer dissemination and metastasis formation may also be increased by ALS treatment, as observed with several tumors (mammary carcinomas, sarcomas, and lymphomas) in mice and hamsters (B. Fisher *et al.*, 1970; E. R. Fisher *et al.*, 1969; Hellmann *et al.*, 1968; Gershon and Carter, 1970; Spreafico and Franchi, 1972). Of interest are also the findings of De Cosse and Gelfant (1968) showing that the abrogation of host immune control induced by ALS can result in the proliferation of noncycling tumor cells and that the incidence of progression from benign skin papillomas to malignancies was enhanced in ALS-treated mice (Haran-Ghera and Lurie, 1971). The incidence of "spontaneous" mammary carcinomas in mice was not significantly influenced by ALS (Hellmann *et al.*, 1968; Monaco, 1970b), whereas the latency period for the appearance of the apparently spontaneous lymphomas of SJL/J mice (Berstein and Allison, 1970), of spontaneous leukemias in AKR mice (Trentin, 1970a), and of malignancies in NZB strain mice (Hirsch, 1970b) was markedly reduced by ALS treatment. Still undefined is the effect of ALS on the incidence of spontaneous tumors; some investigators (Balner, 1970b; Law, 1970a) have observed that the chronic, life-long administration of antiserum has not an observable oncogenic or leukemogenic effect in animals with a natural low incidence of tumors, whereas Allison (1970) and Krueger *et al.* (1971) have observed an increase in the incidence of neoplasms even in such resistant animal strains.

Occasional reports of modest curtailments of tumor growth by ALS have also been published (Bremberg *et al.*, 1967; Woodruff and Smith, 1970), possibly attributable to a mechanism of direct cell toxicity; results analogous in the limited degree and duration of the effects have been obtained in patients with chronic lymphocytic leukemia given ALS infusions (Tsirimbas *et al.*, 1968). In the mechanism by which ALS facilitates tumor development and proliferation, the immunosuppressive activity certainly plays the major role, but other biological activities of the antiserum may also be involved.

The enhanced growth of viruses in ALS-induced lymphoblasts has been discussed—it is known that such blasts can be found also in the blood and tissues of animals treated with ALS (Levey and Medawar, 1966b; Iwasaki *et al.*, 1967; Law, 1970a). The relative importance of the blastogenic and immunosuppressive actions of ALS in the induction of MLV leukemia in mice has been investigated by Law (1970a), who was able to show that when a state of immune tolerance to the virus and virus-specific tumor antigen is induced by neonatal infection, a situation therefore in which immunosuppression would not be acting, the frequency of tumors in ALS-treated animals is not increased as compared with controls.

The possible influence of mechanisms involving immune enhancement in the tumor growth-promoting activity of ALS seems doubtful—absorption of the antiserum with tumor cells does not reduce the activity of ALS (Cerilli and Treat, 1969) which is abolished only by absorption with lymphoid cells. The increased frequency of tumors of lymphoreticular origin in ALS-treated animals (and humans) may also be a consequence of the antiserum activity on this tissue with prolonged cellular proliferation leading to the development of subsequent neoplasia. A similar mechanism has been suggested as responsible for the increased number of tumors in chronic GVH reactions as originally proposed by Schwartz and Beldotti (1965) and recently demonstrated by Krueger *et al.* (1971). Following the observation of chromosomal alterations in bone marrow cells of guinea pigs treated with ALS (Harris *et al.*, 1969), the possibility that direct cell damage by ALS may play a role in the tumor-promoting activity of ALS might additionally be advanced. In conclusion, therefore, ALS immunosuppressive activity can be regarded as sufficient to explain the increased susceptibility of the treated animals to the different oncogenic influences, whereas the possible importance of other biological characteristics of ALS still remain to be clarified.

VI. Evaluation of Immunosuppressive Activity of Antilymphocytic Serum

Ever since the first indications of the immunosuppressive activity of ALS were reported, a great deal of effort has been made to devise tests to evaluate rapidly and objectively the immunosuppressive and toxic activity of the serum, a determination of obvious importance for the clinical use of this agent. Its activity may vary markedly from one batch of material to another even if produced by the same method; the involvement of other problems, such as the best procedure for the production of ALS, has already been mentioned. Since the exact mechanism of the immunosuppressive action of ALS is still unclear, attempts to develop suitable *in vitro* tests have been largely empirical, and it has to be concluded that no totally satisfactory assay has yet been found. In the aim of finding whether or not any correlation existed with *in vivo* activity of the serum, the first to be examined were simple *in vitro* properties of ALS. Soon it was shown that no relation existed between the leukoagglutinating and immunosuppressive properties (Nagaya and Sieker, 1965; Bach *et al.*, 1967; Jeejeebhoy, 1967b; Dormont *et al.*, 1969). It is possible for a serum to show high agglutinin titers and be scarcely active or wholly inactive *in vivo;* the reverse situation, though infrequent, has also been observed (Russe and Crowle, 1965; Bach, 1970b). Some degree of statistical correlation between *in vitro* lymphotoxic and immunosuppressive activities has been found (Bach *et al.*, 1967; Jeejeebhoy, 1967a; Brent *et al.*, 1968; Dormont *et al.*, 1969; Shanfield *et al.*, 1968; Greaves *et al.* 1969), but the predictive value of the lymphotoxic titer is quite limited. Generally, it seems that *in vivo* active sera are also cytotoxic *in vitro* (Jooste *et al.*, 1968), but the most active sera do not necessarily have the highest titers (Perper *et al.*, 1970a); moreover, cases of lymphotoxic but *in vivo* inactive sera have also been described (Jeejeebhoy, 1967b). No relationship has been observed between immunosuppressive and lymphostimulating activities (Greaves *et al.*, 1968); ALS capacity to inhibit PHA-induced lymphotransformation (Mosedale *et al.*, 1968) was reported to correlate rather well with the immunosuppressive activity for rabbit antimouse sera but this observation was not confirmed with antihuman material (Revillard *et al.*, 1970). Inhibition of antigen-induced lymphostimulation was not always correlated with immunosuppressive activity (Greaves *et al.*, 1969; Eysvoogel *et al.*, 1969; Revillard *et al.*, 1970). No indication is given by ALS immunoprecipitating activity with lymphoid organ extracts, immunoglobulins, or other serum fractions (Bach, 1970b). The proposal of Stanbridge and Perkins (1969) to consider the rate of growth of transplantable tumors in animals as an index of ALS immunosuppressive activity, would seem to hold only an experimental interest. Of greater potential might be the assay proposed by Saleh *et al.* (1969) in which the immunosuppressive activity is measured by the inhibition of the GVH reaction mounted by allogeneic lymphocytes injected under the kidney capsule of cyclophosphamide-pretreated rats. A reduction of 40 to 50% in the GVH index after the injection of lymphocytes obtained from ALG-treated subjects correlated with a moderate immunosuppressive activity of the material as judged by skin graft survival (Najarian and Simmons, 1971). Of possible interest as assays but not yet critically evaluated (Southworth *et al.*, 1970) might be the irradiated hamster test of Streilein (1966) and the inhibition of the macrophage migration test described by Al-Askari and Lawrence (1969). By using antimouse sera, Greaves *et al.* (1969) have demonstrated a good correlation between the immunosuppressive activity and the ability of ALS to sensitize lymphocytes for macrophage opsonization. A suggestive correlation has also been reported by Martin and Miller (1969) with the reduction of "homing" to lymphoid organs of labeled lymphocytes after treatment with ALS—an effect which is attributable to the increased susceptibility of the treated cells to phagocytosis by the liver RES. The effect of the pretreatment of rat thymocytes with antirat ALS on the attachment of the cells to monolayers of macrophages permitted the measurement of a titer in cytophilic antibody which correlated quantitatively with the ability of 15 out of 18 sera to prolong skin allograft survival (Bach *et al.*, 1970). Correlation was very good in those cases in which ALS activity was present in the IgG fraction. The test is specific, simple, has marked sensitivity and might easily be automated. If this correlation is also demonstrated with antihuman sera, the opsonization test may be of value, although a measure of toxicity is not obtained and a dose–effect relationship is not defined in this assay since sera diluted so as to be no longer active *in vivo* can still show an opsonizing activity equal to that of active products (Greaves *et al.*, 1969). A correlation has been observed by Möller *et al.* (1970) between the immunosuppressive ability of antihuman sera, as tested in primates, and the capacity of ALS to inhibit the *in vitro* killing of sheep fibroblasts by human lymphocytes stimulated with PHA. Exceptions were, however, observed, e.g., some *in vitro* active sera were not suppressive *in vivo,* therefore this test would not seem to offer advantages over other assays.

Recently the existence has been demonstrated of a good correlation, for antimouse ALS, between the immunosuppressive potency and the capacity to inhibit rosette formation with sheep erythrocytes by spleen cells of nonimmune mice (Bach and Antoine, 1968; Bach *et al.*, 1969a,b). Since human circulating lymphocytes are able to form rosettes and antihuman ALS inhibits this activity, the possible correlation between this *in vitro* inhibitory activity and the immunosuppressive capacity of antihuman preparations as ascertained by the primate assay of Balner, to be described later, has been investigated. Although the data need further confirmation, the results so far obtained indicate a very good correlation (Bach, 1970a; Bach and Dormont, 1971; Bach *et al.*, 1969a). One should, however, also consider the inherent limits of the primate test in measuring immunosuppressive activity and the fact that the type of rosette formation inhibiting antibody in ALS is still unknown. Inhibition of the mixed lymphocyte reaction by ALS has also been proposed as an *in vitro* assay of the immunodepressive activity of the serum, since Revillard *et al.*

(1970) found that a reasonable correlation existed with the rosette inhibitory titer of the sera and their ability to prolong skin allograft survival in monkeys. However, this correlation was not constant, and this assay does not appear to have advantages over the rosette inhibition test. Recently, Thomas *et al.* (1971), by treating human and mouse lymphocytes with appropriate ALS and by applying the indirect immunofluorescence technique, were able to find a high degree of correlation between the observed fluorescence titer and the immunosuppressive activity of the sera.

A different approach, as also proposed by us (Spreafico, 1968, 1970), was made by Perper (1970), based on the measure of the degree and quality of the *in vitro* binding of ALG to lymphocytes. The results given by Perper seem to indicate that such a measure may furnish information on the potency of ALS. Skamene (1970) has found that at least 4% of the total IgG molecules in ALS have to be able to bind specifically to lymphocytes for a preparation to show good immunosuppressive activity.

Of the *in vivo* assays, the one shown to possess some predictive value for antihuman sera is the subhuman primate test described by Balner (Balner *et al.*, 1968a,b, 1969; Balner, 1970a). The rationale for this assay is that apes and monkeys share tissue antigens with man (Balner *et al.*, 1967), thus making these animals, because of the species specificity of ALS, the obvious choice for testing antihuman sera. After evaluation of the immunosuppressive activity by the prolongation of skin allografts exchanged in subhuman primates (rhesus, speciosa, and patas monkeys, baboons, and eventually chimpanzees), the results in animals are compared with the clinical activity of the serum. The assay will permit to obtain also a rough indication of the possible hematological toxicity of the preparation. For many reasons (imperfect standardization of histocompatibility in the animals, economical factors limiting the number of animals that can be tested, problems of toxicity specific to primates, etc.) this assay is far from being satisfactory; moreover, its predictive value for clinical use has not yet been strictly proven—although the test has been shown to have value, contradictory results have also been reported (Najarian and Simmons, 1971). Since ALS is able to inhibit delayed skin reactions to a number of antigens, such as PPD and candidin, in sensitized subjects, ALS activity has also been evaluated in this simple system. However, it is often difficult to evaluate the degree of sensitization of patients, particularly in uremics, in addition the anti-inflammatory activity of the serum, which can be greater than its immunosuppressive potency, by interfering with skin response, makes interpretation of the results quite difficult.

Of interest is the assay used by Najarian and his colleagues (Najarian and Simmons, 1971) in which the immunosuppressive activity of ALS is evaluated by the prolongation of survival of skin grafts exchanged between volunteers with multiple sclerosis. This assay has been shown to correlate with the clinical results in kidney-grafted patients; the practical limitations of this approach are, however, obvious.

VII. Mode of Action of Antilymphocytic Serum

A number of hypotheses has been proposed to explain the immunosuppressive activity of ALS, and an attempt will now be made to discuss the major ones in the light of the available evidence. In spite of the criticism that can be levied on some, many of the postulated mechanisms are, however, not mutually exclusive and may contribute in a greater or lesser degree to the complex biological activity of the serum.

The first theory to be advanced was based on the lymphotoxic activity of ALS *in vitro* and on the evidence that lymphopenia and marked cellular depletion of lymphoid organs could be observed in ALS-treated animals (Monaco *et al.*, 1965b, 1966b; Gray *et al.*, 1966; Lawson *et al.*, 1967). Moreover, it had been noted by some investigators (Sacks *et al.*, 1964; Gray *et al.*, 1966) that the return to a normal immune reactivity after discontinuation of injections was coincident with the reappearance of normal levels of circulating lymphocytes and of normal histology in lymphoid organs. Marked lymphopenia after ALS is not a constant feature nor does its degree have any correlation with the level of immunosuppression induced, and it can be of much shorter duration than the period of immune negativity. Other procedures which give comparable or even greater degrees of lymphopenia, such as steroid injections or thoracic duct drainage (McGregor and Gowans, 1963), do not induce equivalent immunodepression. Furthermore, if ALS acted as an indiscriminate lympholytic agent, its activity should be augmented by other measures, such as thoracic duct cannulation, which also induce a reduction of lymphocytes, but this result has not been observed (Levey and Medawar, 1966c). It has already been pointed out that a general, indiscriminate lymphoid depletion is not a prerequisite nor the characteristic alteration of lymphoid organs after ALS treatment; on the contrary, quite selective lesions are found. Thus, a mechanism of indiscriminate lymphocyte destruction by ALS is no longer considered acceptable.

That ALS may act by interfering with the thymic hormone was advanced by Nagaya and Sieker (1965, 1967) and Russe and Crowle (1965), after they observed that sera raised against thymocytes were more immunosuppressive than those raised against cells of other lymphoid organs.

However, these results have not been confirmed (Wood and Vriesendorp, 1969); *in vivo* active ALabs were shown not to penetrate into the thymus (Spreafico, 1968), and very effective antisera have been produced using pure thymocyte membranes (Levey and Medawar, 1966a; Lance *et al.*, 1968) prepared in such a way as to render it unlikely that any thymic hormone might have been retained to act as an antigen. In addition, the strongest objection that can be raised against this interpretation is that the effects of thymectomy and of ALS are strongly synergistic (Monaco *et al.*, 1965a,b; Jeejeebhoy, 1965b; Lance *et al.*, 1969).

The finding that ALGG as well as ALabs are very powerful immunogens (Clark *et al.*, 1967; Lance and Dresser, 1967; Howard *et al.*, 1968; Spreafico, 1968) has led to consider antigenic competition as a possible mechanism operating in the immunosuppression by ALS. This phenomenon refers to the inhibition of immune responsiveness as the result of the simultaneous or previous introduction of a second, unrelated antigen (Adler, 1964). Related to this mechanism is the "preferential antigen" theory, whereby ALS would act as an obligatory competitor antigen since obviously every lymphocyte bears the receptors to bind it, and antilymphocytic antibody could reach the cell before any other antigen; the lymphocytes thus occupied by this preferential antigen would become incapable of responding to other, less favored stimuli. However, it is difficult to accept the view that the immunosuppressive activity of ALS may be dependent on its antigenicity. In fact, we have shown that nonimmunodepressant doses of ALabs induce the same level of anti-IgG antibody response as *in vivo* active doses (Spreafico, 1968). Moreover, if ALS was to act as an obligatory antigen, it should then be inactive under those conditions where an immune response against it is absent; but it has been shown (Lance and Dresser, 1967) that the induction in animals of tolerance toward the IgG of the antiserum producer species, does not reduce but may actually increase the immunosuppressive potency of ALS.

It was shown by Liacopoulos, 1965; Liacopoulos and Goode, 1964; Liacopoulos *et al.*, 1967, that the injection of animals with high amounts of foreign antigens (protein overloading) can induce a period of nonspecific immune unresponsiveness and that tolerance can be obtained if an antigen is given during this state of unresponsiveness (Liacopoulos *et al.*, 1968). At variance with the Liacopoulos phenomenon which requires high doses of foreign material, ALS is immunosuppressive even in very limited amounts. In addition, negativity with protein overloading is not of rapid beginning and is of finite duration whereas with continuous treatment of ALS, immunosuppression can be indefinite.

Still another mechanism through which ALS may act was proposed by

Levey and Medawar (1967), who suggested that ALS by coating the lymphocyte membrane, might prevent any successive interaction between antigen and its specific receptor thus blocking an essential step of the immune response, i.e., antigenic recognition. It is known that ALS binds to lymphocytes *in vivo* and *in vitro* and that ALS-treated lymphocytes exposed *in vitro* to trypsin, which presumably removes the antibody envelope, regain immune competence (Brent *et al.*, 1968). However, this "blindfolding" hypothesis cannot be reconciled with the observation that immune incompetence after ALS persists in conditions where repeated lymphocyte divisions have occurred (Levey and Medawar, 1967), nor does it explain the nonsuppressive activity of ALS antibody fragments which also coat lymphocytes. The modest and transient localization of specific antibody in lymphoid organs also speaks against this mechanism of action (Lance, 1969a,b).

Another hypothesis about ALS action, which postulated a nondestructive activity on the lymphocytes, is known as the "sterile activation" theory. This theory was proposed by Levey and Medawar (1966a,c) on the basis of the finding that hypertrophic and hyperplastic lymphoid tissues containing blast cells could be found in ALS-treated animals and that ALS has the capacity to induce blast cells "*in vitro*." The theory thus postulates that ALS may induce a generalized but nonimmunologically productive activation of lymphocytes which would result in forestalling any other immunological reactivity. This theory is analogous to that originally proposed to explain the immunosuppressive activity of PHA (Spreafico and Lerner, 1967), an agent which is known to induce a high degree of blast transformation both *in vitro* and *in vivo* (Naspitz and Richter, 1968; Epstein and Smith, 1968). A number of facts militate against this mechanism as being of some importance in the immunosuppressive activity of ALS; in fact, transforming capacity is shared by several agents, none of which approaches the potency and characteristics of ALS (Landy and Chessin, 1969). *In vitro* blast formation by ALS is seen only in the absence of complement which, when present, causes cell death; $F(ab)_2$ antibody fragments are able to provoke transformation but are not immunosuppressive (Anderson *et al.*, 1967, 1968). Moreover, as already discussed, the number of blast cells in lymphoid organs is similar for animals treated with ALS or with normal serum (Monaco *et al.*, 1967b; Van der Werf *et al.*, 1968), a reduction being observable in animals previously rendered tolerant to the foreign IgG (Taub and Lance, 1968a). There results lead to the conclusion that the blast cells and lymphoid hyperplasia which can be seen after prolonged treatment with the antiserum, are the morphological consequence of ALS immunogenicity.

Guttmann and co-workers (1967a,b, 1968) have proposed that the immunosuppressive activity of ALS could be due to the presence in the serum of cross-reacting or antiorgan antibodies which, by binding to the target cell, could block both the afferent and efferent arcs of the immune response, i.e., prevent antigenic recognition as well as protect the grafted organ from attack by sensitized lymphocytes. A similar mechanism of peripheral enhancement could well be the explanation for the prolongation of skin graft survival with antiepidermal serum reported by Levey and Medawar (1966a) and for the longer survival of skin grafts treated *in vitro* with ALS (Raju *et al.*, 1969). In addition to the fact that enhancement could not possibly be operative for immune responses against antigens other than organ allografts, such as proteins and bacteria, against which ALS is also suppressive, this mechanism does not seem to be of great importance even in cases of organ transplantation—skin homografts taken from donors treated with ALS and transplanted to normal recipients are rejected as rapidly as grafts obtained from untreated donors (Lance, 1970a). Furthermore, although ALS is largely species-specific, it can prolong the survival of heterografts across wide barriers such as represented by human skin to mice.

Mention has already been made (Section V, D) of the complex peripheral action of ALS in suppressing both specific and nonspecific inflammatory processes. Although unnecessary to explain the essentials of ALS immunosuppressive activity, the relative importance of such an action on the effector arc of the immune response cannot yet be assessed with certainty.

Evidence has been accumulating in the last few years leading to the conclusion that the mechanism of ALS immunosuppressive activity is mediated through the inactivation of a selected subpopulation of cells, those comprising the recirculating lymphocyte pool. This contention rests on a vast number of functional, histological, and kinetic data which have been very well discussed by Lance (1968a, 1970a,b). It is now well established that lymphocytes do not constitute a homogeneous population as regards their site of origin, function, and life-span. Current knowledge indicates the existence of at least two populations of small lymphocytes: (*a*) the long-lived subpopulation being thymus-derived, with a slow regenerative turnover, continuously and rapidly recirculating via the lymph and blood through the lymphoid organs and the periphery; (*b*) short-lived lymphocytes originating in the bone marrow and having a high turnover with a circulating life-span of not more than a few days (Everett *et al.*, 1970). The recent view that ALS inactivates primarily the members of the long-lived population rests on a substantial number of observations, most of which have already been mentioned in the previous sections; therefore, only the most important of the supportive evidence will now be discussed.

The first indication of how ALS acts was derived from the distinctive morphological alterations of lymphoid organs induced by ALS injection, represented by depletion of cells from the paracortical areas of lymph nodes with preservation of the true cortex, germinal centers, and medulla, by disappearance of lymphocytes from the periarteriolar sheaths in the spleen, but not from the follicular areas, and, finally, by preservation of a normal thymus histology. These very areas had previously been found to be the site of cellular proliferation in cell-mediated immune reactions (Oort and Turk, 1965), a type of reactivity which is preferentially suppressed by ALS. The similarities in the characteristics of ALS immunosuppresion and that induced by thymectomy which also impairs the host's ability to mount cell-mediated immune responses (Miller and Osoba, 1967), the fact that thymectomy strongly synergizes with ALS (Monaco *et al.*, 1969), as well as the finding that the return to normal immune reactivity after serum treatment is slow and thymus-dependent (Lance and Medawar, 1969; Monaco, 1970b) have been mentioned. Thus it is important to emphasize that the same histological modifications induced by ALS are also observed after thymectomy (Parrott *et al.*, 1966; Miller and Osoba, 1967) or after cannulation of the thoracic duct (Gowans and McGregor, 1965), conditions leading to a depletion of the members of the long-lived, recirculating, thymus-dependent lymphocyte pool. In the rat, approximately 90% of thoracic duct lymphocytes are of the long-lived variety (Everett *et al.*, 1970), this organ being one of the main routes of recirculation for this type of cells. Thus it is appropriate to recall that injection of ALS leads to a rapid and profound fall in the cellular output from this source (Agnew, 1968; Tyler *et al.*, 1969). It persists throughout the period of immune nonreactivity, even at a time when the total lymphocyte level in peripheral blood has returned to normal. In addition to the correlation between functional defects and histological lesions, other evidence for the preferential destruction of long-lived lymphocytes can be derived from the findings of Denman *et al.* (1968a,b) and Everett *et al.* (1970). By differential labeling with thymidine-^{3}H of the members of the two lymphoid subpopulations, these authors have shown that ALS causes a selective reduction in the members of the long-lived population both in the organs and in the circulation. Short-lived elements are not affected and, if anything, tend to increase in the blood, possibly to compensate for the drop in the other lymphocyte pool. Also, in accordance with these findings are the observations that after treatment with ALS, blood lymphocytes lose their capacity to respond *in vitro* to PHA (Tursi *et al.*, 1969), a property known to pertain to thymus-derived lymphocytes (Metcalf and Osmond, 1966; Greaves *et al.*, 1968). Moreover, lymphoid cells obtained from serum-treated animals show reduction in elements bearing the θ antigen (Schlesinger and Yron, 1969; Raff, 1969) which is known to be a selective marker of thymus-derived lymphocytes.

The action of ALS in depleting the circulating pool of long-lived lymphocytes, which contains the cells involved in the inductive and effector phases of graft rejection as well as the elements endowed with immunological memory for cellular reactivity, not only explains the inability to mount cell-mediated responses but also the suppressive activity of ALS on only some humoral antibody reactions and the fact that an increase of the antigen dose reduces in some systems the immunosuppressive activity of ALS (Lance, 1970b). Antigens, in fact, may be classified as thymus-dependent (such as sheep erythrocytes) and thymus-independent (such as hemocyanin and pneumococcal polysaccharide)—it is for the former group of antigens that cooperation in antibody production between thymus-derived and marrow-derived lymphocytes has been demonstrated (Miller and Mitchell, 1968). Depletion by ALS of thymus-derived lymphocytes would, therefore, be sufficient to block antibody production to the first class of antigens but would fail to interfere with the reactivity to thymus-independent antigens as observed by Baum *et al.* (1969), Baker *et al.* (1970b), and Kerbel and Eidinger (1971). It has been proposed by Mitchison (1970) that thymus-derived cells cooperate with bone marrow-derived plasma cell precursors by locally concentrating antigen—this could explain the mentioned effect of antigen dosage on the immunosuppressive activity of ALS. The crucial role of timing of ALS administration in relation to antibody production (Berenbaum, 1967) also indicates that antigen-sensitive cells are the most sensitive to the action of the serum (Möller and Zukoski, 1968). Once the response has been triggered, the proliferative and productive phases are unaffected by ALS; and, in fact, proliferation of plasma cells in the medullary cords and at the corticomedullary junction is spared by ALS (Turk, 1970). Antigen-sensitive cells are considered to be members of the recirculating pool (Martin and Miller, 1968; Roitt *et al.*, 1969). Direct evidence of the impairment of thymus-derived lymphocytes has been obtained in the elegant experiments of Martin and Miller (1968) and confirmed by Mitchison (1970), who showed that only thymus cells could restore the immunological reactivity of ALS-treated mice, bone marrow cells being inefficient in this regard.

Other findings relevant to the theory that ALS acts preferentially on the cells of the recirculating pool concern the altered migratory potential of the lymphoid cells after treatment with ALS. Lance and collaborators

(Lance and Taub, 1969; Taub and Lance, 1968b; Taub, 1970) exploiting the tendency of lymph node cells labeled with ^{51}Cr and transferred to syngeneic animals, to home to lymphoid organs, have shown that lymphocytes exposed to ALS *in vitro* or normal lymphocytes injected into serum-treated hosts as well as lymphoid cells taken from ALS-treated animals, localize in lymphoid organs much less than untreated cells. These results again indicate that ALS causes a selective depletion of cells belonging to the recirculating pool, the homing tendency being in fact a specific property of this subpopulation of lymphocytes (Lance and Taub, 1969).

Further evidence in favor of this suggested mode of action of ALS can be obtained from studies on the fate in the organism of injected antilymphocytic antibody, which have shown that factors other than simple antigenic specificity influence the *in vivo* distribution of the material. Using labeled ALabs, it was observed that the antibody is rapidly eliminated from the circulation (Lance, 1969a,b; Spreafico, 1968); whereas the half-life of normal rabbit IgG in mice is approximately 4 to 5 days, in the case of ALabs, 80% of the injected radioactivity is eliminated from the animal in 24 hours (Lance, 1969a). In the first hours after injection the highest level of radioactivity can be found in the blood, then the radioactivity found in the liver increases progressively this organ containing the highest levels from the sixth hour onward (Spreafico, 1968). The antibody hardly penetrates into lymphoid organs (Hintz and Webber, 1965; Denman and Frenkel, 1968a; Lance, 1969a); probably most of the label reaches these organs by attachment to migrant lymphocytes (Lance, 1969a) which are then phagocytized (Everett *et al.*, 1970; Turk, 1970). In lymph nodes, labeled cells are found in the perivascular and paracortical areas with a distribution corresponding to the traffic of the recirculating cells (Lance, 1970a). Thus it appears that ALS poorly destroys lymphocytes after they have migrated into the lymphoid organs, although in the circulation they are susceptible to lysis, with subsequent clearance by the liver (Taub and Lance, 1968b; Taub, 1969).

Based on these findings the following sequence of events can be envisaged to occur after a single or short treatment with ALS. Upon injection relatively high titers of antibody reach the bloodstream, where antibody binds to the circulating lymphocytes lysing them directly through the intervention of complement or indirectly through opsonization and subsequent phagocytosis of the antibody-coated cells by the RES. It is not assumed that ALS makes any distinction in the periphery between long-lived and short-lived lymphocytes, granted access ALS will also inactivate short-lived lymphocytes (Martin, 1969; Everett *et al.*, 1970; Jeejeebhoy, 1970). The preferential activity on long-lived, thymus-derived lymphocytes can be attributed to the physiology of these elements, i.e., to the fact that cells of this type are markedly prevalent in peripheral blood. Their rapid recirculation would explain why there is no need for maintaining high titers for prolonged periods before this subpopulation is substantially reduced in the organs and periphery. In addition, due to their long regeneration time (1–2% per day), ALS effects are prolonged, outlasting its own metabolic lifetime. However, because of the rapid consumption and fall of antibody after a single injection of ALS, rapidly regenerating elements would be expected to overcome in a short time any effect of ALS and to return to their normal levels in peripheral blood. According to this view, cells that are sessile in the lymphoid tissue would be relatively protected because of the poor penetration of ALS into these organs—possibly for no other special reason besides the peripheral consumption of the antibody. This also could give an explanation for the relative insensitivity of the secondary humoral antibody response to the inhibitory activity of ALS. Although ALS may depress both humoral and cell-mediated immune reactions, it is certainly much more effective in interfering with the latter type of reactivity (Levey, 1970), and the difference in sensitivity is especially marked in the secondary response. Although second-set reactions to graft can be easily inhibited and memory abolished, ALS is practically unable to reduce humoral secondary responses and to affect immunological memory (Lance, 1968a,b, 1970b; Lance and Batchelor, 1968). In fact germinal centers, structures which are considered important for secondary humoral antibody production, are unaffected by ALS (Turk, 1970) and by other techniques reducing the recirculating pool, such as thoracic duct drainage or extracorporal irradiation (McGregor and Gowans, 1963; Cronkite *et al.*, 1964), and, thus, could be left to participate in secondary responses. On prolonged treatment, the preferential but not exclusive action of ALS on long-lived lymphocytes would not obviously be expected to be as marked as after shorter courses of administration—a prediction that has been recently confirmed by Jeejeebhoy (1970).

As pointed out before, whether this selective inactivation of thymus-derived lymphocytes is mediated by the action of cytotoxic antibody and complement or by nondirectly cytolytic mechanisms is still the object of controversy. It has been found that survival of allogeneic skin grafts is prolonged by ALS in NZB mice (Martin, 1969) which are genetically deficient in complement components required for cell lysis (Norins, 1965); ALS is equally active in suppressing antibody production in C5-deficient as in C5-competent mice (Barth and Carroll, 1970; Weitzel and Rother, 1970; Cinader *et al.*, 1971). These findings support the contention that complement-dependent cell lysis, which requires C5 (Müller-Eberhard, 1968), it not important in the genesis of ALS immunosuppression. Additional arguments in favor of this view are represented by the fact that the *in vitro* cytotoxic titers do not reflect *in vivo* activity, but, as previously discussed, a measure of ALS opsonizing capacity seems to be a much better indication of immunosuppressive potency. Although opsonins belong to the IgG class, they may be a distinct subclass (Huber and Fudenberg, 1968) and, thus, their level may not parallel the titers of other types of antilymphocytic antibodies. The fact that duck antimouse ALS is not immunosuppressive, has been attributed to an inability of avian antibody to bind mouse complement (Riethmüller, 1967); it has also been shown (Martin, 1969) that duck antibody is not capable of attaching to mouse macrophages. The finding that ALGG $F(ab')_2$ antibody fragments are not immunosuppressive is not in contradiction with the opsonization hypothesis since this finding just indicates that an intact Fc fragment and earlier complement components are necessary. Antilymphocytic serum may also cause immune adherence which is antibody-mediated and requires C1, 4, 2, and 3c, and thereby could promote elimination of lymphocytes by phagocytosis. An analogous result would be obtained from the action of cytophilic antibodies, present in high titers in ALS (Gill, 1969), in which the Fc portion of the molecule links the antibody-coated lymphocyte to macrophages and complement is not required (Berken and Benacerraf, 1965).

VIII. Clinical Uses of Antilymphocytic Serum

The demonstration of the excellent immunosuppressive properties of ALS in animal experiments has prompted early investigations of its possible use in man. Although very encouraging results have been reported, its full potential in human immunosuppressive therapy has not yet been completely ascertained and its use in man is still in an experimental phase. Difficulties in the assessment of its value are various and can be attributed to several factors such as the lack of standardized preparations as regards mode of production, purification, and evaluation of activity and toxicity, lack of information on correct dosages and schedules of treatment, the concomitant use in clinical practice of other immunosuppressive agents which complicates evaluation of effectiveness, and, finally, the still relatively small number of cases investigated and the short duration of the observation periods. A considerable amount of research is still needed along various lines before this agent can be given with confidence more widespread clinical use. The major problems that remain to be solved include: a reliable assay for the prediction of activity and toxicity of the material; choice of the best antigenic source in terms of easy availability and purity; development of methods of immunization giving products with consistently high degrees of immunosuppressive capacity and free from undesirable toxic activity; evolvement of purification methods giving preparations that evoke minimal sensitization; schedules of treatment that minimize toxicity and sensitization and at the same time provide the highest immunosuppression.

The most extensive trial of ALS or its derivatives in human therapy has been in kidney transplantation where it has been used as an adjunct to standard immunosuppressive drugs, generally azathioprine and steroids. The first indication of the beneficial role of ALG in organ transplantation came from the pioneering work of Starzl and associates (1967a,b, 1968, 1969a,b, 1970c) who still now possess the largest casistics of ALS-treated kidney allograft recipients (more than 140 patients in mid-1970). In the first series of patients (Starzl *et al.*, 1969a), ammonium sulfate-precipitated horse globulin was used (Iwasaki *et al.*, 1967), individual doses averaged 1000 leukoagglutinating units/kg/day intramuscularly, the material being given daily starting 5 or 6 days before the operation and for 2 weeks postoperatively. Thereafter injections were given on alternate days for the successive 2 weeks, twice a week in the ensuing 2 months, and, finally, once a week for 1 month. During the period of most intensive therapy the amount of protein administered per week ranged from 20 to 50 mg/kg. On the basis of preliminary experiments in dogs (Starzl *et al.*, 1967a), ALG was given only in conjunction with the purine antagonist, azathioprine (Imuran), given daily from the day before transplantation and continued indefinitely, and with prednisone. The evidence of ALG benefits in these patients can be summarized as follows: (*1*) patients treated with the globulin had the lowest early mortality, and deaths were reduced both in the acute and chronic phase of convalescence; (*2*) loss of function of the graft or death were reduced to 5% at 1 year after operation in the case of intrafamilial exchange compared to 25% in similar patients not treated with ALG. These results were not achieved at the expense of renal function and by using lower dosages of the other immunosuppressive drugs, especially of steroids, the toxicity of which largely contributes to post-transplantation morbidity and mortality (Hill *et al.*, 1967). Analogous results if not better ones have been published by other groups (Traeger *et al.*, 1968a,b, 1969; Pichlmayr *et al.*, 1967, 1968a,b; Calne *et al.*, 1968; Shorter *et al.*, 1967; Woodruff *et al.*, 1969; Russell, 1968). However, none of these early reports was based on controlled clinical trials and in spite of the obvious success of ALG therapy, it is open to question whether these improvements might not, at least in part, be attributed to chance, improved management of donors and recipients, greater experience in the use of immunosuppressive drugs, etc. Moreover, because of improvement in tissue matching, the more recent results in consanguineous kidney transplantation are now very good even without ALG (as high as 95% of success in some series), so that the most stringent test for ALG efficacy would be in cadaveric renal transplantation in which donor and recipient are certainly not identical as regards histocompatibility antigens. Thus, a recently published report by Sheil *et al.* (1971), which describes a careful, controlled trial of ALG as adjuvant treatment in this type of situation, deserves mention. Graft survival after more than 12 months was 83% in ALG-treated patients as compared to 65% in control subjects treated only with azathioprine and steroids; graft failures, as indicated by severely impaired or totally ceased kidney function, was 19% in the ALG group and 41% in controls. Prolonged good function was obtained in 72% of the treated vs. 52% of non-ALG-treated patients; especially impressive was the reduction in the loss of graft function because of rejection: 9% in the treated group compared with 30% in control subjects.

Similarly impressive results were obtained by Najarian and associates (Simmons *et al.*, 1970; Najarian and Simmons, 1971) using an approach which may be representative of the second, more rationalized phase of clinical use of ALS. These investigators used globulin which was purified by forced-flow electrophoresis and raised in horses against a very pure antigen, i.e., *in vitro* cultured human lymphoblasts; the material had previously been assayed in volunteers for its ability to prolong skin allograft survival across histocompatibility differences, and initial dose—response curves were established. On the basis of experimental observations (Simmons *et al.*, 1968; Weil and Simmons, 1968) that an initial, priming course of ALG acted synergistically with the subsequent administration of other immunosuppressants, so that treatment with the globulin need not be to prolonged, and in the hope of avoiding sensitization of the host to the prolonged, and in the hope of avoiding sensitization of the host to the foreign proteins, treatment with ALG by the intravenous route was initiated several hours before operation and continued for only 2 or 3 weeks. Standard dosages of azathioprine and prednisone were also given; donors and recipients in this series of cadaveric kidney transplantation were mis-matched for two or more major histocompatibility antigens. The following results were obtained: rejection was seen in 4 of the 5 patients not treated with ALG within a period of 5 months; out of the 6 recipients given 4 mg/kg/day of ALG, 4 rejected the graft in the first year; in contrast, among the 11 patients receiving 10–20 mg/kg only 1 suffered a rejection in the first year, and in none of the 8 patients injected with 30 mg/kg was graft loss observed.

Thus it can be concluded that ALS plays a very important role in preventing the most common type of kidney rejection which can be observed in the first 3 months after transplantation; in addition, it also seems clear that an improved immunosuppression in the early months after operation, as obtained with ALG, will also inhibit those pathological changes that later develop into chronic rejections (Sheil *et al.*, 1967). The efficacy of ALG in reversing rejection episodes in man is still disputed. In the experience of the majority of the investigators, with the notable exception of Najarian and Simmons (1971) and Mee and Evans (1970), kidney and heart transplants undergoing acute rejection responded well to high doses of ALS, particularly in early rejection with cellular infiltration (Starzl *et al.* 1967a, 1968; James, 1969; Pichlmayr, 1970; Traeger *et al.*, 1971; Cooley *et al.*, 1969a); a special indication seems to exist in those patients for whom other immunosuppressive drugs have to be interrupted because of toxicity. An additional value of ALS in the treatment of these conditions may be seen also in the fact that any reduction in the high doses of steroids called for in the management of these episodes, reduces the risks of infectious complications.

Results on the use of antilymphocytic antibody in the clinical transplantation of other organs are still too limited to permit any reasonable conclusion; however, there are some indications that this material is of value in cases of heart (Cooley *et al.*, 1969a,b; Stinson *et al.*, 1970), bone marrow (Mathé *et al.*, 1970; Amiel *et al.*, 1970), and liver allografts; (Mikaeloff and Calne, 1969; Starzl *et al.*, 1970b).

Evidence of immunosuppressive activity of ALS in humans has also been given by Monaco *et al.* (1967b) who were able to prolong skin allograft survival. A similar study has recently been performed by Simmons *et al.* (1970) who showed that the number of incompatibilities between donor and recipient had no effect on the length of skin allograft prolongation for a given dose of of ALG. This prolongation is directly related to the ALG dose injected: a doubling of median survival time has been obtained with 20 mg/kg/day of ALG given for 7 to 14 days. Preexisting delayed hypersensitivity to a number of antigens (mumps, *Trichophyton*, *Monilia*, PPD, toxoplasmin, candidin, and streptokinase) is also suppressed by ALS (Starzl *et al.*, 1967a,b; Monaco *et al.*, 1967b; Traeger *et al.*, 1968a,b).

The capacity of ALS to interfere with autoimmune diseases in animals has stimulated interest on the effects of this material in the treatment of similar human conditions, such as multiple sclerosis, dermatomyositis, myasthenia gravis, temporal arteritis, pemphigus, malignant glomerulonephritis, nephrotic syndromes, sympathetic ophthalmia, and chronic hepatitis (Pirofsky *et al.*, 1969; Brendel *et al.*, 1970; Traeger *et al.*, 1970; Trepel *et al.*, 1968; Melli and Mazzei, 1970; Fuchs, 1960; Frick *et al.*, 1971; Gateau, 1971). Although amelioration has been observed in some cases, any conclusion on the merits of this type of treatment would be unwarranted; it should be recalled, however, that the animal experiments have failed to reveal a marked influence of ALS on already established disesaes (Denman, 1969 ; Kalden *et al.*, 1969a,b; Jasin and Ziff, 1970).

IX. Complications of Antilymphocytic Serum Therapy

Injection of antilymphocytic antibody in man is associated with a number of practical and theoretical hazards that pose serious limitations to its clinical use. The observed side effects may be broadly divided into those derived from the immunosuppression itself and those that are the consequences of antigen–antibody interaction. After intramuscular injection, local pain almost invariably occurs, accompanied by erythema, induration, tenderness, and itching; the degree of pain varies but occasionally it is so severe as to require narcotics. The majority of investigators agree that pain usually declines with the prolongation of therapy, but this does not seem to be a general feature. Although diminuition of the local reactions can be obtained with antihistaminics and possibly with inhibitors of kinin release (Mowbray, 1970), pain at the site of injection together with the difficulty of giving adequate doses in reasonable volumes, were among the reasons that prompted the current use of the intravenous route. It is noteworthy that local pain was not observed with ALS produced in goats (Pirofsky *et al.*, 1969; Sheil *et al.*, 1971). In the majority of patients a rise in temperature occurred, occasionally accompanied by hypotension; with advancing experience in the production of more refined globulin preparation and the use of the intravenous route, fever has become less prominent; however, it is probable that its total avoidance will not be achieved especially when active preparations are employed, fever being caused at least in part, by the action of cell breakdown products. A rather high incidence of thrombocytopenia, which on occasion was responsible for the discontinuance of treatment, was recorded in the first trials with ALG (Woodruff *et al.*, 1969; Kashiwagi *et al.*, 1968); this phenomenon, attributable to the presence of contaminating and cross-reacting antibodies as well as to the consumption of platelets in intravascular clotting, as described experimentally by Andersson and Wood (1970), has been of less importance with the use of more purified antigen sources (Najarian and Simmons, 1971).

Some of the most serious complications of chronic ALG administration are derived from the recipient's immunization to the xenogeneic protein: in 40% of the patients treated beyond 2 weeks, clinical signs of allergic reactivity developed despite concurrent immunosuppressive treatment (Najarian and Simmons, 1971), and acute anaphylactic episodes and one or more of the clinical manifestations of serum sickness have been reported with relatively high frequency (Starzl *et al.*, 1968; Kashiwagi *et al.*, 1968; Monaco *et al.*, 1967b; Gewurz *et al.*, 1970). Most of the acute reactions occurring within an hour of injection respond well to standard treatment; however, sensitization has made it necessary to discontinue treatment in a substantial number of patients (Starzl *et al.*, 1968) or to employ ALG prepared in other animal species. However cross-reactivity between animal globulins (specially horse and goat) has been documented (Amemiya *et al.*, 1970), which limits the usefulness of switching to a second-line agent. Differences in the dosages, the length of treatment, and purity of the material make it difficult to assess the real frequency of sensitization. In a series of 40 patients treated by Starzl (Starzl *et al.*, 1970a), 36 developed antibodies against horse proteins, mostly against α- and β-globulin contaminants of the antilymphocytic globulin preparation (Kashiwagi *et al.*, 1968). Similar incidences have been found by Butler *et al.* (1969) and Weksler *et al.* (1970). Najarian and Simmons (1971), on the other hand, contend that, even with a prolonged course of intravenous ALG, 60% of the patients showed no allergic reactivity nor were antibodies to horse globulin detectable. Moreover, despite laboratory evidence of sensitization (elevated antihorse globulin titers, low serum levels of horse globulin, and immune elimination of radiolabeled foreign globulin), not all patients exhibited allergic phenomena such as urticaria, skin rashes, hives, fever and chills, arthralgia, myalgia, and dyspnea (Moberg *et al.*, 1970a; Weksler *et al.*, 1970; Wolf *et al.*, 1971).

One of the most disquieting potential complication of clinical ALG administration is the development of damage to the kidney, an obviously undesirable possibility particularly in renal transplantation. This nephrotoxic effect can theoretically be due either to the direct presence of anti-kidney antibodies or to circulating antigen–antibody complexes, which could give origin to a nephrotixic serum nephritis or to an immune complex nephritis respectively, according to the mechanisms discussed by Unanue and Dixon (1967). The presence of antibody reacting with glomerular basement membrane was observed in approximately two-thirds of some sixty ALG preparations against human thymus, spleen or lymph node antigens (Taylor, 1970b) ; it was also observed that not all horses given the same type of antigen will of necessity produce these antimembrane antibodies, and experiments have been made (Taylor, 1970b) to determine the practical feasibility of absorbing this antibody from the sera. It is quite probable that the antigen provoking the formation of this antibody is represented by reticulin, therefore, less toxic ALG should be obtained by employing purer antigenic preparations. In fact antisera raised against thoracic duct lymphocytes or against *in vitro* cultured lymphoblasts did not show *in vivo* binding to glomerular basement membranes (Najarian and Simmons, 1971) nor deposition of horse globulin in the glomeruli of patients.

The importance of the host immune response against the foreign horse proteins in causing renal damage, in analogy with the autologous phase of experimental glomerulonephritis (Feldman *et al.*, 1963), is still unclear, and further investigations of renal lesions in recipients who are tolerant to ALG is necessary before this mechanism can be assessed. Many preparations of ALS contain considerable amounts of antibody against plasma proteins (James *et al.*, 1970); after absorption they may also contain soluble immune complexes. Deposition in the glomerulus of preformed or *in vivo* formed immune complexes may thus produce immune complex nephritis, which may also occur with subcutaneous injection (Lance, 1968a). Circulating immune complexes have been observed in patients by Weksler *et al.* (1970), and immune complex nephritis has been documented during ALG therapy in man (Gewurz *et al.*, 1970) and in animals (Lindquist *et al.*, 1969).

Fortunately, however, the kidney lesions so far observed in patients receiving ALG have not been of great importance. The modifications observed consist of deposits of heterologous and autologous proteins (mostly IgM and β_1C globulins) in the subendothelial space with focal alterations of epithelial, endothelial, and mesangial cells and fusion of foot processes, thickening of glomerular basement membrane, increase of the mesangial matrix, and intimal thickening of the small vessels (Starzl *et al.*, 1967a,b). Traeger's earlier data (Traeger *et al.*, 1968a) are in substantial agreement with these results pointing to reasonable safety for the kidney of ALG. Later observations with more purified antisera have also failed to show functional or histological signs of organ impairment on prolonged treatment, even in patients treated with ALG for nephrotic syndromes (Traeger *et al.*, 1970). A recent report by the same group (Fries *et al.*, 1970) on the pathology observed in functional renal allografts, followed for more than 3 months after continuous ALG treatment, indicates that the type of lesions observed (cellular infiltration of the interstitium, increase in mesangial fibrosity, thickening of glomerular basement membrane) was similar to that found in patients not given ALG, but in the latter group the incidence of vascular and glomerular changes was decreased: IgM and IgG deposits were seen in 30% and 10% of the biopsies, respectively, and no subepithelial deposits from circulating complexes could be found. Clinical status, improved by ALG, did not correlate with the pathological changes, suggesting that good renal function might be an insensitive index of renal damage. The risks of renal lesions will probably be lessened with the increasing refinement and specificity of the material now being employed and with treatments of shorter duration, with more "blitzkrieg"-like schedule as is generally now preferred.

The effect of circulating antibody to the foreign globulin and the resulting rapid clearance of ALG from the recipient's serum on the immunosuppressive potency is still uncertain. In animals the induction of tolerance to the xenogeneic globulins has been shown to potentiate immunosuppressive activity. In order to avoid the risks of host sensitization and possibly to increase ALG effectiveness, attempts have been made also in man to induce a state of specific unresponsiveness to horse globulins prior to their therapeutic administration. Studies of Taub *et al.* (1969), Butler *et al.* (1969, 1970), and Weksler *et al.* (1970) suggest that the immunological response of patients to ALG could be prevented by pretreatment with aggregate-free γ-globulin. Others were unable to obtain the same result (Moberg *et al.*, 1970b; Wolf *et al.*, 1971); pretreatment did not significantly improve the incidence of clinical or serological nonreactivity over that observed in patients therapeutically given ALG intravenously, a route of administration which is considered to be less immunogenic than direct injection into the tissues. Furthermore, in patients unprotected by the concurrent administration of other immunosuppressants, pretreatment with aggregate-free horse γ-globulin could result in earlier allergic responsiveness. The described failures, however, do not rule out the possibility of attaining this goal, possibly through refinements of the procedure; the recent findings of Butler *et al.* (1971a) that tolerance to horse globulin could be induced by the concurrent use of cyclophosphamide and prednisone are of interest in this connection. The comparative immunogenicity for man of ALS raised in various species has not yet been investigated. Earlier experience from treatment of diphteria or pneumonia indicates that rabbit antisera give lower incidence of allergic reactions as compared with horse antisera.

Infections are frequent in subjects treated with the common combination of azathiorpine and steroids, and even in patients given only steroids (Fulginiti *et al.*, 1968). Infections with unusual microorganisms, particularly fungal and protozoan or viruses still represent a serious problem in many transplantation centers; however the use of ALG has certainly not worsened this situation; on the contrary, reduction in these complications having been observed (Najarian and Simmons, 1971). The diminution of rejection episodes and consequent reduction in the frequency and amounts of the other immunosuppressants are among the reasons for this improved result; evidence has been previously presented for the conclusion that ALS-treated animals are not more susceptible to bacteria present in the normal environment because their humoral response is not significantly impaired.

The most threatening complication of immunosuppressive therapy in man is represented by the development of malignancy. In view of the already discussed effects of antilymphocytic antibody on tumor induction and growth in animals and of some clinical findings, such as the insurgence of a reticulum cell sarcoma at the intramuscular site of ALG injection (Deodhar *et al.*, 1969), the question has been raised whether ALS might be regarded as more dangerous in this respect than other immunosuppressive agents. This problem has acquired lately greater importance since the number of *de novo* malignant neoplasms developing in long-term survivors after organ transplantation is steadily increasing. According to a recent survey, in some 5000 kidney recipients throughout the world, 28 epithelial and 24 mesenchymal tumors have been observed (Schneck and Penn, 1971); among 184 renal homograft recipients surviving their operation for at least 4 months and which have been observed for the past 8 years, the incidence of neoplasms was 6% (Penn *et al.*, 1971). The overall frequency for all malignancies is, thus, far greater than that seen in the population at large, and even higher when the general population is age-adjusted to the average age of the transplanted patients, most of whom are under 40 years (McKhann, 1969). Among all types of tumors, lymphomas have been observed in the highest number (22/52), an incidence which is startingly greater than in the general population (0.9/100,000). A number of hypotheses could be put forward to explain the high prevalence of neoplasms in homograft recipients as well as in patients with diseases associated with immunological deficiency (Good, 1967; Miller, 1968), such as continuous stimulation of the host immune system by the homograft antigens (Schwartz and Beldotti, 1965), chromosome damage by immunosuppressive agents (Jensen, 1967; Friedrich and Zenthen, 1970), loss of immune surveillance mechanisms responsible for quelling neoplastic mutant cells (Burnet, 1967), and the unhindered action of oncogenic viruses (Law, 1970a). In this context it is interesting to correlate the high frequency in these patients of apparently primary brain tumors, with the knowledge that this organ is immunologically a relatively privileged site. As regards the possible greater oncogenicity of ALS in comparison with other commonly used immunosuppressants, an examination of tumor incidence in various transplantation centers before and after the advent of clinical ALG therapy has shown that at the present time it is not warranted to consider ALS as specifically more dangerous than other agents (Starzl *et al.*, 1970a). It does appear that a higher incidence of tumor is the price to be paid for better immunosuppression, irrespective of the treatment employed to reach this goal.

Acknowledgment

The invaluable assistance of Miss Scalvini and Miss Gönczy is gratefully acknowledged.

References

Abaza, H. M., Nolan, B., Watt, J. G., and Woodruff, M. F. A. (1966). *Transplantation* **4,** 618.

Abbott, W. M., Otherson, H. B., Monaco, A. P., Simmons, R. L., Wood, M. L., and Russell, P. S. (1966). *Surg. Forum* **17,** 228.

Abbott, W. M., Monaco, A. P., and Russell, P. S. (1969). *Transplantation* **7,** 291.

Adler, F. L. (1964). *Progr. Allergy* **8,** 41.

Agnew, H. D. (1968). *J. Exp. Med.* **128,** 111.

Al-Askari, S., and Lawrence, H. S. (1969). *Transplant. Proc.* **1,** 400.

Alexander, J. W. (1970). Personal communication.

Al-Falluji, M. M., Minton, J. P., and Dodd, M. C. (1969). *Fed. Proc. Fed. Amer. Soc. Exp. Biol.* **28,** 768.

Allen, J., Friedman, H., and Mills, L. (1969). *Transplant. Proc.* **1,** 436.

Allison, A. C. (1967). *Brit. Med. Bull.* **23,** 60.

Allison, A. C. (1970). *Fed. Proc. Fed. Amer. Soc. Exp. Biol.* **29,** 167.

Allison, A. C., and Law, L. W. (1968a). *Proc. Soc. Exp. Biol. Med.* **127,** 207.

Allison, A. C., and Law, L. W. (1968b). *Proc. Soc. Exp. Biol. Med.* **127,** 797.

Allison, A. C., Berman, L. D., and Levey, R. H. (1967). *Nature (London)* **215,** 185.

Amemiya, H., Kashiwag, N., Putnam, C. W., and Starzl, T. E. (1970). *Clin. Exp. Immunol.* **6,** 279.

Amiel, J. L., Mathé, G., Schwarzenberg, L., Schneider, M., Choay, J., Trolard, P., Hayat, M., Schlumberger, J.-R., and Jasmin, C. (1970). *Presse Med.* **78,** 1727.

Anderson, N. D., and Wood, S. (1970). *Fed. Proc. Fed. Amer. Soc. Exp. Biol.* **29,** 145.

Anderson, N. F., and Dalton, R. G. (1971). *Transplantation* **12,** 54.

Anderson, N. F., James, K., and Woodruff, M. F. A. (1967). *Lancet* **1,** 1126.

Anderson, N. F., Clark, J. G., James, K., Reid, B. L., and Woodruff, M. F. A. (1968). *In* "Advances in Transplantation" (J. Dausset, J. Hamburger, and G. Mathé, eds.), p. 103 Munksgaard, Copenhagen.

Anigstein, L., Anigstein, D. M., Rennels, E. G., and O'Steen, W. K. (1966). *Cancer Res.* **26,** 1867.

Anigstein, L., Anigstein, D. M., and Rennels, E. G. (1967). *Tex. Rep. Biol. Med.* **25,** 214.

Arbesman, C. E., Kantor, S. Z., Rose, N. R., and Witebsky, E. (1960). *J. Allergy* **31,** 257.

Atai, M., and Kelly, W. D. (1967). *Surg. Gynecol. Obstet.* **125**, 13.

Bach, F. H., and Bach, M. L. (1970). *Fed. Proc. Fed. Amer. Soc. Exp. Biol.* **29**, 130.

Bach, J. F. (1970a). *Fed. Proc. Fed. Amer. Soc. Exp. Biol.* **29**, 120.

Bach, J. F. (1970b). *Rev. Eur. Etud. Clin. Biol.* **15**, 28.

Bach, J. F., and Antoine, B. (1968). *Nature (London)* **217**, 658.

Bach, J. F., and Dormont, J. (1971). *Transplantation* **11**, 96.

Bach, J. F., Neveu, T., Kline, M., Watchi, J. M., Dardenne, M., and Antoine, B. (1967). *In* "Cell Bound Immunity with Special Reference to Antilymphocyte Serum and Immunotherapy of Cancer" (Z. M. Bacq, A. Castermans, and G. Lejeune, eds.), Volume 43, p. 103. Edition de l'Université de Liége, Liége.

Bach, J. F., Dardenne, M., Dormont, J., and Antoine, B. (1969a). *Transplant. Proc.* **1**, 403.

Bach, J. F., Dormont, J., Dardenne, M., and Balner, H. (1969b). *Transplantation* **8**, 265.

Bach, M. K., Brashler, J. R., and Perper, R. J. (1970). *Transplantation* **9**, 49.

Baker, P. J., Barth, R. F., Stashak, P. W., and Amsbaugh, D. F. (1970a). *J. Immunol.* **104**, 1313.

Baker, P. J., Stashak, P. W., Amsbaugh, D. F., Prescott, B., and Barth, R. F. (1970b). *J. Immunol.* **105**, 1581.

Balner, H. (1970a). *Fed. Proc. Fed. Amer. Soc. Exp. Biol.* **29**, 117.

Balner, H. (1970b). *Fed. Proc. Fed. Amer. Soc. Exp. Biol.* **29**, 181.

Balner, H., and Dersjant, M. (1967). *Antilymphocytic Serum, Ciba Found. Symp.* p. 85.

Balner, H., and Dersjant, M. (1969). *Nature (London)* **224**, 376.

Balner, H., VanLeeuwen, A., Dersjant, M., and VanRood, J. (1967). *Transplantation* **5**, 624.

Balner, H., Eysvoogel, V. P., and Cleton, F. J. (1968a). *Lancet* **1**, 19.

Balner, H., Van Bekkum, D. W., DeVries, M. J., Dersjant, M., and VanPutten, L. M. (1968b). *In* "Advances in Transplantation" (J. Dausset, J. Hamburger, and G. Mathé, eds.), p. 449. Munksgaard, Copenhagen.

Balner, H., Dersjant, M., and Van Bekkum, D. W. (1969). *Transplantation* **8**, 281.

Barnes, A. D. (1969). *Nature (London)* **223**, 1059.

Baroni, C., Kimball, J. W., Ward, E. N., and Wagar, R.D. (1969). *Transplantation* **7**, 303.

Barth, R. F., and Carrol, G. F. (1970). *J. Immunol.* **104**, 522.

Barth, R. F., Southworth, J., and Burger, G. M. (1968). *J. Immunol.* **101**, 1282.

Barth, R. F., Friedman, R. M., and Malmgren, R. A. (1969). *Lancet* **ii**, 723.

Baum, J. G., Lieberman, G., and Frenckel, E. P. (1969). *J. Immunol.* **102**, 187.

Bennet, B., and Bloom, B. R. (1968). *Proc. Nat. Acad. Sci. U.S.* **59**, 756.

Berenbaum, M. C. (1967). *Nature (London)* **215**, 1481.

Berken, A., and Benacerraf, B. (1965). *J. Exp. Med.* **123**, 119.

Berstein, N. A., and Allison, A. C. (1970). *Nature (London)* **224**, 1139.

Bert, G., Lajolo di Cossano, D., Pecco, P., and Mazzei, D. (1970). *Lancet* **i**, 365.

Besredka, A. (1900). *Ann. Inst. Pasteur* **14**, 390.

Betel, I., Appelman, A. W. M., and Balner, H. (1970). *Transplantation* **9**, 431.

Betuel, H., Richard, G. B., and Colobert, L. (1970). *Nature (London)* **225**, 459.

Billingham, M. E. J., Robinson, B. V., and Robson, J. M. (1969). *Brit. Med. J.* **ii**, 93.

Billingham, M. E. J., Robinson, B. V., and Gaugas, J. M. (1970). *Nature (London)* **227**, 276.

Binns, R. M., Simpson, E., Nehlsen, S. L., and Ruszkiewicz, M. (1971). *Transplant. Proc.* **3**, 784.

Boak, J. L., Fox, M., and Wilson, R. E. (1967). *Lancet* **i**, 750.

Boak, J. L., Dagher, R. K., Corson, J. M., and Wilson, R. E. (1968). *Clin. Exp. Immunol.* **3**, 801.

Boyse, E. A., Old, L. J., Stockert, E., and Shigeno, N. (1968). *Cancer Res.* **28**, 1280.

Brambilla, A., Davis, J. S., Spreafico, F., Tonda, G., and Torrigiani, G. (1968). *Boll. Ist. Sieroter. Milan.* **47**, 86.

Bremberg, S., Klein, E., and Stjernsward, J. (1967). *Cancer Res.* **27**, 2113.

Brendel, W., Land, W., and Pichlmayr, R. (1970). *In* "Pharmacological Treatment in Organ and Tissue Transplantation" (A. Bertelli and A. P. Monaco, eds.), p. 208. Excerpta Med., Amsterdam.

Brent, L., and Kilshaw, P. J. (1970). *Nature (London)* **227**, 898.

Brent, L., Courtenay, T., and Gowland, G. (1967). *Nature (London)* **215**, 1461.

Brent, L., Courtenay, T., and Gowland, G. (1968). *In* "Advances in Transplantation" (J. Dausset, J. Hamburger, and G. Mathé, eds.), p. 117. Munksgaard, Copenhagen.

Brunstetter, F. H., and Claman, H. N. (1968). *Transplantation* **6**, 485.

Bunting, C. H. (1903). *Univ. Pa. Med. Bull.* **16**, 200.

Burnet, F. M. (1967). *Lancet* **i**, 1171.

Butler, W. T., Rossen, R. D., Hensh, E. M., De Bakey, M. E., and Driethrich, E. B. (1969). *Nature (London)* **224**, 856.

Butler, W. T., Rossen, R. D., Morgen, R. O., Trentin, J. J., Judd, K. P., and Knight, V. (1970). *Fed. Proc. Fed. Amer. Soc. Exp. Biol.* **29**, 194.

Butler, W. T., Rossen, R. D., Reisberg, M. A., Marow, J. B., Trentin, J. J., and Judd, K. P. (1971a). *J. Immunol.* **106**, 1.

Butler, W. T., Rossen, R. D., and Reisberg, M. A. (1971b). *Transplant. Proc.* **3**, 733.

Cachera, J. P., Lacombe, M., Bui-Mong-Hung, Lacassagne, J. P., Crepin, Y., Hattaway, A., Halpern, B., and Dubost, C. (1968). *Presse Med.* **76**, 1557.

Calne, R. Y., Evans, D. B., and Herbertson, B. M. (1968). *Brit. Med. J.* **ii**, 404.

Carraz, M., Traeger, J., Fries, D., Perrin, J., Saubier, E., Brochier, J., Veysseyre, C., Prevot, J., Bryon, P., Jouvanceaux, A., Archimbaud, J. P., Bonnet, P., Manuel, Y., Bernhardt, J. P., and Traeger-Bouillat, Y. (1967). *Rev. Inst. Pasteur Lyon* **1**, 17.

Caspary, E. A., Field, E. J., and Woodruff, M. F. A. (1971). *Transplantation* **11**, 170.

Cerilli, G. J., and Treat, R. C. (1969). *Transplantation* **8**, 774.

Chew, W. B., and Lawrence, J. S. (1937). *J. Immunol.* **33**, 271.

Christian, H. A., and Leen, T. F. (1905). *Boston Med. Surg. J.* **152**, 397.

Cinader, B., Jeejeebhoy, H. F., Koh, S. W., and Rabbatt, A. G. (1971). *J. Exp. Med.* **133**, 81.

Clark, J. G., James, K., and Woodruff, M. F. A. (1967). *Nature (London)* **215**, 869.

Clarke, J. A., Salsbury, A. J., and Willoughby, D. A. (1968). *J. Pathol. Bacteriol.* **96**, 235.

Clunie, G. J., Nolan, B., James, K., Watt, J. G., and Woodruff, M. F. A. (1968). *Transplantation* **6**, 459.

Cochrane, C. G., and Dixon, F. J. (1969). *In* "Textbook of Immunopathology (P. A. Miescher and H. J. Müller-Eberhard, eds.), p. 94. Grune & Stratton, New York.

Cohen, C., and Sell, K. (1970). *Fed. Proc. Fed. Amer. Soc. Exp. Biol.* **29**, 133.

Cohen, J., De Vries, M. J., Van Noord, M. J., and Lubbe, F. H. (1970). *Transplantation* **10**, 1.

Collste, L. G., Groth, C. G., Kashiwagi, N., and Schantz, B. (1971). *Transplantation* **12**, 91.

Colobert, L. (1970). *C. R. Acad. Sci., Ser. D* **271**, 726.

Cooley, D. A., Bloodwell, R. D., and Hellmann, G. L. (1969a). *Ann. Surg.* **169**, 892.

Cooley, D. A., Nora, J. J., Trentin, J. J., Hellmann, G. L., Bloodwell, R. D., and Leachman, R. D. (1969b). *Transplant. Proc.* **1,** 703.

Cronkite, E. P., Jansen, C. R., Cottier, H., Rai, K., and Sipe, C. R. (1964). *Ann. N.Y. Acad. Sci.* **113,** 566.

Cruickshank, A. H. (1941). *Brit. J. Exp. Pathol.* **22,** 126.

Currey, H. L., and Ziff, M. (1966). *Lancet* **ii,** 889.

Currey, H. L., and Ziff, M. (1968). *J. Exp. Med.* **127,** 185.

Dalton, R. G., Touraine, J. L., Anderson, N. F., and Woodruff, M.F.A. (1970). *Nature (London)* **225,** 1140.

Darrow, C. C., La Fontaine, G. S., Smith, J. J., Martin, D. P., Sell, K., and Kayhoe, D. E. (1971). *Transplant. Proc.* **3,** 730.

David, J. R. (1966). *Proc. Nat. Acad. Sci. U.S.* **61,** 1250.

Davis, R. C., Glasgow, A. H., Williams, L. F., Nabseth, D. C. Olsson, C. A., Schmitt, G. W., Idelson, B. A., Cooperband, S. R., Harrington, J. T., and Mannick, J. A. (1971). *Transplant. Proc.* **3,** 766.

Davis, R. C., Cooperband, S. R., and Mannick, J. A. (1969). *Surgery* **66,** 58.

De Cosse, J., and Gelfant, S. (1968). *Science* **162,** 698.

De Mesteer, T. R., Anderson, N. D., and Shaffer, C. F. (1968). *J. Exp. Med.* **127,** 731.

Denman, A. M. (1969). *Clin. Exp. Immunol.* **5,** 217.

Denman, A. M., and Frenkel, E. P. (1967). *J. Immunol.* **99,** 498.

Denman, A. M., and Frenkel, E. P. (1968a). *Immunology* **14,** 107.

Denman, A. M., and Frenkel, E. P. (1968b). *Immunology* **14,** 115.

Denman, A. M., Denman, E. J., and Holborow, E. J. (1966). *Lancet* **ii,** 841.

Denman, A. M., Denman, E. J., and Holborow, E. J. (1966). *Lancet* **ii,** 841.

Denman, A. M., Denman, E. J., and Holborow, E. J. (1967). *Lancet* **i,** 1084.

Denman, A. M., Denman, E. J., and Embling, P. H. (1968a). *Lancet* **i,** 321.

Denman, A. M., Denman, E. J., and Holborow, E. J. (1968b). *Nature (London)* **217,** 177.

Denman, A. M., Russell, A. S., Loewi, G., and Denman, E. J. (1971). *Immunology* **20,** 973.

Deodhar, S. D., Crile, G., and Schofield, P. T. (1968). *Lancet* **i,** 168.

Deodhar, S. D., Kurlinka, A. G., Vidt, D. G., Robertson, A. L., and Hazard, J. B. (1969). *New Engl. J. Med.* **280,** 1104.

Di Carlo, F. J., Beach, V. L., Hagnes, L. J., Silver, N. J., and Steinetz, B. G. (1963). *Endocrinology* **73,** 170.

Dicke, K. A., Tridente, G., and Van Bekkum, D. W. (1969). *Transplantation* **8,** 422.

Di Luzio, N. R., and Pisano, J. C. (1970). *Lancet* **i,** 309.

Doak, P. B., Dalton, N. T., Meredith, J., Montgomerie, J. Z., and North, J. D. K. (1969). *Brit. Med. J.* **iv,** 522.

Domingo, E. O., and Warren, K. S. (1968). *Amer. J. Pathol.* **52,** 613.

Donawick, W., Shaffer, C. F., Dodd, D. C., Buchanan, J. W., and Fregin, G. F. (1971). *Transplant. Proc.* **3,** 551.

Dormont, J., Eyquem, A., Laveragne, M., Bach, J. F., Dimictriu, D., Watchi, J. M., Lamy, R., and Raynaud, M. (1969). *Pathol. Biol.* **17,** 807.

Dubernard, J. M., Bonneau, M., Bomel, J., Montagard, J., Blitz, M., Latour, M., Blanc-Brunat, N., Fries, D., Brochard, J. C., Bansillon, V., Bansillon, G., and Capodicasa, G., (1971). *Transplant. Proc.* **3,** 545.

Dumonde, D. C., Wolstencroft, R. A., Panayi, G. S., Mathew, M., Morley, J., and Howson, W. T. (1969). *Nature (London)* **224,** 38.

Edelman, R., and Wheelock, E. F. (1968). *Lancet* **i,** 771.

Eysvoogel, V. P., Du Bois, M. J. G., and Van Loghem, J. J. (1969). *Transplant. Proc.* **1**, 408.

Epstein, L. B., and Smith, C. W. (1968). *J. Immunol.* **100**, 421.

Everett, N. B., Schwartz, M. R., Tyler, R. W., and Perkins, W. D. (1970). *Fed. Proc. Fed. Amer. Soc. Exp. Biol.* **29**, 212.

Falcoff, E. (1970). *C. R. Acad. Sci., Ser. D* **271**, 545.

Fateh-Moghadam, A., Pichlmayr, R., VonSchweden, H. W., and Knedel, M. (1967). *Klin. Wochenschr.* **45**, 578.

Feldman, J. D., Hammer, D., and Dixon, F. J. (1963). *Lab. Invest.* **12**, 748.

Field, E. J. (1969). *Brit. Med. J.* **iii**, 758.

Field, E. O., and Gibbs, J. E. (1968). *Nature (London)* **217**, 561.

Fisher, B., Soliman, O., and Fisher, E. R. (1970). *Cancer Res.* **30**, 2035.

Fisher, E. R., and Fisher, B. (1970). *Proc. Soc. Exp. Biol. Med.* **133**, 1342.

Fisher, E. R., Soliman, O., and Fisher, B. (1969). *Nature (London)* **221**, 227.

Flexner, S. (1902). *Univ. Pa. Med. Bull.* **15**, 287.

Floersheim, G. L. (1969). *Transplantation* **8**, 392.

Floersheim, G. L., and Ruszkiewicz, M. (1969). *Nature (London)* **222**, 854.

Foerster, J., Lamelin, J. P., Green, I., and Benacerraf, I. (1969). *J. Exp. Med.* **129**, 295.

Fox, M., Diethelm, A. G., Orr, W. M., Gassock, R. J., and Murray, J. E. (1967). *Surg. Forum* **18**, 272.

Franchi, G., and Van Bekkum, D. W. (1969). Personal communication.

Frick, E., Angstwurm, H., and Spath, G. (1971). *Muenchen. Med. Wochenschr.* **113**, 221.

Friedrich, U., and Zenthen, E. (1970). *Humangenetik* **8**, 289.

Fries, D., Blanc-Brunat, N., and Traeger, J. (1970). *Transplantation* **10**, 20.

Fuchs, J. (1969). *Klin. Monatsbl. Augenheilk.* **154**, 777.

Fulginiti, V. A., Scribner, R., Groth, C. G., Putnam, C. W., Brettschneider, L., Gilbert, S., Porter, K. A., and Starzl, T. E. (1968). *New Engl. J. Med.* **279**, 619.

Gateau, P. (1971). *Presse Med.* **79**, 51.

Gaugas, J. M. (1968). *Nature (London)* **220**, 1246.

Gaugas, J. M., and Rees, R. J. W. (1968). *Nature (London)* **219**, 408.

Gaugas, J. M., Chesterman, F. C., Hirsch, M. S., Rees, R. J. W., Harvey, J. J., and Gilchrist, C. (1969). *Nature (London)* **221**, 1033.

Gershon, A. K., and Carter, R. (1970). *Nature (London)* **226**, 369.

Gewurz, H., Clark, D. S., Finstad, J., Kelly, W. D., Varco, R. L., Good, R. A., and Gabrielsen, A. E. (1966). *Ann. N.Y. Acad. Szi.* **129**, 673.

Gewurz, H., Pickering, R. J., Moberg, A., Simmons, R. L., and Good, R. A. (1970). *Int. Arch. Allergy Appl. Immunol.* **39**, 210.

Gill, P. G. (1969). *J. Immunol.* **102**, 1329.

Gill, P. G., and Gotjamanos, T. (1969). *Lancet* **ii**, 645.

Good, R. A. (1967). *Immunopathol. Int. Symp., 5th* (P. A. Miescher and P. Grabar, eds.), p. 366. Grune and Stratton, New York.

Govallo, V. I., and Kosmiadi, G. A. (1968). *Folia Biol. (Prague)* **14**, 293.

Gowans, J. L., and McGregor, D. D. (1965). *Progr. Allergy* **9**, 1.

Gozzo, J. J., Wood, M. L., and Monaco, A. P. (1971). *Transplant. Proc.* **3**, 779.

Gozzo, J. J., Rule, A. H., and Gentile, J. P. (1969). *Transplantation* **8**, 338.

Grabar, P., Tadjebacke, H., and Buffe, D. (1968). *Ann. Inst. Pasteur* **114**, 159.

Grant, G. A., and Roe, F. J. (1969). *Nature (London)* **223**, 1060.

Grasbeck, R., Nordman, C., and De La Chapelle, A. (1964). *Acta Med. Scand. Suppl.* **412**, 39.

Gray, J. G., Monaco, A. P., and Russell, P. S. (1964). *Surg. Forum* **15**, 142.

Gray, J. G., Monaco, A. P., Wood, M. L., and Russell, P. S. (1966). *J. Immunol.* **96**, 217.

Greaves, M. F., Roitt, I. M., Zamir, R., and Carnaghan, R. B. A. (1967). *Lancet* **ii**, 1317.

Greaves, M. F., Roitt, I. M., and Rose, M. E. (1968). *Nature* (*London*) **220**, 293.

Greaves, M. F., Tursi, A., Playfair, J. H. L., Torrigiani, G., Zamir, R., and Roitt, I. M. (1969). *Lancet* **i**, 68.

Green, J. A., Cooperband, S. R., and Kibrick, S. (1969). *Science* **164**, 1415.

Grogan, J. B. (1969). *J. Reticuloendothel. Soc.* **6**, 411.

Grogan, J. B. (1970). *J. Reticuloendothel. Soc.* **8**, 561.

Grogan, J. B., and Hardy, J. D. (1967). *Surgery* **62**, 352.

Gunnarson, A., Moberg, A. W., and Gewurz, H. (1969). *Surg. Forum* **20**, 263.

Guttmann, R. D., Carpenter, C. B., Lindquist, R. R., and Merrill, J. P. (1967a). *J. Exp. Med.* **126**, 1099.

Guttmann, R. D., Carpenter, C. B., Lindquist, R. R., and Merrill, J. P. (1967b). *Lancet* **i**, 248.

Guttmann, R. D., Carpenter, C. B., Lindquist, R. R., and Merrill, J. P. (1968). *In* "Advances in Transplantation" (J. Dausset, J. Hamburger, and G. Mathé, eds.), p. 141. Munksgaard, Copenhagen.

Guttmann, R. D., Lindquist, R. R., and Ockner, S. A. (1969). *Transplantation* **8**, 837.

Halpern, B. N., Cachera, J. P., Lacombe, M., Hattaway, A., Crepin, V., Hung, B., Laurent, D., and Dubost, C. (1969). *Transplant. Proc.* **1**, 467.

Haran-Ghera, N., and Lurie, M. *J. Nat. Cancer Inst.* **46**, 103.

Hardy, M. A., Quint, J., and Monaco, A. P. (1979a). *Transplantation* **9**, 487.

Hardy, M. A., Quint, J., and Monaco, A. P. (1970b). *Ann. Surg.* **171**, 51.

Harris, P. F., Archer, J. F., and Hugler, J. H. (1969). *J. Anat.* **105**, 206.

Harris, S., and Harris, T. N. (1966). *J. Immunol.* **96**, 478.

Hayes, C. R., Willard, L. F., and Wilson, R. E. (1970). *Transplantation* **9**, 343.

Heise, E. R., and Weiser, R. S. (1970). *J. Immunol.* **104**, 704.

Hellmann, K., Hawkins, R. T., and Whitecross, S. (1968). *Brit. Med. J.* **ii**, 533.

Herman, A. H., and Schloerb, P. R. (1967). *Transplantation* **5**, 732.

Hill, R. B., Dahrling, B. E., Starzl, T. E., and Rifkind, D. (1967). *Amer. J. Med.* **42**, 327.

Hintz, B., and Webber, M. M. (1965). *Nature* (*London*) **208**, 797.

Hirsch, M. S. (1970a). *Fed. Proc. Fed. Amer. Soc. Exp. Biol.* **29**, 169.

Hirsch, M. S. (1970b). *Fed. Proc. Fed. Amer. Soc. Exp. Biol.* **29**, 175.

Hirsch, M. S., and Murphy. F. A. (1968a). *Nature* (*London*) **218**, 478.

Hirsch, M. S., and Murphy, F. A. (1968b). *Lancet* **ii**, 37.

Hirsch, M. S., Nahmias, F. A., Murphy, F. A., and Kramer, J. H. (1968). *J. Exp. Med.* **127**, 327.

Hirsch, M. S., Black, P. H., Wood, M. L., and Monaco, A. P. (1970). *Proc. Soc. Exp. Biol. Med.* **134**, 309.

Hoehn, R. J., and Simmons, R. L. (1967). *Transplantation* **5**, 1409.

Holm, G. (1969). *Antibiot. Chemother.* (*Basel*) **15**, 295.

Holm, G. and Perlman, P. (1969). *Transplant. Proc.* **1**, 420.

Holt, J. L., Ling, N. R., and Stanworth, D. R. (1966). *Immunochemistry* **3**, 359.

Hook, W. A., Chirigos, M. A., and Chan, S. P. (1969). *Cancer Res.* **29**, 1008.

Howard, R. R. S., Asfis, N., and Woodruff, M. F. A. (1968). *Nature* (*London*) **220**, 816.

Huber, H., and Fudenberg, H. H. (1968). *Int. Arch. Allergy Appl. Immunol.* **34**, 18.

Hughes, D. (1970). *Brit. Med. J.* **iii**, 710.

Huntley, R. T., Taylor, P. D., Iwasaki, Y., Marchioro, T. L., Jeejeebhoy, M. F., Porter, K. A., and Starzl. T. E. (1966). *Surg. Forum* **17,** 2330.
Inderbitzen, T. (1956). *Int. Arch. Allergy Appl. Immunol.* **8,** 150.
Iwahashi, H., Nagaya, H., Sealy, W. C., and Sieker, H. O. (1970). *Transplantation* **9,** 558.
Iwasaki, Y., Porter, K. A., Amend, J. R., Marchioro, T. L., Zulke, V., and Starzl, T. E. (1967). *Surg. Gynecol. Obstet.* **124,** 1.
James, K. (1969). *Progr. Surg.* **7,** 140.
James, K. (1970). *Fed. Proc. Fed. Amer. Soc. Exp. Biol.* **29,** 128.
James, K., and Anderson, N. F. (1967). *Nature (London)* **213,** 367.
James, K., and Anderson, N. F. (1968). *Clin. Exp. Immunol.* **3,** 227.
James, K., and Jubb, V. S. (1967). *Nature (London)* **215,** 367.
James, K., and Medawar, P. B. (1967). *Nature (London)* **214,** 1052.
James, K., and Milne, I. (1971). *Transplantation* **12,** 109.
James, K., Pullar, D. M., and James, V. S. (1968). *Clin. Exp. Immunol.* **3,** 963.
James, K., James, V. S., and Pullar, D. M. (1969). *Clin. Exp. Immunol.* **4,** 93.
James, K., Pullar, D. M., James, V. S., Wood, A., Epps, H. B. G., and Rahr, L. (1970). *Transplantation* **10,** 208.
Jandasek, J. (1970). *Acta Virol. (Prague)* **14,** 467.
Jasin, H. E., and Ziff, M. (1970). *Fed. Proc. Fed. Amer. Soc. Exp. Biol.* **29,** 177.
Jasin, H. E., Lennard, D., and Ziff, M. (1969). *Fed. Proc. Fed. Amer. Soc. Exp. Biol.* **28,** 768.
Jeejeebhoy, H. F. (1965a). *Immunology* **9,** 417.
Jeejeebhoy, H. F. (1965b). *Lancet* **ii,** 106.
Jeejeebhoy, H. F. (1967a). *Transplantation* **5,** 273.
Jeejeebhoy, H. F. (1967b). *Transplantation* **5,** 1121.
Jeejeebhoy, H. F. (1970). *J. Exp. Med.* **132,** 963.
Jeejeebhoy, H.F., and Vela-Martinez, J. M. (1968). *Transplantation* **6,** 149.
Jeejeebhoy, H. F., Rabbat, A. G., and Vela-Martinez, J. M. (1968). *Transplantation* **6,** 765.
Jensen, K. M. (1967). *Acta Med. Scand.* **182,** 445.
Jooste, S. V., Lance, E. M., Levey, R. H., Medawar, P. B., Ruszkiewicz, M., Sharman, R., and Taub, R. N. (1968). *Immunology* **15,** 697.
Judd, K. P., and Trentin, J. J. (1971). *Transplantation* **11,** 303.
Judd, K. P., Allen, C., Guiberteau, M., and Trentin, J. J. (1969). *Transplant. Proc.* **1,** 470.
Kalden, J., James, K., Williamson, W. G., and Irvine, W. J. (1969a). *Clin. Exp. Immunol.* **5,** 597.
Kalden, J., James, K., Williamson, W. G., and Irvine, W. J. (1969b). *Clin. Exp. Immunol.* **5,** 973.
Kamoun, P. P., and Hamburger, J. (1970). *Transplantation* **10,** 53.
Kashiwagi, N., Brantigan, C. O., Brettscheider, L., Groth, G., and Starzl, T. E. (1968). *Ann. Intern. Med.* **68,** 275.
Kassai, T., Szepes, G., Réthy, L., and Toth, G. (1968). *Nature (London)* **218,** 1055.
Kerbel, R. S., and Eidinger, D. (1971). *J. Immunol.* **106,** 917.
Kinnaert, P., Penneman, R., and Dirk, M. (1969). *Lancet* **ii,** 1250.
Kinne, D. W., and Simmons, R. L. (1967). *J. Immunol.* **98,** 251.
Klein, G., and Oettgen, H. F. (1969). *Cancer Res.* **29,** 1741.
Knight, S., and Ling, N. R. (1967). *Immunology* **12,** 537.
Kolb, W. P., and Granger, G. A. (1968). *Proc. Nat. Acad. Sci. U.S.* **61,** 1250.
Koumans, R. K. J., and Burke, J. F. (1969). *Surgery* **66,** 89.
Krueger, G. R. F., Malmgren, R. A., and Berard, C. W. (1971). *Transplantation* **11,** 138.

Kubista, T. P., Shorter, R. G., and Hallenbeck, G. A. (1967). *Cancer Res.* **27**, 2072.
Lance, E. M. (1968a). *In* "Advances in Transplantation" (J. Dausset, J. Hamburger, and G. Mathé, eds.), p. 107. Munksgaard, Copenhagen.
Lance, E. M. (1968b). *Nature (London)* **217**, 557.
Lance, E. M. (1969a). *J. Exp. Med.* **130**, 49.
Lance, E. M. (1969b). *Antibiot. Chemother. (Basel)* **15**, 310.
Lance, E. M. (1970a). *Clin. Exp. Immunol.* **6**, 789.
Lance, E. M. (1970b). *Fed. Proc. Fed. Amer. Soc. Exp. Biol.* **29**, 209.
Lance, E. M. (1970c). *J. Immunol.* **105**, 108.
Lance, E. M., and Batchelor, R. (1968). *Transplantation* **6**, 490.
Lance, E. M., and Dresser, D. W. (1967). *Nature (London)* **215**, 488.
Lance, E. M., and Medawar, P. B. (1968). *Lancet* **i**, 1174.
Lance, E. M., and Medawar, P. B. (1969). *Proc. Roy. Soc., Ser. B* **173**, 447.
Lance, E. M., and Medawar, P. B. (1970a). *Lancet* **i**, 167.
Lance, E. M., and Medawar, P. B. (1970b). *Fed. Proc. Fed. Amer. Soc. Exp. Biol.* **29**, 151.
Lance, E. M., and Taub, R. N. (1969). *Nature (London)* **221**, 841.
Lance, E. M., Ford, P. J., and Ruszkiewicz, M. (1968). *Immunology* **15**, 571.
Lance, E. M., Levey, R. H., and Medawar, P. B. (1969). *Proc. Nat. Acad. Sci. U.S.* **64**, 1356.
Lance, E. M., Ford, P. J., and Ruszkiewicz, M. (1970). *Fed. Proc. Fed. Amer. Soc. Exp. Biol.* **29**, 106.
Land, W., Frick, E., and Roscher, R. (1969). *Klin. Wochenschr.* **47**, 633.
Landy, M., and Chessin, L. M. (1969). *Antibiot. Chemother. (Basel)* **15**, 199.
Landy, M., Sanderson, R. P., and Jackson, A. L. (1965). *J. Exp. Med.* **122**, 483.
Law, L. W. (1970a). *Fed. Proc. Fed. Amer. Soc. Exp. Biol.* **29**, 171.
Law, L. W. (1970b). *Fed. Proc. Fed. Amer. Soc. Exp. Biol.* **29**, 175.
Law, L. W., Ting, R. C., and Allison, A. C. (1968). *Nature (London)* **220**, 611.
Lawrence, J. S., Barnett, E. V., and Graddock, C. G. (1968). *Transplantation* **6**, 70.
Lawson, R. K. (1967). *Transplantation* **5**, 1137.
Lawson, R. K., Ellis, L. R., Kirckeim, D., and Hodges, G. V. (1967). *Transplantation* **5**, 169.
Ledney, G. D. (1967). *Exp. Hematol.* **14**, 42.
Ledney, G. D. (1969). *Transplantation* **8**, 127.
Ledney, G. D., and Van Bekkum, D. W. (1968). *In* "Advances in Transplantation" (J. Dausset, J. Hamburger, and G. Mathé, eds.), p. 441. Munksgaard, Copenhagen.
Ledney, G. D., and Van Bekkum, D. W. (1969). *J. Nat. Cancer Inst.* **42**, 633.
Leibowitz, S., Rennedy, L. A., and Lessoff, M. H. (1968). *Clin. Exp. Immunol.* **3**, 753.
Lejeune, G., Degiovanni, G., Haeven-Severynes, A. M., Bovillenne, C., and Broc-teur, G. (1970). *Symp. Ser. Immunobiol. Stand.* **16**, 61.
Lernor, R. E. (1970). *Amer. J. Ophthalmol.* **69**, 453.
Leuchars, E., Wallis, V. J., and Davies, A. J. S. (1968). *Nature (London)* **219**, 1325.
Levey, R. H. (1970). *Fed. Proc. Fed. Amer. Soc. Exp. Biol.* **29**, 156.
Levey, R. H., and Medawar, P. B. (1966a). *Proc. Nat. Acad. Sci. U.S.* **56**, 1130.
Levey, R. H., and Medawar, P. B. (1966b). *Proc. Nat. Acad. Sci. U.S.* **58**, 470.
Levey, R. H., and Medawar, P. B. (1966c). *Ann. N.Y. Acad. Sci.* **129**, 164.
Levey, R. H., and Medawar, P. B. (1967). *Antilymphocytic Serum, Ciba Found. Symp.* p. 72.
Liacopoulos, P. (1965). *Tex. Rep. Biol. Med.* **23**, 63.
Liacopoulos, P., and Goode, J. H. (1964). *Science* **146**, 1305.

Liacopoulos, P., Merchant, B., and Harrell, B. E. (1967). *Proc. Soc. Exp. Biol. Med.* **125,** 958.

Liacopoulos, P., Herlem, G., and Perrament, M. F. (1968). *In* "Advances in Transplantation" (J. Dausset, J. Hamburger, and G. Mathé, eds.), p. 183. Munksgaard, Copenhagen.

Liebermann, G., Baum, J., and Frenkel, E. P. (1967). *Fed. Proc. Fed. Amer. Soc. Exp. Biol.* **26,** 417.

Lindquist, R. R., Guttmann, D., Carpenter, C. B., and Merrill, J. P. (1969). *Transplantation* **8,** 545.

Ling, N. R., Knight, S., Hardy, D., Stanworth, D. R., and Holt, P. H. L. (1967). *Antilymphocytic Serum, Ciba Found. Symp.* p. 57.

Lolecka, S., Dray, S., and Gotoff, S. P. (1970). *J. Immunol.* **104,** 296.

Lucke, J. N., Immelman, E. J., Symes, M. O., and Himt, A. C. (1968). *Nature (London)* **217,** 560.

Lundgren, G. (1969). *Clin. Exp. Immunol.* **5,** 381.

McGregor, D. D., and Gowans, J. L. (1963). *J. Exp. Med.* **117,** 303.

McIntyre, K. R., Sell, S., and Miller, J. F. A. P. (1964). *Nature (London)* **204,** 151.

Mackaness, G. B., and Blanden, R. V. (1967). *Progr. Allergy* **11,** 89.

Mackaness, G. B., and Hill, M. (1969). *J. Exp. Med.* **129,** 993.

McKhann, C. F. (1969). *Transplantation* **8,** 209.

MacLaurin, B. P., and Humm, J. A. (1970). *Clin. Exp. Immunol.* **6,** 125.

MacSween, R. N. M., Ono, K., Bell, P. R., Thomason, C. M., and Starzl, T. E. (1970). *Clin. Exp. Immunol.* **6,** 273.

Mandel, M. A., and Asofsky, R. (1968). *J. Immunol.* **100,** 1319.

Mandel, M. A., and De Cosse, J. J. (1969). *J. Immunol.* **103,** 1288.

Marshall, V. R., and Knight, R. (1969). *J. Immunol.* **102,** 1498.

Martin, W. J. (1969). *J. Immunol.* **103,** 990.

Martin, W. J., and Miller, J. F. A. P. (1968). *J. Exp. Med.* **128,** 865.

Martin, W. J., and Miller, J. F. A. P. (1969). *Int. Arch. Allergy Appl. Immunol.* **35,** 163.

Mathé, G., Amiel, J. L., Schwarzenberg, L., Choay, J., Trolard, P., Schneider, M., Hayat, M., Schlumberger, J. R., and Jasmin, C. (1970). *Brit. Med. J.* **ii,** 131.

Mee, A. D., and Evans, D. B. (1970). *Lancet* **ii,** 16.

Melli, G., and Mazzei, D. (1970). *Minerva Med.* **61,** 3064.

Metcalf, W. R., and Osmond, D. G. (1966). *Exp. Cell Res.* **41,** 669.

Metchnikoff, E. (1898). *Ann. Inst. Pasteur* **12,** 263.

Metchnikoff, E. (1899). *Ann. Inst. Pasteur* **13,** 737.

Miale, J. B. (1947). *Blood* **2,** 175.

Mikaeloff, P. and Calne, R. Y. (1969). *Progr. Surg.* **7,** 253.

Mikaeloff, P., Pichlmayr, R., Rassat, J. P., Messmer, K., Bomel, J., Tidow, G., Etiennemartin, M., Malluret, J., Belleville, P., Jouvenceau, A., Falconnet, J., Descotes, J., and Brendel, W. (1967). *Presse Med.* **75,** 1967.

Milgrom, F. (1970). *Fed. Proc. Fed. Amer. Soc. Exp. Biol.* **29,** 114.

Miller, J. F. A. P., and Mitchell, G. F. (1968). *J. Exp. Med.* **128,** 801.

Miller, J. F. A. P., and Osoba, D. (1967). *Physiol. Rev.* **47,** 437.

Miller, R. W. (1968). *J. Nat. Cancer Inst.* **40,** 1079.

Mitchell, R. M., Sheil, A. G. R., Slafsky, S. F., and Murray, J. E. (1966). *Transplantation* **3,** 323.

Mitchison, N. A. (1964). *Proc. Roy. Soc., Ser. B* **161,** 275.

Mitchison, N. A. (1968). *Immunology* **15,** 509.

Mitchison, N. A. (1970). *Fed. Proc. Fed. Amer. Soc. Exp. Biol.* **29,** 222.

Moberg, A. W., Gewurz, H., and Jetzer, T. (1970a). *Surgery* **68,** 862.
Moberg,.A. W., Gewurz, H., Simmons, R. L., and Najarian, J. S. (1970b). *Lancet* **ii,** 214.
Möller, G. (1970). *Immunology* **19,** 583.
Möller, G., and Zukoski, C. (1968). *J. Immunol.* **101,** 325.
Möller, G., Lundgren, G., and Balner, H. (1970). *Transplantation* **9,** 166.
Monaco, A. P. (1970a). *Fed. Proc. Fed. Amer. Soc. Exp. Biol.* **29,** 114.
Monaco, A. P. (1970b). *Fed. Proc. Fed. Amer. Soc. Exp. Biol.* **29,** 153.
Monaco, A. P., and Franco, D. J. (1969). *Transplantation* **7,** 73.
Monaco, A. P., Wood, M. L., and Russell, P. S. (1965a). *Surg. Forum* **16,** 209.
Monaco, A. P., Wood, M. L., and Russell, P. S. (1965b). *Science* **149,** 432.
Monaco, A. P., Wood, M. L., and Russell, P. S. (1966a). *Ann. N.Y. Acad. Sci.* **129,** 190.
Monaco, A. P., Wood, M. L., Gray, J. G., and Russell, P. S. (1966b). *J. Immunol.* **96,** 229.
Monaco, A. P., Abbott, W. M., and Otherson, H. B. (1966c). *Science* **153,** 1264.
Monaco, A. P., Wood, M. L., and Russell, P. S. (1967a). *Transplantation* **5,** 1106.
Monaco, A. P., Wood, M. L., Van Der Werf, B. A., and Russell, P. S. (1967b). *Antilymphocytic Serum, Ciba Found. Symp.* p. 111.
Monaco, A. P., Franco, D. J., and Wood, M. L. (1969). *Antibiot. Chemother. (Basel)* **15,** 328.
Moorhead, T. G. (1905). *Practitioner* **75,** 733.
Morris, P. J., and Burke, J. F. (1967). *Nature (London)* **214,** 1138.
Mosedale, B., Felstead, R. J., and Parke, J. A. C. (1968). *Nature (London)* **218,** 983.
Mowbray, J. F. (1970). *Proc. Roy. Soc. Med.* **63,** 1067.
Moynihan, P. C., Grogan, J. B., and Hardy, J. D. (1967). *Surg. Forum* **18,** 235.
Müller-Eberhard, H. J. (1968). *Advan. Immunol.* **8,** 1.
Muschel, L. M., Gustafson, L., and Atai, M. (1968). *Immunology* **14,** 285.
Nagaya, H., and Sieker, H. O. (1965). *Science* **150,** 1181.
Nagaya, H., and Sieker, H. O. (1967). *Proc. Soc. Exp. Biol. Med.* **127,** 131.
Nagaya, H., McKenzie, W. N., Jr., Kilburn, K. H., and Sieker, H. O. (1970). *J. Immunol.* **104,** 511.
Nahmias, A. J., Hirsh, M. S., Kramer, J. H., and Murphy, F. A. (1969). *Proc. Soc. Exp. Biol. Med.* **132,** 696.
Najarian, J. S., and Simmons, R. L. (1971). *New Engl. J. Med.* **285,** 158.
Najarian, J. S., Merkel, F. R., Moore, G. E., Good, R. A., and Aust, J. C. (1969). *Transplant. Proc.* **1,** 460.
Najarian, J. S., Simmons, R. L., Gewurz, H., Moberg, A., Merkel, F., and Moore, G. E. (1970). *Fed. Proc. Fed. Amer. Soc. Exp. Biol.* **29,** 197.
Naspitz, L. R., and Richter, M. (1968). *Progr. Allergy* **12,** 1
Nehlsen, S. L. (1971). *Transplant. Proc.* **3,** 811.
Nelson, D. S. (1970). *Pathology* **2,** 183.
Norins, L. C. (1965). *J. Immunol.* **94,** 437.
Nossa, L., Muresan, T., Marcu, A., and Abrudeanu, O. (1969). *Nature (London)* **222,** 1082.
Ogburn, C. A., Harris, T. N., and Harris, S. (1969). *Transplantation* **7,** 112.
Oliver, C. B., and Feldman, J. D. (1971). *Transplantation* **11,** 412.
Ono, K., Bell, D., Kashiwagi, N., and Starzl, T. E. (1969a). *Surgery* **66,** 698.
Ono, K., De Witt, C. W., Wallace, J. M., and Lindsey, E. S. (1969b). *Transplantation* **7,** 122.
Oort, J., and Turk, J. L. (1965). *Brit. J. Exp. Pathol.* **46,** 197.

Osler, A. G. (1961). *Advan. Immunol.* **1**, 131.
Otte, M., and Grosjean, D. (1967). *C. R. Soc. Biol.* **161**, 738.
Pappenheimer, A. M. (1917a). *J. Exp. Med.* **25**, 633.
Pappenheimer, A. M. (1917b). *J. Exp. Med.* **26**, 163.
Parrott, D. M. V., De Sousa, M. B., and East, J. (1966). *J. Exp. Med.* **123**, 191.
Pearson, C. M., and Wood, F. D. (1964). *J. Exp. Med.* **120**, 547.
Pekarek, R. J., Svejcar, J., and Johanovski, J. (1971). *Immunology* **20**, 895.
Penn, I., Halgrimson, C. G., and Starzl, T. E. (1971). *Transplant. Proc.* **3**, 773.
Perper, R. J. (1970). *Fed. Proc. Fed. Amer. Soc. Exp. Biol.* **29**, 123.
Perper, R. J., Glenn, E. M., and Monovich, R. E. (1969). *Nature (London)* **223**, 86.
Perper, R. J., Lyster, S. C., Monovich, R. E., and Bowersox, B. E. (1970a). *Transplantation* **9**, 447.
Perper, R. J., Monovich, R. E., and Bowersox, B. E. (1970b). *J. Immunol.* **104**, 1063.
Phillips, B., and Gazet, J. C. (1967). *Nature (London)* **215**, 548.
Phillips, B., and Gazet, J. C. (1968). *Nature (London)* **220**, 1140.
Phillips, B., and Gazet, J. C. (1969). *Nature (London)* **222**, 1292.
Phillips, B., and Gazet, J. C. (1970). *Nature (London)* **228**, 369.
Phondke, G. P., Sundaram, K., and Sundaresan, P. (1970). *Nature (London)* **225**, 79.
Pichlmayr, R. (1967). *Z. Ges. Exp. Med.* **143**, 161.
Pichlmayr, R. (1970). *Fed. Proc. Fed. Amer. Soc. Exp. Biol.* **29**, 111.
Pichlmayr, R., Brendel, W., and Zenker, R. (1967). *Surgery* **61**, 774.
Pichlmayr, R., Brendel, W., and Zenker, R. (1968a). *Muenchen. Med. Wochenschr.* **110**, 893.
Pichlmayr, R., Brendel, W., Mikaeloff, P., Wiebecke, B., Rassat, J. P., Pichlmayr, I., Bomel, J., Fateh-Moghadam, A., Thierfelder, S., Messmer, K., Descotes, J., and Knedel, M. (1968b). *In* "Advances in Transplantation" (J. Dausset, J. Hamburger, and G. Mathé, eds.), p. 147. Munksgaard, Copenhagen.
Pirofsky, B., Bardana, E. J., Bayracki, C., and Porter, G. A. (1969). *J. Amer. Med. Ass.* **210**, 1059.
Pisano, J. C., Patterson, J. T., and Di Luzio, N. R. (1969). *Proc. Soc. Exp. Biol. Med.* **132**, 517.
Porter, K. A. (1967). *J. Clin. Pathol.* **20**, Suppl., 518.
Possanza, G. J., and Stewart, P. B. (1971). *Clin. Exp. Immunol.* **6**, 291.
Poste, G. (1970). *Transplantation* **10**, 106.
Potworoski, E. F., and Nairn, R. C. (1967). *Immunology* **13**, 597.
Putnam, C. W., Kashiwagi, N., Iwasaki, Y., Terasaki, P. I., Marchioro, T. L., and Starzl, T. E. (1967). *Surgery* **61**, 951.
Rabbat, A. G., and Jeejeebhoy, H. F. (1970). *Transplantation* **9**, 164.
Raff, M. (1969). *Nature (London)* **224**, 378.
Raju, S., and Grogan, J. B. (1969). *Transplantation* **8**, 695.
Raju, S., Grogan, J. B., and Hardy, J. D. (1969). *J. Surg. Res.* **9**, 327.
Ranløv, P., and Hardt, F. (1970). *Transplantation* **10**, 438.
Reif, A. E. (1963). *J. Immunol.* **91**, 557.
Revillard, J. P., Brochier, J., Treeger, J., and Balner, H. (1970). *Transplantation* **9**, 592.
Richtie, W. T. (1908). *J. Pathol. Bacteriol.* **12**, 140.
Ricketts, H. T. (1902). *Trans. Chicago Pathol. Soc.* **5**, 178.
Riethmüller, G. (1967). *Lancet* **ii**, 1210.
Riethmüller, G., Riethmüller, D., Stein, H., and Hausen, P. (1968). *J. Immunol.* **100**, 969.

Rodriguez-Paradisi, E., Thierfelder, S., Götze, D., Eulitz, M., and Beil, L. (1971). *Clin. Exp. Immunol.* **8,** 107.
Roitt, I. M., Greaves, M. F., Torrigiani, G., Brostoff, J., and Playfair, J. H. L. (1969). *Lancet* **ii,** 367.
Rook, G. A. W., and Webb, H. E. (1970). *Brit. Med. J.* **iv,** 210.
Rosenberg, J. C., Hawkins, E., and Rector, F. (1971). *Transplantation* **11,** 151.
Rule, A. H., and Judd, K. P. (1968). *Transplantation* **6,** 970.
Russe, H. P., and Crowle, A. J. A. (1965). *J. Immunol.* **94,** 74.
Russell, P. S. (1968). *Amer. J. Med.* **44,** 776.
Russell, P. S., and Monaco, A. P. (1967). *Transplantation* **5,** 1086.
Sacks, J. H., Filipone, D. R., and Hume, D. M. (1964). *Transplantation* **2,** 60.
Saleh, W., MacLean, L. D., Gordon, J., and Lamoureaux, G. (1969). *Transplantation* **8,** 525.
Schlesinger, M., and Yron, I. (1969). *Science* **164,** 1412.
Schneck, S. A., and Penn, I. (1971). *Lancet* **i,** 983.
Schrek, R., Preston, F. W., and Dietz, A. A. (1969). *Blood* **33,** 555.
Schwartz, R. S., and Beldotti, L. (1965). *Science* **149,** 1511.
Sell, S. A. (1969). *Ann. Intern. Med.* **71,** 177.
Seller, M. J., and Polani, P. E. (1969). *Lancet* **i,** 18.
Shanfield, I., Ladaga, L. G., Wren, S. F. G., Blennerhasset, J. B., and MacLean, L. D. (1968). *Surg. Gynecol. Obstet.* **127,** 29.
Sheagren, J. N., Edlin, J. B., Barth, R. F., and Melmgrem, R. A. (1970). *J. Immunol.* **106,** 634.
Sheil, A. G. R., Dammin, G. J., Mitchell, R. M., and Murray, J. E. (1967). *Brit. J. Surg.* **54,** 12.
Sheil, A. G. R., Kelly, G. E., Storey, B. G., May, J., Kalowski, S., Mears, D., Rogers, J. M., Johnson, J. R., Charlesworth, J., and Stewart, J. M. (1971). *Lancet* **i,** 359.
Shellam, G. R. (1969). *Immunology* **17,** 267.
Shigeno, H., Hämmerling, K., Old, J. D., and Boyse, P. B. (1968). *Lancet* **ii,** 320.
Shorter, R. G., and Elveback, L. R. (1970a). *Transplantation* **9,** 253.
Shorter, R. G., and Elveback, L. R. (1970b). *Transplantation* **10,** 435.
Shorter, R. G., Spencer, R. J., and Hallenbeck, G. A. (1967). *J. Amer. Med. Ass.* **202,** 845.
Shorter, R. G., Hallenbeck, G. A., Nava, C., O'Kane, H. O., De Weerd, J., and Johnson, W. J. (1968). *Arch. Surg. (Chicago)* **97,** 323.
Simmons, R. L., Ozerkis, A. J., and Hoehn, R. J. (1968). *Science* **160,** 1127.
Simmons, R. L., Moberg, A. W., and Gewurz, H. (1970). *Surgery* **68,** 62.
Sinclair, N. R. St. C., and Elliot, E. V. (1968). *Immunology* **15,** 325.
Skamene, E. (1970). *Fed. Proc. Fed. Amer. Soc. Exp. Biol.* **29,** 126.
Skamene, E., and Russell, P. S. (1971). *Clin. Exp. Immunol.* **8,** 195.
Smith, R. T. (1968). *New Engl. J. Med.* **278,** 1207.
Smolin, G., and Okimoto, M. (1968). *Amer. J. Ophthalmol.* **66,** 804.
Southworth, J. G., Oharrian, S. H., Plate, J. M., and Amos, D. B. (1970). *Fed. Proc. Fed. Amer. Soc. Exp. Biol.* **29,** 101.
Spira, D. T., Silverman, P. H., and Gaines, C. (1970). *Immunology* **19,** 759.
Spreafico, F. (1968). *Proc. Int. Symp. Transplant. Immunol., Padua Acta Med. Patavina.* **28,** 914.
Spreafico, F. (1970). *Transplantation* **10,** 227.
Spreafico, F. (1971). Unpublished results.
Spreafico, F., and Franchi, G. (1972). In preparation.

Spreafico, F., and Lerner, E. M. (1967). *J. Immunol.* **98,** 407.

Spreafico, F., Morselli, P. L., and Marc, V. (1972). In preparation.

Stanbridge, E. J., and Perkins, F. T. (1969). *Nature (London)* **221,** 80.

Starzl, T. E., Marchioro, T. L., Porter, K. A., Iwasaki, Y., and Cerilli, G. J. (1967a). *Surg. Gynecol. Obstet.* **124,** 301.

Starzl, T. E., Porter, K. A., Iwasaki, Y., Marchioro, T. L., and Kashiwagi, N. (1967b). *Antilymphocytic Serum, Ciba Found. Symp.* p. 4.

Starzl, T. E., Groth, G., Terasaki, P. I., Putman, C. W., Brettschneider, L., and Marchioro, T. L. (1968). *Surg. Gynecol. Obstet.* **126,** 1023.

Starzl, T. E., Groth, G., Brettschneider, L., Smith, G. V., Penn, I., and Kashiwagi, N. (1969a). *Antibiot. Chemother. (Basel)* **15,** 349.

Starzl, T. E., Brettschneider, L., Penn, I., Schmidt, R. W., Bell, P., Kashiwagi, N., Townsend, C. M., and Putman, C. W. (1969b). *Transplant. Proc.* **1,** 448.

Starzl, T. E., Penn, I., Brettschneider, L., Ono, K., and Kashiwagi, N. (1970a). *Fed. Proc. Fed. Amer. Soc. Exp. Biol.* **29,** 191.

Starzl, T. E., Brettschneider, L., and Putnam, C. W. (1970b). *Progr. Liver Dis.* **3,** 495.

Starzl, T. E., Porter, K. A., and Andres, G. (1970c). *Ann. Surg.* **172,** 437.

Statsny, P., Stenbridge, V. A., Vischer, T., and Ziff, M. (1965). *J. Exp. Med.* **122,** 681.

Sterling, W. A., Elveback, L. R., and Shorter, R. G. (1970). *Transplantation* **10,** 297.

Stewart, P. B., and Bell, R. (1970). *Nature (London)* **227,** 278.

Stewart, P. B., and Cohen, V. (1969). *Science* **164,** 1083.

Stinson, E. B., Griepp, R. B., and Clark, D. A. (1970). *J. Thorac. Cardiovasc. Surg.* **60,** 303.

Streilein, J. W. (1966). *Ann. Intern. Med.* **65,** 511.

Strom, T. B., Levin, B. S., Dohrmann, G. J., and Pollack, V. E. (1968). *Proc. Soc. Exp. Biol. Med.* **129,** 261.

Sutthiwan, P., Shorter, R. G., Hallenbeck, G. A., and Elveback, L. R. (1969). *Transplantation* **8,** 249.

Suvatte, V., Githens, J. M., and Colofiore, J. (1968). *Transplantation* **6,** 826.

Taub, R. N. (1969). *Antibiot. Chemother. (Basel)* **15,** 250.

Taub, R. N. (1970). *Fed. Proc. Fed. Amer. Soc. Exp. Biol.* **29,** 142.

Taub, R. N., and Lance, E. M. (1968a). *J. Exp. Med.* **128,** 1281.

Taub, R. N., and Lance, E. M. (1968b). *Immunology* **15,** 633.

Taub, R. N., Brown, S. M., Kochwa, S., Rubin, A. D., and Dameshek, W. (1969). *Lancet* **ii,** 521.

Taylor, H. E. (1970a). *Fed. Proc. Fed. Amer. Soc. Exp. Biol.* **29,** 114.

Taylor, H. E. (1970b). *Transplant. Proc.* **2,** 413.

Taylor, R. B., and Wortis, H. H. (1968). *J. Exp. Med.* **128,** 927.

Tevethia, S. S., Dreesman, G. R., Lausch, N., and Rapp, F. (1968). *J. Immunol.* **101,** 1105.

Thomas, D., Mosedale, B., and Zola, H. (1971). Personal communication.

Thorsby, E., and Lie, S. (1968). *Vox Sang.* **15,** 44.

Torrigiani, G., and Roitt, I. M. (1965). *J. Exp. Med.* **122,** 181.

Traeger, J., Perrin, J., Fries, D., Saubier, E., Carraz, M., Bonnet, P., Archimbaud, J. P., Bernhardt, J. P., Brochier, J., Betuel, H., Veysseyre, C., Bryon, P., Prevot, J., Jouvanceau, A., Bansillon, V., Zech, P., and Rollet, A. (1968a). *Lyon Med.* **219,** 307.

Traeger, J., Perrin, J., Fries, D., Saubier, E., Carraz, M., Bonnet, P., Archimbaud, J. P., Bernhardt, J. P., Brochier, J., Betuel, H., Veysseyre, C., Bryon, P., Prevot, J., Jouvancreau, A., Bansillon, V., Zech, P., and Rollet, A. (1968b). *Presse Med.* **76,** 1517.

Traeger, J., Fries, D., Perrin, J., Carraz, M., Saubier, E., Bonnet, P., Archimbaud, J. P.,

Barnhardt, J. P., Betuel, H., Veysseyre, C., and Prevot, J. (1969). *E.D.T.A. Proc., Excerpta Med.* **5,** 140.

Traeger, J., Durix, A., Blanc, N., Brochier, J., and Rivillard, J. P. (1970). *Symp. Ser. Immunobiol. Stand.* **16,** 67.

Traeger, J., Touraine, J. L., Fries, D., and Berthoux, F., (1971). *Transplant. Proc.* **3,** 749.

Trainin, N., and Linker-Israeli, M. (1970). *J. Nat. Cancer Inst.* **44,** 893.

Trentin, J. J. (1970a). *Fed. Proc. Fed. Amer. Soc. Exp. Biol.* **29,** 114.

Trentin, J. J. (1970b). *Fed. Proc. Fed. Amer. Soc. Exp. Biol.* **29,** 175.

Trepel, F., Pichlmayr, R., Rimura, J., Brendel, W., and Begemann, H. (1968). *Klin. Wochenschr.* **46,** 856.

Tridente, G., and Van Bekkum, D. W. (1969). *In* "Lymphocytic Tissue and Germinal Centers in Immune Response" (L. Fiore-Donati and M. G. Hanna, eds.), p. 371. Plenum, New York.

Tsirimbas, A. D., Psisterer, H., Hornung, B., Thierfeder, S., and Stich, N. (1968). *Klin. Wochenschr.* **46,** 583.

Turcotte, J. G., Haines, R. F., Niederhuber, J. E., and Gikas, P. W. (1971). *Transplant. Proc.* **3,** 814.

Turk, J. L. (1970). *Fed. Proc. Fed. Amer. Soc. Exp. Biol.* **29,** 136.

Turk, J. L., and Polak, L. (1969). *Lancet* **i,** 130.

Turk, J. L., and Willoughby, D. A. (1967). *Lancet* **i,** 249.

Turk, J. L., and Willoughby, D. A. (1969). *Antibiot. Chemother. (Basel)* **15,** 267.

Turk, J. L., Willoughby, D. A., and Stevens, J. E. (1968). *Immunology* **14,** 683.

Tursi, A., Greaves, M. F., Torrigiani, G., Playfair, J. H. L., and Roitt, I. M. (1969). *Immunology* **17,** 801.

Tyler, R. W., Everett, N. B., and Schwartz, M. R. (1969). *J. Immunol.* **102,** 179.

Unanue, E. R., and Dixon, F. J. (1967). *Advan. Immunol.* **6,** 1.

Van Bekkum, D. W., Ledney, G. D., Balner, H., Van Putten, L. M., and De Vries, M. J. (1967). *Antilymphocytic Serum, Ciba Found. Symp.* p. 97.

Van Bekkum, D. W., Heysteck, G. A., and Marguat, R. L. (1969). *Transplantation* **8,** 678.

Vandeputte, M. (1968). *Life Sci.* **7,** 855.

Vandeputte, M. (1970). *Transplant. Proc.* **1,** 100.

Van Der Werf, B. A., Monaco, A. P., Wood, M. L., and Russell, P. S. (1968). *In* "Advances in Transplantation" (J. Dausset, J. Hamburger, and G. Mathé, eds.), p. 133. Munksgaard, Copenhagen.

Varet, B., Levy, J. P., Leclerc, J. C., and Senik, A. (1968). *Int. J. Cancer* **3,** 727.

Volkert, M., and Lundstedt, C. (1968). *J. Exp. Med.* **127,** 327.

Vredevoe, D. L., and Hays, E. F. (1969). *Cancer Res.* **29,** 1685.

Wagner, J. L., and Haughton, G. (1971). *J. Nat. Cancer Inst.* **46,** 1.

Waksman, B. H., Arbouys, S., and Arnason, B. G. (1961). *J. Exp. Med.* **114,** 997.

Ward, P. A. (1968). *J. Exp. Med.* **128,** 1201.

Warnatz, H., Scheiffarth, F., and Baier, F. (1969). *Transplantation* **8,** 347.

Weigand, H., and Hotchin, J. (1961). *J. Immunol.* **86,** 401.

Weil, R., and Simmons, R. L. (1968). *Ann. Surg.* **167,** 239.

Weitzel, R. H., and Rother, K. (1970). *Eur. Surg. Res.* **2,** 310.

Weksler, M. E., Bull, G., Schwartz, G. H., Stenzel, K. H., and Rubin, A. L. (1970) *J. Clin. Invest.* **49,** 1589.

White, R. G., Jenkins, G. C., and Wilkinson, P. C. (1963). *Int. Arch. Allergy Appl Immunol.* **22,** 156.

Wilhelm, R. E., Fisher, J. P., and Cooke, R. A. (1958). *J. Allergy* **26,** 493.

Wilkinson, P. C., and White, R. G. (1966). *Immunology* **11,** 229.
Willoughby, D. A., Bowghton, B., Spector, W. G., and Schild, H. O. (1963). *Immunology* **6,** 484.
Willoughby, D. A., Walters, M. N., and Spector, W. G. (1965). *Immunology* **8,** 578.
Winn, H. J., and Daddi, G. (1970). *Fed. Proc. Fed. Amer. Soc. Exp. Biol.* **29,** 104.
Woiwod, A. J. (1970). *Proc. Roy. Soc. Med.* **63,** 949.
Woiwod, A. J., Courtenay, J. S., Edwards, D. C., Epps, H. B., Knight, R. R., Mosedale, B., Phillips, A. W., Rahr, L., Thomas, D., Woodroffe, J. G., and Zola, H. (1970). *Transplantation* **10,** 173.
Wolf, R. E., Remmers, A. R., Sarles, H. E., Fish, J. C., and Lindley, J. D. (1971). *Transplantation* **11,** 418.
Wood, M. L. (1970). *Transplantation* **9,** 122.
Wood, M. L., and Vriesendorp, H. M. (1969). *Transplantation* **7,** 522.
Woodruff, M. F. A. (1960). "The Transplantation of Tissues and Organs." Thomas, Springfield, Illinois.
Woodruff, M. F. A. (1967). *Antilymphocytic Serum, Ciba Found. Symp.* p. 108.
Woodruff, M. F. A., and Anderson, N. A. (1963a). *Nature* (*London*) **200,** 702.
Woodruff, M. F. A., and Anderson, N. A. (1963b). *J. Clin. Pathol.* **20,** 466.
Woodruff, M. F. A., and Anderson, N. A. (1964). *Ann. N.Y. Acad. Sci.* **120,** 119.
Woodruff, M. F. A., and Smith, L. H. (1970). *Nature* (*London*) **225,** 377.
Woodruff, M. F. A., Forman, B., and Fraser, K. B. (1951). *J. Immunol.* **67,** 57.
Woodruff, M. F. A., Reid, B. L., and James, K. (1967). *Nature* (*London*) **216,** 758.
Woodruff, M. F. A., Nolan, B., Robson, J. S., and McDonald, M. K. (1969). *Lancet* **i,** 6.
Woods, D. A. (1969). *Nature* (*London*) **224,** 276.
Yussman, M. A. (1969). *Surg. Forum* **20,** 404.
Zisman, B., Hirsh, M. S., and Allison, A. C. (1970). *J. Immunol.* **104,** 1155.
Zola, H., Mosedale, B., and Thomas, D. (1970). *Transplantation* **9,** 259.
Zola, H., Thomas, D., Mosedale, B., and Courtenay, J. S. (1971). *Transplantation* **12,** 49.

Selective Multiphase Cancer Therapy: Conceptual Aspects and Experimental Basis

MANFRED VON ARDENNE

Forschungsinstitut Manfred von Ardenne
Dresden-Weisser Hirsch
Deutsche Demokratische Republik

I. Introduction

This report is an attempt to condense in limited space the theoretical basis and the results of experimental procedure of a new approach to cancer therapy correlating with the conditions in the treatment of human neoplastic disease. It represents the laboratory and clinical experience of almost 10 years of research during which, in collaboration with a group of coworkers, I have tried to elucidate the multifaceted aspects of cancer and cancer therapy.

The details of these studies are published in the form of a book (von Ardenne, 1971b) which consists of a collection of 107 papers. They should be consulted by the interested reader for information on the guiding principles and technical essentials of procedure and evaluation.

Two general principles should be mentioned here.

1. The complexity of the problem has been approached by mathematical analysis of pathophysiological processes—by analyzing and controlling measurement, i.e., by applying the methods of exact natural science.

2. Multiphase cancer therapy is characterized by "the combination of several weak agents on particularly sensitive systems of the cancer cell." The combination of the individual approaches has been established for the purpose of selectively enhancing therapeutic action and reducing toxic effects, it comprises the following steps (therapeutic measures):

(a) Marked increase in tumor cell glycolysis by a 30-hour rise of blood glucose concentration until stationary concentrations are reached (selective increase of the tumor cell glycolysis in the tumor tissue).

(b) Temporary increase of body temperature to, e.g., 40°C.

(c) Temporary increase of the concentration of particular intrinsic substances and cell organelles in the organism with respect to the tumor tissue (e.g., retinol and lysosomal content of tumor cells).

(d) Initiation of the natural cellular lytic mechanisms of the cancer cells by an activating stimulus with respect to a combination of therapeutic measures.

(e) Extension of the lytic mechanism under the labilizing influence of measures a, b, and c to a chain reaction leading to cell damage, similar to the processes occurring in inflammatory tissues. The resulting selective amplification of primary cancer cell damage (by measure d) represents the basic mechanism of the therapy concept.

(f) Stimulation and amplification of natural or artificial immunomechanisms to damage cancer cells near the capillaries, which are difficult to reach by measure a.

The single steps of the treatment procedure and their combination will be described in the following sections.

II. The Individual Phases—Their Selective Mechanism and Combination

A. Physical Aspects of the Selectivity Problem in Cancer Therapy

As is known, a cure for cancer at an advanced (metastatic) stage can only be expected if it is possible to damage the cells in all the cancer tissues of the body in such a way that out of a million cancer cells at most only a few survive. At the same time, only a small number of normal cells may be killed in healthy tissue. This is a task that can only be solved by highly selective treatment. Physics, and more especially electronics, offer examples of approaches for the development of procedures with this high degree of selectivity. In this connection, of prime importance are the principle of coupling (multiple use) of selective elements and, particularly, the mechanism of chain reactions (theoretically identical with the feedback mechanism). In our 10-year investigation devoted to the development of multiphase cancer therapy (von Ardenne, 1971b), we have attempted to introduce these two physical principles into the pathophysiology of the disease and to bring about their concrete realization.

B. Lasting Increase in Tumor Glycolysis with Optimized Hyperacidity as the Main Selective Element of Multiphase Cancer Therapy

Aerobic glycolysis of cancer cells, discovered about five decades ago (Warburg 1930), made it possible for us to induce a very useful element of selectivity between cancerous and normal tissue by optimizing the hyperacidity of cancer tissues (von Ardenne, 1965a) on the basis of calculations (von Ardenne and Rieger, 1966) and measurements (von Ardenne *et al.*, 1969a) [pH difference (Δ pH) = almost 1 pH unit]. These findings were the result of the following investigations.

1. It was found that in both animals and humans it was possible to elevate the blood glucose concentration [$c_{\mathrm{Gk(C)}}$] during therapy practically without risk from $c_{\mathrm{Gk(C)}} \approx 100$ (normal) to 400 mg/100 ml and thereby to achieve intensification of fermentation and hyperacidity of cancer tissue (von Ardenne, 1965a; von Ardenne *et al.*, 1970d). By stimulating fermentation we ran contrary to efforts that had met with failure for decades, namely, to cure cancer by inhibiting fermentation.

2. Cells of the brain, the retina, and the peripheral nervous system also reveal appreciable aerobic glycolysis *in vivo* as a condition of their activity, as can be seen in Table I. With a normal blood glucose concentration there is no utilizable pH difference between healthy nerve tissue and cancer tissue (both have pH values around 7.0 to 7.1). The selective element, that is to say, the pH difference between cancer tissue and normal tissue, only results from the increase in the blood glucose concentration over a prolonged period of time. That the hyperacidity of the various tissues of the nervous system remains practically unaltered while the blood glucose concentration is increased (von Ardenne and Reitnauer, 1970a) is due to natural physiological barriers that limit the transport of glucose. These

TABLE I

In Vivo Aerobic Glycolysis of Cancer Cells and Absence of Aerobic Glycolysis in Normal Cells as the Fundamental Difference in Metabolism of These Two Cell Types[a,b]

Cells	Proportion N_c of aerobic glycolysis *in vivo* in glucose metabolism	Tissue parameters *in vivo*: $c_{Gk(C)}$ = 100 mg/100 ml		Tissue parameters *in vivo*: $c_{Gk(C)}$ = 400 mg/100 ml	
		$c_{Gk(C)}$ (mg/100 ml)	pH[e]	$c_{Gk(C)}$ (mg/100 ml)	pH
1. Normal cells					
Liver	0	50	7.35	200	7.35
Embryonic tissue	0	50	7.35	200	7.35
Red bone marrow	0	50	7.35	200	7.35
Brain (special case)	0.085[c]	6 (BBB)	7.05	6 (BBB)	7.05
Retina (special case)	0.085[c]	≈6 (BBB)	7.1	≈6 (BBB)	7.0
Nerves (special case)	—	(BNB)	6.8 (Unstimulated)	(BNB)	6.8 (Unstimulated)
2. Cancer cells					
Morris hepatoma 5123; slight deviation (doubling time T_c = 15 days)	0.32 (With anaerobic glycolysis portion)	20 (High value due to low glucose consumption)	7.2	80	≈**6.8**
Hepatoma	≈0.35[d] (With anaerobic glycolysis portion)	1–5	7.0	4–20	6.0
DS-carcinosarcoma	≈0.35 (With anaerobic glycolysis portion)	1–5	7.0	4–20	**6.0**
Walker carcinoma	0.35[d] (With anaerobic glycolysis portion)	1–5	7.0	4–20	**6.0**

[a] Taken from Warburg, 1930.

[b] This difference in metabolism is the foundation of the multiphase cancer therapy concept and is further reflected by *in vivo* pH values for $c_{Gk(C)} = 400$ mg/100 ml in cell Types 1 and 2. The boldface pH values in the last column show that the pH difference necessary for therapeutic selectivity between cancer tissue and normal tissue ($\Delta pH \approx 1.0$ unit) is only produced by the multiplication of the blood glucose concentration in conjunction with the natural barriers [blood–brain barrier (BBB) and blood–nerve barrier (BNB)] of nerve tissue.

[c] In normal cells with this amount of partial aerobic fermentation, a limit is given *in vivo* to the glucose metabolism (hyperacidity), for instance by the BBB in the case of brain cells. Cells of this type, therefore, represent a special case (functional exception). Since the BBB and the BNB are not fully developed in fetuses, there is a labile situation, particularly in diabetes mellitus, which can easily lead to damage.

[d] This small proportion of the lactic acid fermentation established from *in vivo* measurements can only explain the high tumor hyperacidity obtained if the time constant of lactic acid exchange is assumed to be about 3 times larger than the time constant of glucose exchange. By assuming the same value for the two time constants, for the sake of simplicity roughly correct tumor acidity values were predicted. This owing to the fact that at the same time the proportion of lactic acid fermentation in the glucose metabolism was estimated considerably too high, at ≈ 0.9 (compensation of both errors). For the difference in the two time constants, see Rieger, 1970.

[e] For a review on intra- and extracellular pH of various tissues, see Waddel and Bates, 1969. Agreement of pH value for intra- and extracellular milieu is around 6.3 to 6.8. (In some cases doubtful measured values are taken from the literature.)

are the blood–brain barrier (BBB) (Quadbeck, 1967) and the recently discovered blood–nerve barrier (BNB) (von Ardenne, 1970a).

3. The mathematical study of *in vivo* fermentation of cancerous tumors and especially the equation of tumor hyperacidity (von Ardenne and Rieger, 1966) revealed that *in vivo*, once stable concentration ratios have become established, the hyperacidity of the cancer cells is virtually independent of the time constant of the glucose–lactic acid exchange. This means that, for instance, cancer cells in the poorly vascularized inner part of a tumor are hyperacidified to almost exactly the same degree as cancer cells that lie closer to the capillaries of the border zone of the tumor. This astonishing finding is explained by the fact that, on the one hand, the cell regions with a poor blood supply inside the tumors have access to much less glucose, but, on the other hand, the small amount of lactic acid which is formed flows out much more slowly. The observation that, as a first approximation all cancer tissues are homogeneously hyperacidified satisfies an additional postulate for the utilization of the pH difference as a selective element.

4. Because of the good hydrogen ion exchange found across the outer membrane of the cancer cells (von Ardenne and Reitnauer, 1970b) and because of the need to combat metastases, it was necessary to measure the dependence of the attainable pH decrease upon the number of cancer cells in metastases or micrometastases after elevation of the blood glucose concentration to 400 mg/100 ml. Figure 1 shows the results. It is apparent

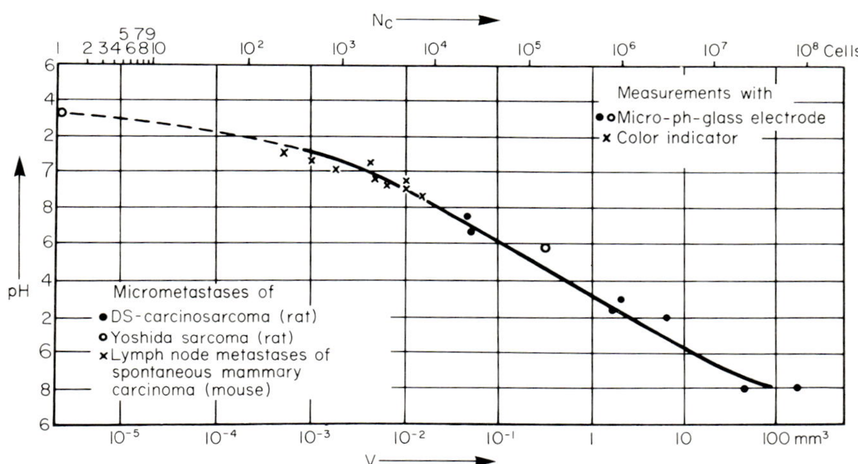

FIG. 1. Activity range of host defense increased nonspecifically by single BCG inoculation and after 3 days, 100 minutes, 40°C hyperthermia. Plot of pH values of metastases as a function of volume V and cell number N_c. (BCG) Bacillus Calmette-Guérin.

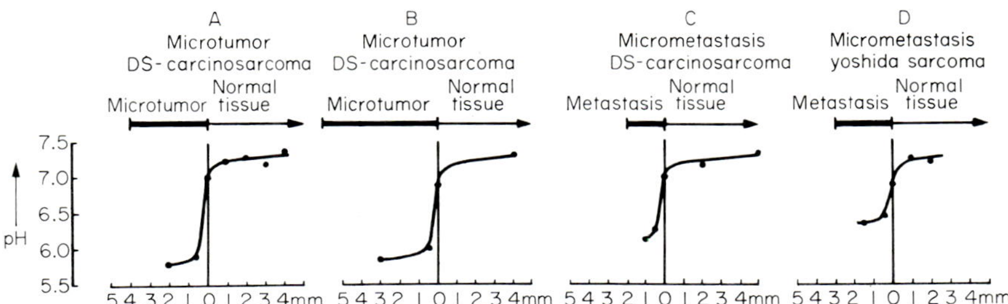

FIG. 2. Profiles of pH values in and near various hyperacidified microtumors and micrometastases, as measured by micro-pH glass electrode with a free tip of ~80 μm.

from this figure that micrometastases with cells numbering $N_c > 10^6$ can be adequately hyperacidified. This would be an additional reason for using the pH difference as a selective element. However, with cells numbering $N_c < 10^6$ only the stimulation of the natural defenses is achieved (see Chapter A.31.2, von Ardenne, 1971b; von Ardenne *et al.*, 1969a; von Ardenne and Chaplain, 1970). The measurements were obtained with an especially developed micro-pH glass electrode with the measuring tip only 80 μm in length (von Ardenne *et al.*, 1969b). As is shown in Fig. 2 this micro-pH glass electrode made it possible to record the pH profile inside and close to optimally acidified micrometastases (von Ardenne *et al.*, 1970a). These measurements showed that the low pH value almost reaches the "dividing line" between cancer tissue and healthy tissue. The transition to the normal pH of healthy tissue occurs only in a thin layer of a few tenths of a millimeter. The narrow confines of our therapy based on optimized hyperacidity lie in this thin transitional layer, the limits of which are indicated in Fig. 3 in a sectional view of a tumor border zone. This observation led to introducing the immunological approach as a definite component of the concept of multiphase cancer therapy (von Ardenne and Chaplain, 1971), for, as is suggested by the sectional view, it could be directed quite specifically against (possibly surviving) cancer cells in this transitional layer close to the capillaries which are more difficult to hyperacidify.

5. In the past many attempts were made, without any therapeutic objectives, to intensify the hyperacidity of solid tumors by the infusion of glucose (Ashby, 1966; Rauen and Norpoth, 1967). In literature, usually duration of the glucose infusion does not exceed 60 minutes and, indeed, as a rule is considerably shorter (glucose injections). The time constant for the glucose–lactic acid exchange for tumors is about ($\tau \approx 50$ minutes (von Ardenne and Rieger, 1966). As is known, the concentration only becomes stationary after a period corresponding to 3 times the time constant

of exchange, in other words, in this instance only after (3 × 50 =) 150 minutes. The limiting value of tumor hyperacidity can thus only be expected 150 minutes after increasing the blood glucose concentration to 400 mg/100 ml, that is, about 240 minutes after the beginning of the infusion with the appropriate dose of glucose. The measurement shown in Fig. 4 of a rat DS carcinosarcoma is in excellent accord with these estimates. Within 60 minutes after the beginning of the glucose infusion the pH value dropped from 7.0 to 6.61. Upon continuation of the glucose infusion until a stationary concentration was reached, that is, until time t = 240 minutes, the tumor pH value dropped to 6.22. The pH change resulting simply from waiting for the establishment of a stationary concentration was thus almost 0.4 pH units. This finding is a decisive factor for the success of therapy. To distinguish this approach from earlier experiments with a short duration of infusion, the term "optimized tumor hyperacidity" is introduced to the procedure of treatment. The pH measurement was made with a glass electrode, the sensitive tip of which had a relatively large measuring surface. Thus, because of the amount of normal tissue measured at the same time, which is fairly considerable, this measurement may even be considered as a determination of a mixed pH value. In the present case it was possible to reconstruct the actual pH limit for pure tumor tissue at the site of the measurement from microtome sections showing the profile of the tip of the

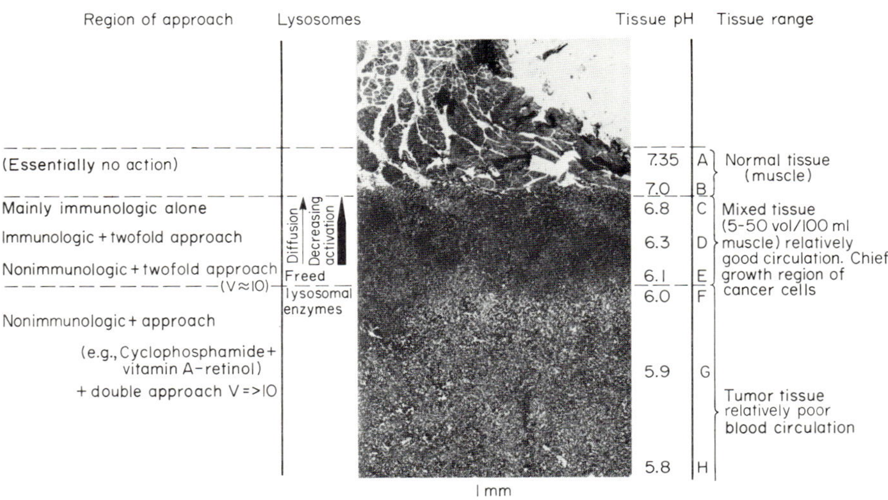

FIG. 3. Photomicrograph of a section of border zone between rat DS-carcinosarcoma and adjacent normal tissue under conditions of hyperacidification. (V) volume.

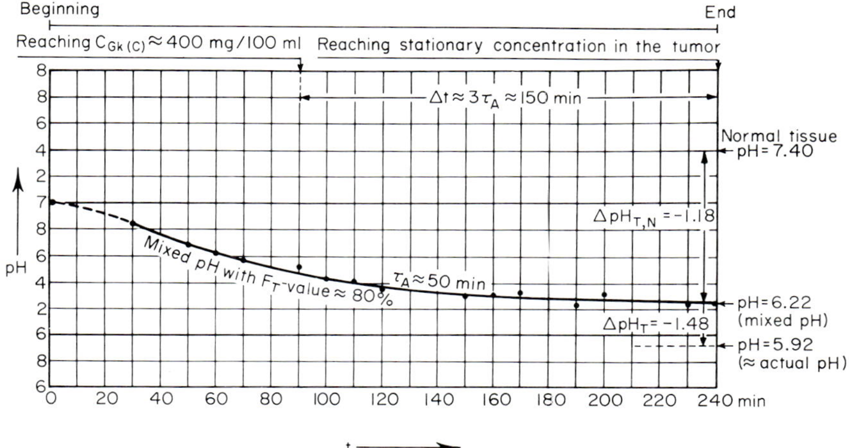

FIG. 4. Plot of pH of rat DS-carcinosarcoma as a function of attainment of stationary value after intravenous (i.v.) glucose infusion at a dosage rate of $Dt^{-1}{}_A = 5.5$ gm kg^{-1}/100 minutes. (Meinsberg GA 70-type glass electrode with $F \sim 100$ mm^2.)

glass electrode in the tissue and, thus, revealing the cancer tissue–normal tissue region of the surface measured. The value was found to be pH 5.92.

From this and numerous other pH measurements on tumors and metastases (von Ardenne *et al.*, 1969g; von Ardenne *et al.*, 1969f; von Ardenne *et al.*, 1970a), it follows that with the method of optimized tumor hyperacidity all cancer tissues in the organism with a number of cells (N_c) $> 10^6$ can be brought selectively to pH values that are about 1 pH unit lower than the lowest pH value of normal tissue. This result furnished an element of very high selectivity between cancer and normal tissue.

C. 40°C Hyperthermia as an Additional Selective Element in Multiphase Cancer Therapy

Selective weakening of cancer cells, or more specifically of essential structural proteins of cancer cell membranes, can be achieved *in vivo* not only by optimized hyperacidity of tumors, but also by overheating cancer cells. The difference between the heat sensitivity of cancer cells and the most heat-sensitive normal cells is relatively slight (Cavaliere *et al.*, 1967), so that the contribution of hyperthermia in improving the overall selectivity of therapy is smaller by far than the contribution of optimized hyperacidity. Nevertheless, the hyperthermia step cannot be omitted at present because it can also contribute appreciably to the deterioration of the essential structural proteins of the cell membranes. By introducing hyperthermia, even a slight decrease in pH [a reduction of 0.3 pH units at 40°C—150 minutes hyperthermia compared to 37°C (von Ardenne, 1971b)] is sufficient to achieve the weakening of cancer cells necessary for therapy, so as to render the therapeutic process well tolerated even for older patients in a poor state of health. Generally speaking, the temperature is not raised above 40°C in total-body hyperthermia. Higher temperatures ($\Delta T = +1°$ to $+3°$C) are only used locally upon additional topical hyperthermia of tumors suitable for this purpose.

The twofold approach of optimized tumor hyperacidity plus 40°C hyperthermia discloses the fundamental process of the multiphase therapy of cancer discussed in the next section.

D. Mechanism of Lysosomal Cytolysis and the Following Cytolytic Chain Reaction

It was pointed out in the Introduction that from the physical standpoint particularly high expectations are attached to the chain reaction mechanism in solving the problem of selectivity in cancer therapy. That Nature should keep such a chain reaction in readiness in the live organism and that this chain reaction takes place not only in the extremely rare cases of spontaneous cures, but also in the more common spontaneous tumor regressions following therapeutic measures, has already been suggested by this author (von Ardenne, 1965b). Some months later (von Ardenne, 1965a) the principal conditions for eliciting the chain reaction were actually realized: elevation of the blood glucose concentration, thereby artificially stimulating fermentation and hyperacidity of the tumor tissue, which in combination with hyperthermia, raises, in turn, the toxic effect of cellular breakdown products of the cancer cells in the tissue with a lower pH value. Investigations lasting up to 1968 finally led to the disclosure of the finer details of the mechanism of lysosomal cytolytic chain reaction (von Ardenne and Reitnauer, 1968a; von Ardenne *et al.*, 1969d).

A chain reaction of cell killing is attained when a milieu exists in which substances (lytic enzymes) liberated from a dying cell contribute to the death of neighboring cells during the process. In the chain reaction theory (Friedman, 1952), three distinct states are recognized.

1. *Subcritical States*

In this phase the amount of substances liberated from a dying cell, related to the reaction volume during the period of the process, is only sufficient for the death of a certain small number of other cells (mean multiplication factor of chain reaction k).

In the subcritical course which generally takes place during therapy, the chain reaction acts as enhancer: it gives rise to the increase of a primary cell-killing rate, produced by appropriate measures, by a multiplication factor k.

2. *Transition to the Critical State*

In this phase the substances liberated from a dying cell cause the death of all cells in the reaction volume during the process. The multiplication factor k of the chain reaction reaches the value of the number of cells in the volume. A critical course can be brought about by a strong artificial reduction of the pH value of the medium. The limiting value for the second state, in the case of Ehrlich mouse ascites cancer (EMAC) cells as a function of temperature and time of action of the combination of hyperacidity and hyperthermia can be seen (von Ardenne and Reitnauer, 1968a).

3. *Supercritical State*

In this phase there is no need for any primary activating stimulus because the parameters present in the reaction volume already elicit the dying of cells, the death of which then leads to killing of all the other tumor cells.

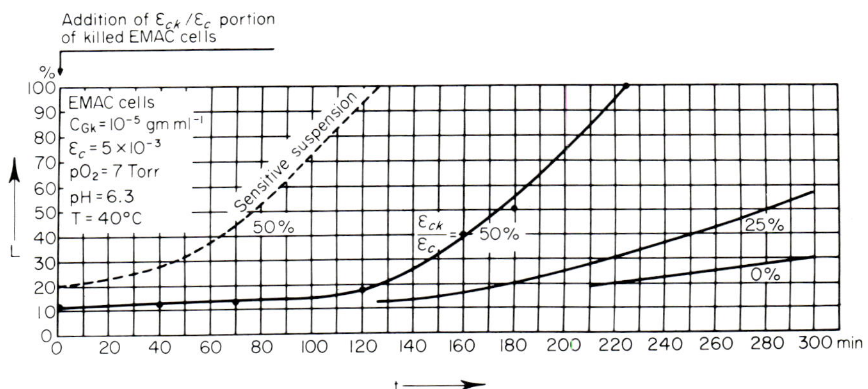

FIG. 5. Cell killing by twofold approach (pH = 5.5, 42°C, 100 minutes) at C_{Gk} = 10^{-5} gm ml^{-1} and pO_2 = 7 mm Hg, directly before addition. Damage of cancer cells by added dead cancer cells that where killed by hyperacidification and hyperthermia: Trypan blue staining, L, as a function of action time, t, of dead cancer cells killed at pH 6.3 and T = 40°C. LY medium (Warburg, 1962); *in vitro* measurements. (EMAC) Ehrlich mouse ascites tumor cells.

That substances liberated from killed cancer cells can really contribute to the death of other cancer cells is demonstrated by the *in vitro* experiment on the elementary process of cytolysis chain reaction summarized in Fig. 5. In the figure the trypan blue-staining, L, of EMAC cells is plotted as a function of the time of action, t, of EMAC cells that have just been killed (E_{ck}) at pH 6.3 and $T = 40°C$. The glucose concentration c_{GK} in the cell suspension with a cell density ϵ_c and partial oxygen pressure pO_2 simulated conditions in a tumor. This experiment, which corresponds to a subcritical chain reaction, shows that the cells are stainable (killed off) after a time t which is the shorter, the higher the percentage of cytolyzed cancer cells added at time $t = 0$. The broken-line curve, which reveals particularly

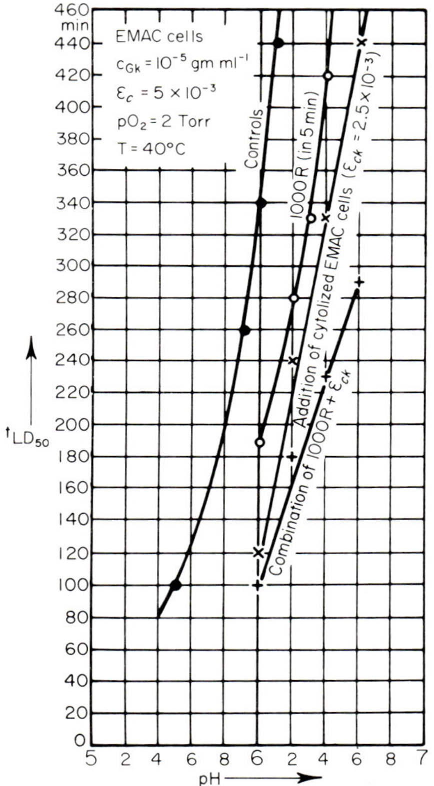

FIG. 6. *In vitro* measurements of $t_{LD/50}$ as a function of pH in cancer cells after short 1000 R irradiation and addition of 0.5 ϵ_c cytolyzed EMAC cells.

rapid killing due to the addition of 50% cytolyzed EMAC cells, resulted from a cell suspension with a greater sensitivity (greater liberation of lysosomes and higher lysosome content; see further below).

Figure 6 shows a further *in vitro* measurement in which a comparison is made between the increase in cell damage due to the addition of 33% lysed EMAC cells and the action of an X-ray dose of $D = 1000$ R in an EMAC cell suspension subjected to therapeutic measures. The ordinate gives the time $t_{LD}/_{50}$ for 50% of the cells to be stained by trypan blue as a function of the pH value of the medium adjusted with lactic acid at a temperature of $T = 40°C$. The lysed EMAC cells were obtained in this case by brief incubation with 0.1% Triton X. The left curve designated "controls" shows the cytolysis chain reaction turning critical ($k = \infty$). Furthermore, it is shown that at pH 6.3 and $T = 40°C$, after 330 minutes, 50% of the EMAC cells become stainable (are killed off) if the suspension is irradiated with an X-ray dose of $D = 1000$ R. At this dose the damage rate is $L_1 \approx 24\%$ of the EMAC cells strongly weakened by pH 6.3 and $T = 40°C$. From comparative measurements of this type, it was possible to determine numerically the degree of selective intensification I resulting from weakening of the cancer cells and from the multiplication factor k, with its great dependence upon the pH value (see below).

As to the nature of substances liberated from dying cells and contributing to the death of neighboring cells, it was reasonable to suppose that the lysosomal enzymes exercise this key function. Ten years ago Ch. de Duve (1959) isolated characteristic cell organelles by density gradient ultracentrifugation, examined them in the electron microscope, and investigated their biochemical properties. These studies (de Duve, 1961) showed that the lytic enzymes of the cell were bound in cell organelles, the lysosomes, and were separated from the rest of the cellular space by a particularly labile membrane. The structural proteins of the lysosomal membranes form the main target in the concept of the multiphase therapy of cancer. Since 1959, some forty different lysosomal enzymes have been found. The spectrum and relative frequency of these enzymes vary, for instance as a function of cell type (cells of various organs) and of the environmental conditions (e.g., supply of substances that are to undergo pinocytosis). The pH optimum of most lysosomal enzymes is in the strongly acid region, as a rule around pH ≈ 5.0.

In the case of individual lysosomal enzymes, for instance acid phosphatases, the increase in enzymic activity between pH $= 7.1$ (about the lowest pH value of normal tissue, such as in the brain, retina, peripheral nerves, and heavily used muscles) and the 6.0 to 6.3 attainable in cancer tissues, as shown in Fig. 7, is only relative enzymic activity $A_{rel} \approx 2$, and

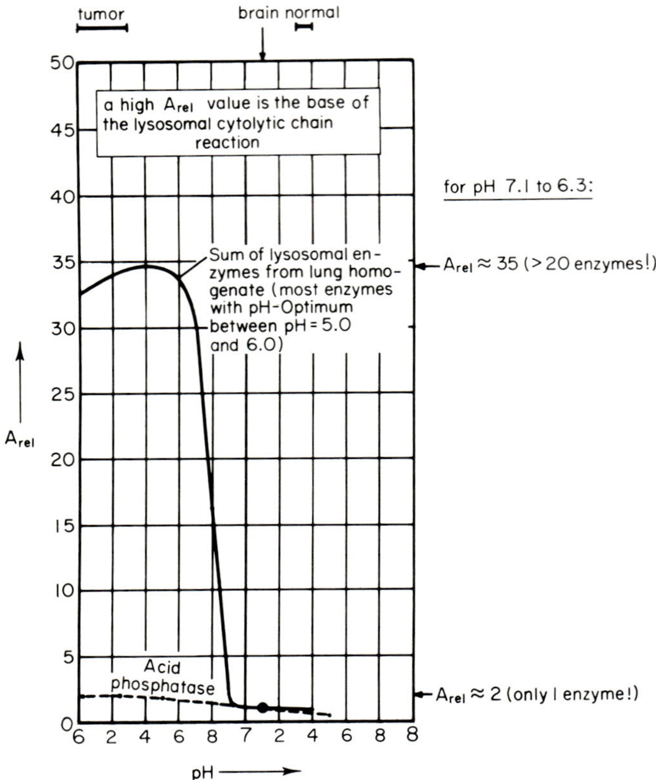

FIG. 7. Relative enzymic activity A_{rel} of acid phosphatase alone and of sum of lysosomal enzymes in units of enzymic activity at pH = 7.1 (pH of brain) as a function of pH. Tissue at a blood glucose level of 4×10^{-3} gm ml^{-1}. (Solid curve data from Druckrey *et al.*, 1959; broken curve data from Shaw, 1966.)

in other enzymes measured individually at the most, 3. Thus, a factor which is of the greatest importance for the chain reaction mechanism is that upon interaction between the many lysosomal enzymes with their pH optima close to 5.0 the relative enzymic activity increases to an extraordinary degree, for instance to values around $A_{rel} \approx 35$. At the same time, as is shown by the solid curve in Fig. 7, there is an extremely steep drop in enzymic activity as soon as the pH value rises above about 6.9.* In this

* Further biochemical investigations on the $A_{rel} = f(\text{pH})$ curve of lysosomal enzymes and groups of these enzymes are in progress.

example, practically the maximal activity of all the lysosomal enzymes is found at pH 6.6. The potentiation of action and its pH dependence in a group of many enzymes with about the same pH optimum is a discovery of which the fundamental biological importance reaches far beyond the therapeutic problems discussed here. This extraordinarily strong and steep increase at pH below 6.9 in the relative enzymic activity is an essential condition in bringing about the cytolysis chain reaction. The activation of all the lysosomal enzymes at values with pH < 6.3 is so strong that the portion of these enzymes finally reaching the extracellular space from a dying cell contributes to a considerable degree to the destruction caused to adjacent cells. In addition to the extracellular effect discussed, the great increase in the activity of all the lysosomal enzymes in the acid range also contributes to a higher rate of intracellular liberation of lysosomal enzymes. A single selective element, the pH difference between cancer tissue and normal tissue, will, therefore, often be used in our therapeutic concept (von Ardenne and Rieger, 1967); this is the basis of the weakening of the

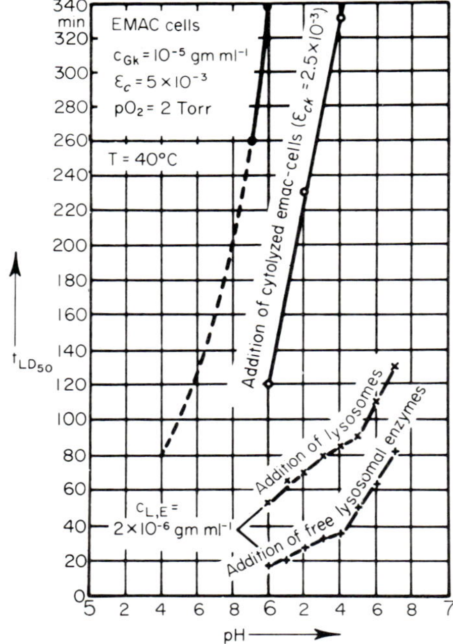

FIG. 8. *In vitro* measurements of $t_{LD/50}$ as function of pH upon addition of free and bound lysosomal enzymes. $t_{LD/50}$ = time for 50% staining with trypan blue; LY medium; pH controlled by lactic acid additions. (EMAC) Ehrlich mouse ascites tumor cells.

cancer cells and, in particular, their lysosomal membranes, the increased rate of liberation of lysosomal enzymes, and a very strong increase in the activity of lysosomal enzymes.

Using the same method of presentation as in Fig. 6, a comparison is made in Fig. 8 for the case of an EMAC cell suspension kept under antineoplastic conditions, between the increased cell damage caused by the addition of 33% cytolyzed EMAC cells and the action of added isolated lysosomes or added liberated lysosomal enzymes from EMAC cells (von Ardenne *et al.*, 1969d).

The lysosomes were isolated by isopyknic zonal ultracentrifugation, and the free lysosomal enzymes were obtained with an ultrasonic field so strong that the lysosomal membranes were destroyed. In order to simulate the high density of the *in vivo* situation, the lysosomes or the liberated lysosomal enzymes were preincubated with EMAC cells in a small volume of solution (2 ml) at 20°C for 5 minutes. This ensures almost complete adsorption.

The lysosomal enzyme content of EMAC cells is relatively low, amounting to about 2×10^{-9} mg/cell. The concentrations of lysosomes (c_L) and lysosomal enzymes ($c_E = 2 \times 10^{-6}$ gm ml^{-1} taken as basis for curves compared with one another correspond to a lysosomal content or a free lysosomal enzyme content of 5×10^{-3} gm ml^{-1} EMAC cells (according to the EMAC cell density ϵ_c used in the measurement in Fig. 8). The concentrations for lysosomes or lysosomal enzymes, therefore, are selected for the *in vitro* measurements in Fig. 8 so that they correspond to a primary lethality rate of $L_1 = 50\%$. From the *in vitro* measurement one can see a very pronounced destructive effect caused by the addition of free lysosomal enzymes and a pronounced damaging effect caused by the addition of an equivalent quantity of lysosomes. That this strong effect is already present at pH < 6.7 is in accord with the shape of the solid curve in Fig. 7. Furthermore, the *in vitro* measurement also shows a considerable increase in the effect with further lowering of the pH. An appreciable contribution to this accelerated lethality is provided by weakening of the cancer cells which becomes intensified with falling pH and at 40°C.

Proof that the membranes of the lysosomes (their structural proteins) represent the actual target in the concept of multiphase cancer therapy and that the liberation of lysosomal enzymes inside the cell represents the primary process of cell damage is provided by the measurement shown in Fig. 9. A lysosomal enzyme which can readily be investigated by known methods (Thomas and Aldridge, 1966) is acid phosphatase. The relative concentration of acid phosphatase in the intracellular and extracellular spaces as a function of the time of action t of combined therapeutic attack

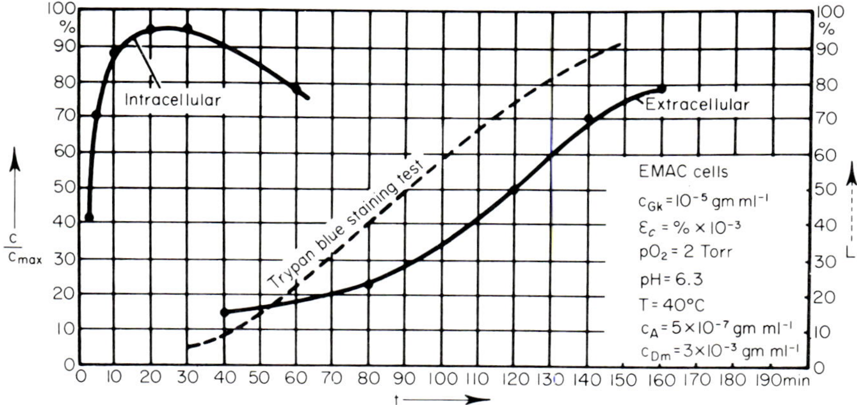

FIG. 9. Relative concentration C/C_{max} of acid intracellular and extracellular phosphatase as function of action time t of combined therapeutic measures (pH 6.3 + 40°C hyperthermia) + vitamin A (A) + dimethylsulfoxide (Dm). (EMAC) Ehrlich mouse ascites tumor cells.

[(pH 6.3 + 40°C hyperthermia temperature) + (vitamin A–retinol, $c_A = 5 \times 10^{-7}$ gm ml^{-1}) + dimethylsulfoxide (DMSO), $c_{DM} = 3 \times 10^{-3}$ gm ml^{-1}] was measured. This combination corresponds to a possible variation of our therapeutic concept. An almost identical result was obtained with phospholipase as indicator enzyme. A few minutes after establishing the active combination, the liberation of lysosomal indicator enzymes set in and after about a time interval $t = 20$ minutes the maximum intracellular concentration was reached by both lysosomal enzymes. The lysosomal enzymes (indicator enzymes) appear much later in the extracellular space, only when the trypan blue color test indicates pore formation of the external cell membrane. The shape of the two concentration curves shows that the intracellular liberation of lysosomal enzymes actually takes place much earlier than the destruction of the outer cell membrane. The mechanism of lysosomal cytolysis chain reaction may be largely explained by the measurements described in this section.

E. Lysosomal Cytolysis and the Following Chain Reaction as a Universal Biomechanism

It is both the object and the result of multiphase cancer therapy to elicit the natural mechanism of cytolysis of the cells localized strictly in cancer tissues. It should be mentioned in passing that the same chain reaction mechanism takes place topically in inflammation in the focus of inflammation (von Ardenne *et al.*, 1969d), in the brain in death due to narcosis or to hyperglycemic coma (von Ardenne *et al.*, 1970c), in the heart muscle in cardiac infarction (see Chapter A.12. in von Ardenne, 1971b), in the skin in radiation erythema and vitamin A erythema (von Ardenne and Reitnauer, 1970c), and in the entire body in general autolysis after the onset of death (von Ardenne, 1970b).

F. Selective Intensification of Primary Cancer Cell Destruction by Weakening the Cancer Cells Mediated by the Subcritical Lysosomal Chain Reaction

Because of the rapid decrease of the relative enzymic activity as soon as pH 6.7 is reached, the cytolysis and the following chain reaction immediately breaks off as soon as healthy tissue is reached. Since the pH value in the tissues of the larger vessels in tumors comes close to the normal value of pH 7.35, these vessels remain untouched by the destructive mechanism, and, thus, the danger of internal hemorrhaging is much reduced in multi-

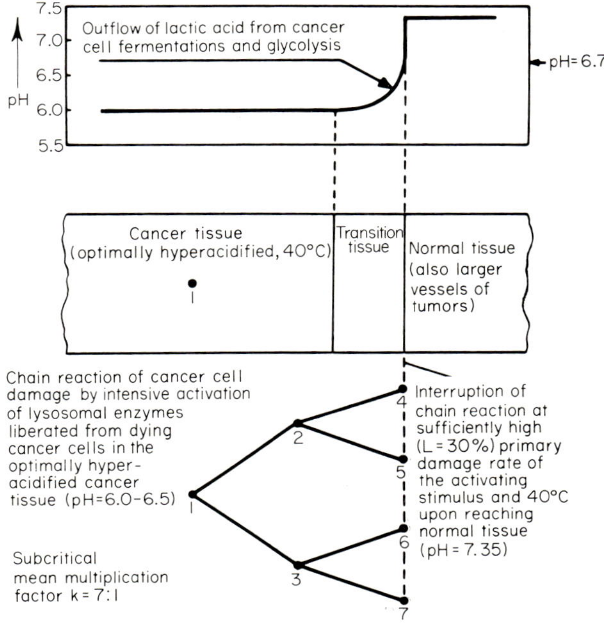

Fig. 10. Schematic presentation of experimental finding that the discovered chain reaction under specified conditions also damages a high percentage of nearby living cancer cells.

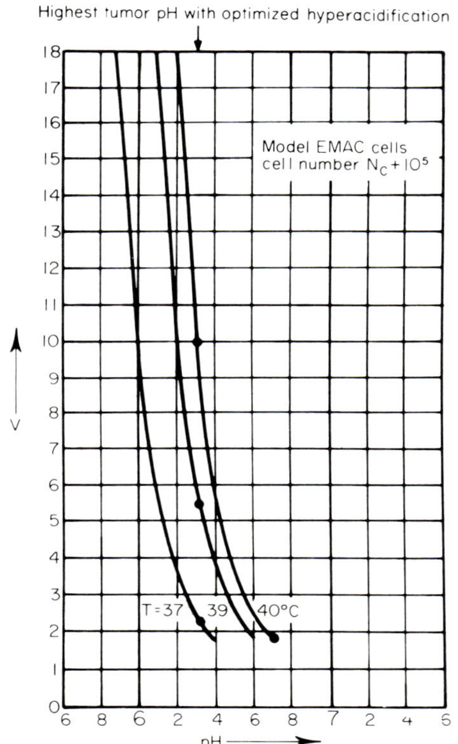

FIG. 11. Selective reinforcement V (volume) of cancer cell damage as function of pH with 300 minutes twofold approach at various hyperthermia temperatures. (EMAC) Ehrlich mouse ascites tumor cells.

phase therapy of cancer. As is indicated by Fig. 10, the chain reaction mechanism has a strong effect even in the critical transitional tissue between cancerous and normal tissue. During the process lasting several 100 minutes the lysosomal enzymes liberated into the strongly hyperacidified cancer tissue reaches as far as the normal tissue by diffusion and convection. Since the lysosomal enzymes are fully activated until they reach pH 6.7 (Fig. 7), it may be expected that up to this pH value the cytolysis chain reaction is fully active in the transitional tissue. But this layer lies close to the border adjacent to the normal tissue (Fig. 3), so that only a few cancer cells have a chance of survival. As was already stated in Section II, B, 4 the immunological measures included in the concept of multiphase cancer therapy are directed against these few cells.

With increasing hyperacidity of the cancer tissue, as has been shown, the weakening of the cancer cells, particularly their lysosomal membranes, and at the same time the activation of the liberated lysosomal enzymes, rapidly increases. Increase of these two factors causes a very rapid rise in the multiplication factor of the cytolysis chain reaction. In this interaction the pH dependence described leads to an extraordinarily steep rise in the selective intensification factor of cancer cell damage as soon as the pH drops under about 6.5 at 40°C (or under about 6.2 at 37°C). Figure 11 shows the determining values for this rise, obtained from *in vitro* measurements (see Section II, D). The shape of the curves and the extremely steep rise in the intensification factor of cancer cell damage reveals the decisive importance of optimized tumor hyperacidity and its combination with 40°C hyperthermia (twofold approach). It is apparent from Fig. 11 that under these conditions a difference (advance) of a few tenths of pH units can decide the success or failure of therapy in hyperacidification of cancer tissue.

Using one of the most favorable (most selective) cancerostatic agents known at present, it is possible to kill about 30 to 70% of the cancer cells

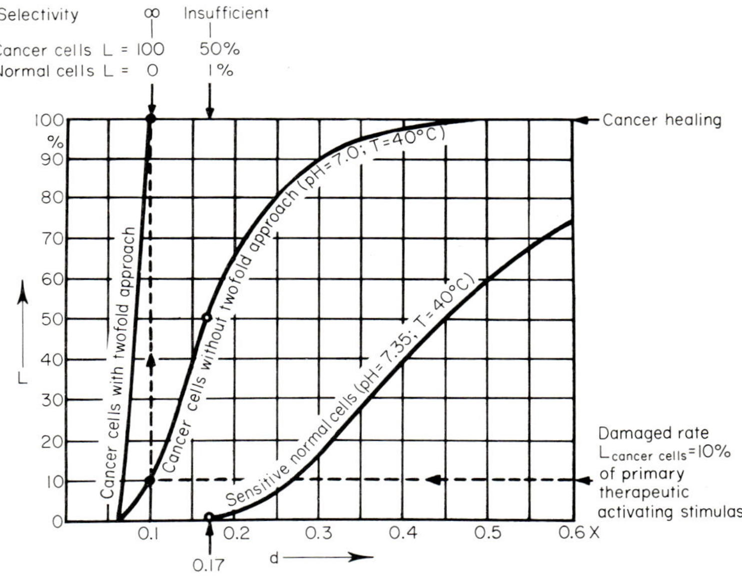

FIG. 12. Quantitative representation of multiphase cancer therapy. Action of selective twofold approach, optimized tumor hyperacidification + 40°C hyperthermia, on the shape of cell damage $L = f$ (dosage d) curves, by a factor of 10 = chain reaction contribution 4 times cell labilization 2.5. x = the stimulating agent.

at one stroke if the dose applied is so selected that there is no critical accompanying damage to the sensitive normal cells of the organism at the same time. This is why so far, in general, a cure for cancer could not be achieved by cancerostatics alone, which can merely delay temporarily the growth of the tumor. This situation roughly corresponds to a dose value $d = 0.17x$ and the points plotted on the two curves on the right side of Fig. 12. Successful selective intensification of cancer cell damage leads to a fundamental change in the situation, as is shown by the left curve of Fig. 12, plotted for the case of volume $V = 10$ times intensification. Upon tenfold intensification the lower dose $d = 0.1x$ is sufficient:sensitive normal cells are no longer damaged and a primary cancer damage of $L_1 = 10\%$ to destroy 100% of the cancer cells in the tumors is attained. Every primary therapeutic approach (activating stimulus) which brings about a damage rate of $L_1 > 10\%$ in cancer tissues could, thus, theoretically lead to a cure of the cancer or at any rate make it possible to live with the cancer with periodical application of therapy.

With ionizing radiation as the activating stimulus, radiation multiphase therapy is in the form of single focal doses, $D = 300$–$1000\ R$ (von Ardenne and Chaplain, 1968; von Ardenne and Reitnauer, 1968c) without critical associated damage to healthy tissue. Due to the low focal dose, it becomes possible to irradiate larger segments of the body and therewith in many cases to combat metastases by radiology.

The selective intensification of cancer cell damage in combination with the many classic procedures would also provide a satisfactory solution to cancer therapy in that the many years of experience of oncologists and radiation therapists would be fully utilized. Every cancer physician can essentially keep his tried and proved methods. He need not change present therapeutic procedures to make use of the new methods described, but, on the contrary, the effects of his treatment can be enhanced by the process of selective intensification.

G. *In Vitro* Experiments with Strict Simulation of the *in Vivo* Conditions in Formulating a Multiphase Cancer Therapy Concept

In investigations to formulate a cancer therapy consisting of many single steps the number of necessary experiments grows to an extraordinary degree because the possible combinations multiply rapidly with increasing number of steps. The position is thus entirely different from that with the simple screening test on tumor-bearing laboratory animals (average duration of experiments about 100 days). The clarification of the very complex problems in the course of a time-span of a few years held out some hope of success if it were possible to reduce the number of experiments

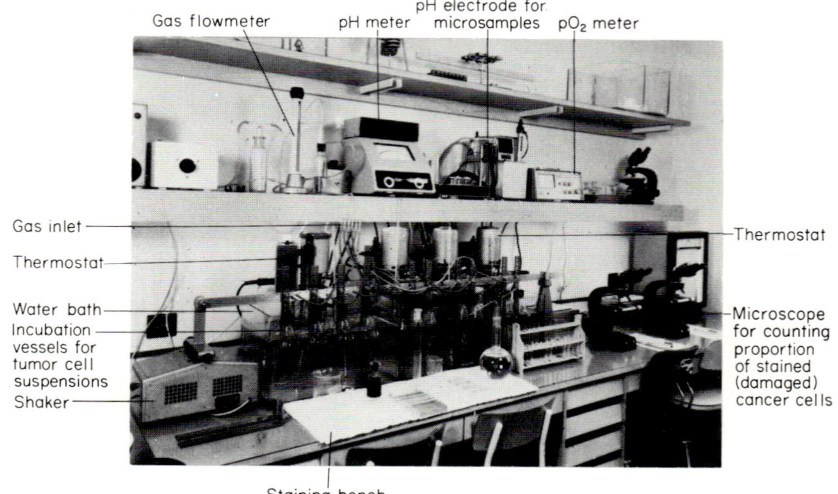

FIG. 13. View of apparatus for rapid measurement of cancer cell damage under ten different conditions (pH, temperature, glucose concentration, pO_2, agent concentration, agent combination) using trypan blue stain as an indicator.

considerably by developing strategic focal points (von Ardenne, 1971b) and by using rapid *in vitro* measuring procedures based on guiding theoretical aspects. Figure 13 shows the apparatus, installed during this phase of our research, for the rapid measurement of cancer cell damage under ten different conditions, using trypan blue as an indicator. The *in vitro* measurements, as a rule, on suspensions of EMAC cells which can readily be reproduced, were invariably carried out with strict simulation of all important *in vivo* parameters of cancer tissues and of the therapeutic variant to be tried (von Ardenne *et al.*, 1967a). By this strict simulation and by directing the therapeutic approach against essential molecules of the cell (reduction of the influence of biological variability of its environment), our *in vitro* experiments allowed definite conclusions to be drawn as to the *in vivo* situation, the correctness of which was confirmed during a later phase of the work.

If larger systems of cells were selected as the therapeutic target in these *in vitro* experiments, in agreement with theoretical ideas (von Ardenne *et al.*, 1967b, von Ardenne and Reitnauer, 1968b), there was a scattering in the effect far too great for clinical application, as shown in Fig. 14B. In this case the combination of many therapeutic approaches not only led to an intensification of the effect, but also to an increased scattering of the effect. A slight permissible scattering effect was always observed, as shown in Fig. 14A. Here the structural protein of the lysosomal membrane, in other words, a molecule, was the primary therapeutic target for damage, based on the concept of multiphase cancer therapy, by a combination of steps (hyperacidity + hyperthermia + activating stimulus with lysosome weakener). Such a molecule changes as soon as the necessary conditions (pH value, temperature, time of action of these values, etc.) exist in the cancer cells or in the cancer tissues, irrespective of the type of cancer cell, type of tumor, or site of the cell in the tumor involved. This leads to the hope of a universal therapy against all cancer tissues in which the processes of molecular damage can be applied. The slight variation in effect which remains according to Fig. 14 can probably be attributed to a residual influence of biological variability (e.g., the cell cycle of the cancer cells and their lysosomes or lysosomal enzyme contents).

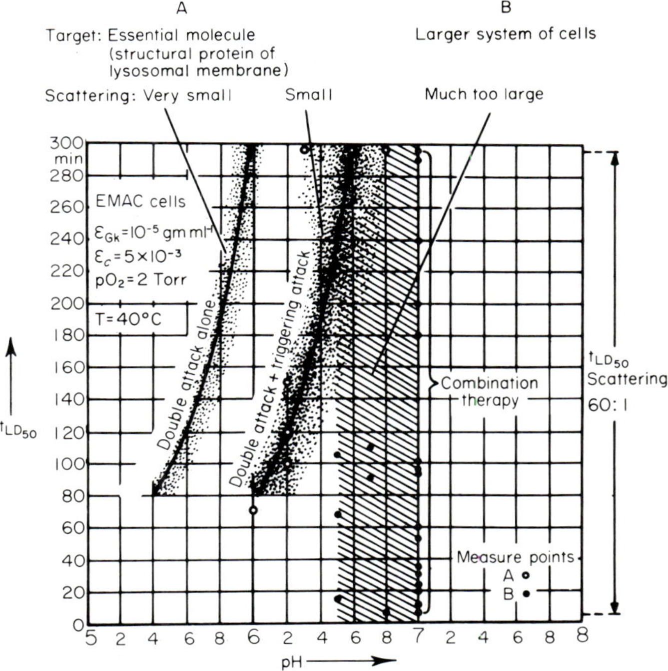

FIG. 14. Values for scatter regions for time $t_{LD/50}$ (50% trypan blue staining) as function of pH under conditions of (A) multiphase cancer therapy and (B) combination therapy. (Data for part B taken from Fig. 14 of von Ardenne, 1970c.) (EMAC) Ehrlich mouse ascites tumor cells.

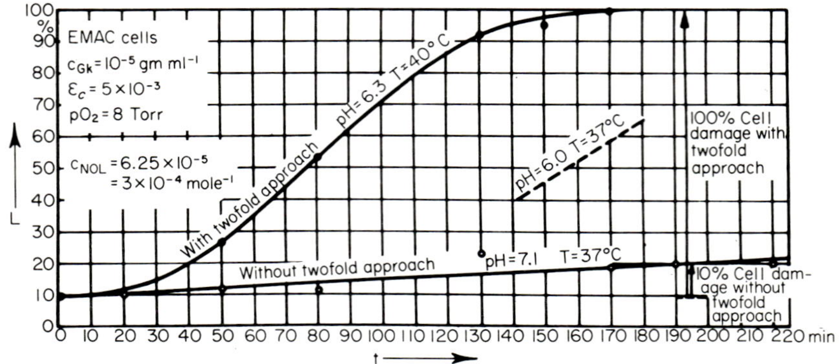

FIG. 15. *In vitro* measurements of damage L as function of action time t by N-oxide mustard of concentration C_{NOL}, with and without twofold approach (optimized tumor hyperacidification + 40°C hyperthermia); LY medium. (EMAC) Ehrlich mouse ascites tumor cells.

In vitro measurements of cancer cell damage after implementation of the chain reaction and intensification process are shown in Fig. 15. As has already been discussed above, in this measurement the important parameters existing in cancer tissues are strictly simulated. After 200 minutes action of the cytostatic, N-oxide mustard (Mitomen, NSC 10,107) in the given concentration, under normal tumor conditions (pH 7.1, $T = 37$°C), there is a 10% damage to the cancer cells. This damage by the activating stimulus increases to 100%, that is, to say there is an intensification of the cancer cell damage by a factor of 10, if, under otherwise identical conditions, a pH of 6.3 is maintained in this experiment by furnishing lactic acid and if the temperature is adjusted to $T = 40$°C.

Once the concept of multiphase cancer therapy had been elaborated on the basis of the interaction of several thousand *in vitro* series of experiments with pH determinations in optimally hyperacidified cancer tissues, it was then possible to test the important variants of the therapeutic concept, allowing for the long duration of the experiments on laboratory animal tumors.

H. Analysis of Different Variants of Multiphase Cancer Therapy by *in Vivo* Experiments on Highly Resistant Laboratory Animal Tumors

From the middle of 1968 to the end of 1970 (von Ardenne *et al.*, 1969a,b,c; 1971; von Ardenne and Chaplain, 1969a,b, 1970; von Ardenne and Reitnauer, 1970a,b) an experimental program was started on almost 2000 laboratory animals (tumor-bearing mice and rats) using the device for continuous infusions illustrated in Fig. 16, with simultaneous hyperthermia. A report is given (von Ardenne, 1971a) on therapeutic experiments on about 1000 laboratory animals, corresponding to about 50% of the total animal program encompassed so far. The experiments were based on the concept of multiphase cancer therapy with seven different variants of the activating stimulus: weak local X-ray dose, or cyclophosphamide, or cyclophosphamide + vitamin A + DMSO, or Na deoxycholate, or isophosphamide, or EMAC antiserum, or (and) Bacillus Calmette-Guérin vaccination. These therapeutic experiments were made on seven different mouse and rat tumor types: Ehrlich ascites carcinoma (mouse); mammary carcinoma Ma 21224 (mouse); solid ascites carcinoma (mouse); Jensen sarcoma (rat); Walker carcinosarcoma 256 (rat); Druckrey hepatoma (rat); and DS-carcinosarcoma (rat). This large-scale experiment showed the extraordinary increase in the therapeutic effect with the lysosomal cytolysis chain reaction (i.e., use of the double approach consisting of optimized

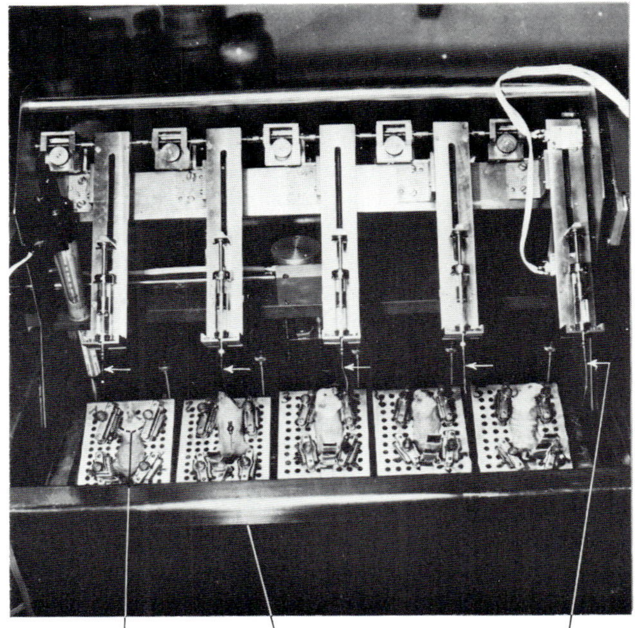

FIG. 16. Apparatus for conducting infusions of laboratory animals in combination with hyperthermia.

hyperacidity of the tumors + hyperthermia). If the primary (activating) stimulus was administered in a low dose so that it alone did not result in any curative effect, addition of the twofold approach gave rise to curative rates between 24 and 85%. The *in vitro* result shown in Fig. 15, therefore, was fully confirmed *in vivo*.

A further result of all laboratory experiments carried out so far is the observation that in all seven tumor types listed above, it is possible to achieve a high rate of cure with multiphase cancer therapy. This indicates the expected universality of the therapy, resulting from selection of a molecule, such as structural protein of the lysosomal membrane, as the therapeutic target.

With the two tumor types (mammary carcinoma Ma 21224 of the mouse and DS-carcinosarcoma of the rat) which yielded the poorest results in our large-scale experiment, a special experiment was undertaken with more than 500 animals. The programming and the results of this multiphase cancer therapy experiment on highly resistant laboratory animal tumors with various versions of the activating stimulus combination are summarized in Table II. The therapeutic effect of the individual approaches on mammary carcinoma of the mouse only (size of tumor from 6 to 7 mm in diameter at the time of the main therapeutic process) can be seen from the series of measurements given in Table II, Experiments 1 to 3. In the case of this tumor model, which probably corresponds to the conditions existing in many tumor types treatment with cyclophosphamide (Experiment 1) alone, despite its high dosage of 80 mg kg^{-1} did not lead to cure nor even to delay of tumor growth. Administration of subtoxic doses of vitamin A (Experiment 2) again did not lead to cure, but to a somewhat more pronounced delay in growth. Of the therapeutic measures, the most effective when used alone is the twofold approach consisting of optimized tumor hyperacidity plus hyperthermia. The dose of hyperthermia was 41°C for 70 minutes; the 40°C equivalent dose was, therefore, somewhat lower than that actually used on humans. With the twofold approach alone (Experiment 3), which, in this series of experiments, increased damage to cancer cells by endogenous defenses, no cures could be achieved. Even the combination of cyclophosphamide with the twofold approach (Experiment 4) did not lead to cure in the case of this extraordinarily therapy resistant tumor. There is a sudden increase in the therapeutic effect up to a cure rate of 42% upon additional administration of vitamin A (Experiment 6). This cure rate was obtained despite the fact that, in this series of experiments, the dose of cyclophosphamide was reduced from 80 to 25 mg kg^{-1}. According to our concept this result reflects the strong weakening of the lysosomal membrane by vitamin A (alcohol) and the

TABLE II

RESULTS OF MULTIPHASE CANCER THERAPY ON HIGHLY RESISTANT LABORATORY ANIMALS BY USING VARIOUS VERSIONS OF THE ACTIVATING STIMULUS COMBINATION[a]

		Activating stimulus combination						Delay in growth (%)			
Tumor (species)[b]	Experiment No.	Cyclophosphamide (mg kg^{-1})	Vitamin A	Ionizing radiation (R)	Stimulation of natural defenses	Twofold approach	Stimulation of natural defenses after treatment	4–7 days	8–14 days	15–21 days	Cures (%)
Mammary carcinoma Ma 21224 (ϕ = 6–7 mm)	1	80	—	—	—	—	—	0	0	0	**0**
	2	—	Standard	—	—	—	—	35	8	0	0
	3	—	—	—	—	Standard	By twofold approach	63	13	0	0
	4	80	—	—	—	Standard	By twofold approach	4.2	25	0	0[d]
	6	25	Standard	—	—	Standard	By twofold approach	0	12	16	42[d]
	8	25	Standard	—	By BCG inoculation[c]	Standard	By twofold approach	3.5	3.5	7	**85**
DS-carcinosarcoma (rat), m_T < 5 gm	10	60	—	—	—	Standard	By twofold approach	0	25	75	**0**
	12	50	Standard	500 (focus)	By tuberculin inoculation	Standard	By twofold approach	0	0	0	100

[a] Experiments with more than 500 laboratory animals. Because of the good tolerance of the process found in human cancer patients, the percent values are related to the total number of animals having survived the process.

[b] (ϕ) diameter; (m_T) tumor mass.

[c] BCG, Bacillus Calmette-Guérin.

[d] Influence additional lysosomal labilization with vitamin A: jump in cure rates from 0 (Experiment 4) to 42% (Experiment 6) although the cyclophosphamide dose was reduced from 80 to 25 mg kg^{-1}.

resulting intensification of the lysosomal cytolysis chain reaction. This result impressively demonstrates the importance of vitamin A (several days of subtoxic doses of vitamin A) within the concept of multiphase cancer therapy. The increase of the cure rate from 42 to 85% by using in addition immunological defenses (Experiment 8) is also in good accord with the ideas explained above. The immunological effect, according to von Ardenne and Chaplain (1970) is brought about by stimulation of unspecific natural defenses with the aid of BCG vaccination. The use of BCG in the immunotherapy of transplantable or chemically induced animal tumors (Zbar and Tanaka, 1971; Simmons and Rios, 1971; Bekierkunst, 1971) and in human malignancies (Mathé *et al.*, 1969; Morton *et al.*, 1970) seems to gain increasing recognition. Further immunological procedures using antiaggutinins of the albumin gland of *Helix pomatia* (von Ardenne *et al.*, 1969e; von Ardenne *et al.*, 1970b) are under investigation.

In summary it may be stated that even in the case of highly resistant laboratory animal tumors, cure rates that are close to or equal to 100% can be achieved upon a single treatment based on the concept of the multiphase cancer therapy. This favorable outcome of the *in vivo* experiments led us in 1970 to make preparations for clinical application of multiphase cancer therapy.

I. Increasing the Tolerance of Multiphase Cancer Therapy as an Important Condition for Clinical Application of the Treatment Program

Since 1965 our research has aimed at rendering multiphase cancer therapy process tolerable even to humans at a very advanced age and in a poor general state of health. A large segment of the road to our goal was covered once it became possible to reduce the temperature necessary for the hyperthermia step to 40°C. In animal experiments, allowances could be made without further thought for a moderate death rate which occurred even at 40°C, since the high hyperthermia sensitivity of laboratory animals in comparison with humans is generally known (von Ardenne and Reitnauer, 1968c, Fig. 3) and since in humans there is no need for the prolonged anesthesia during the process, which represents a considerable stress. The anesthesia necessary in animal experiments must actually be regarded as contraindicated when carrying out the process on humans (von Ardenne *et al.*, 1970c). Despite the far more favorable situation with humans, observations and results of measurements in carrying out the twofold approach of multiphase cancer therapy on healthy persons (von Ardenne *et al.*, 1970d) showed the need for further measures to increase tolerance of the therapeutic process. By making use of the principle of the two-

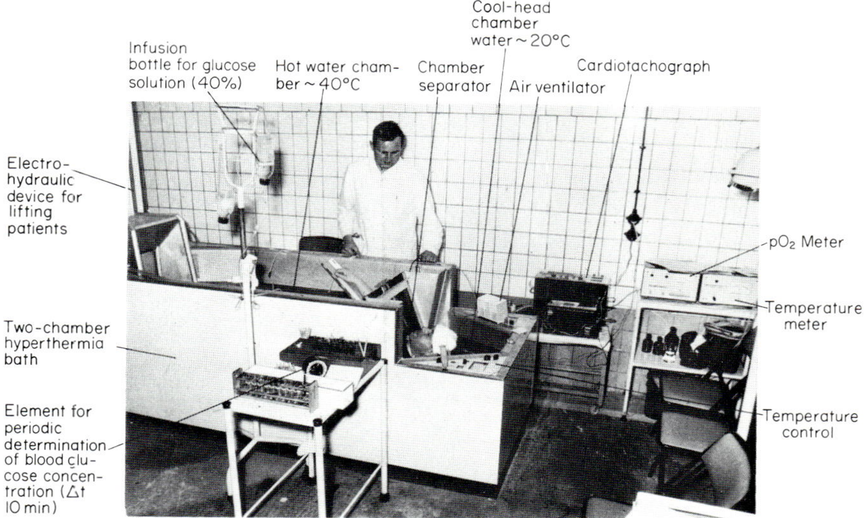

FIG. 17. Arrangement of two-chamber hyperthermia device for carrying out twofold approach multiphase cancer therapy in man.

chamber hyperthermia tank with a cooling head chamber (von Ardenne, 1965a, 1971b; von Ardenne *et al.*, 1970d), illustrated in Fig. 17, placing the patient in a horizontal position with limbs slightly elevated, and applying other technical aids, the stress on the patient can be considerably reduced as compared to earlier hyperthermia procedures (Lampert, 1948). Nevertheless, in the final phase of the process, precollapse or collapse states are invariably observed after about 200 or 300 minutes of hyperthermia at 40°C in humans in their middle years, and after about 120 minutes at 40°C in humans at an advanced age, when the cardiac and circulatory reserves are practically used up by the considerable excess stress, as shown in Fig. 18. Before transferring multiphase cancer therapy to clinical use, it will, therefore, be necessary to make the process tolerable even for old persons in a poor state of health. We have been engaged in investigations on the solution of this problem.

The principal development as to increasing the tolerance of multiphase cancer therapy was furnished by investigations on the position and direction of the oxygen–hemoglobin (Hb) binding curves for older persons at temperatures of 37° and 40°C (von Ardenne and Lippmann, 1970). Whereas in middle-aged persons an oxygen pressure value of $pO_2 \approx 92$ mm Hg is found in the arterial blood (37°C), in older persons (≥ 65 years) this value

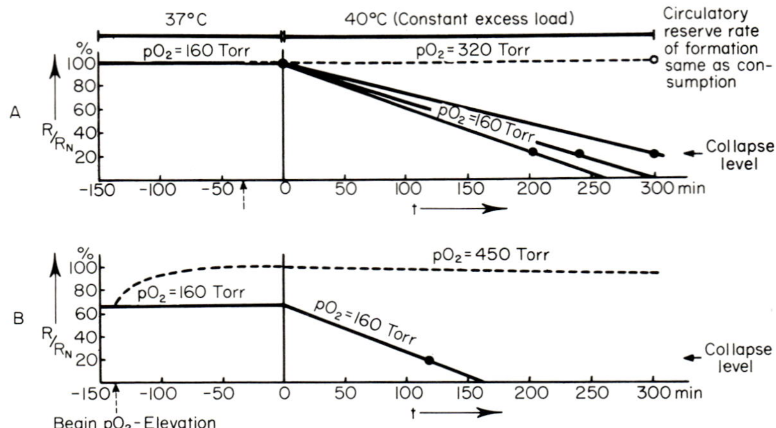

FIG. 18. Representation of magnitude of circulatory reserve R/R_N as function of 40°C treatment time t with and without raising pO_2 of inhaled air before and during treatment, for humans of middle (A) and advanced (B) age. RS = normal circulatory reserve of a 24-year-old man at 37°C.

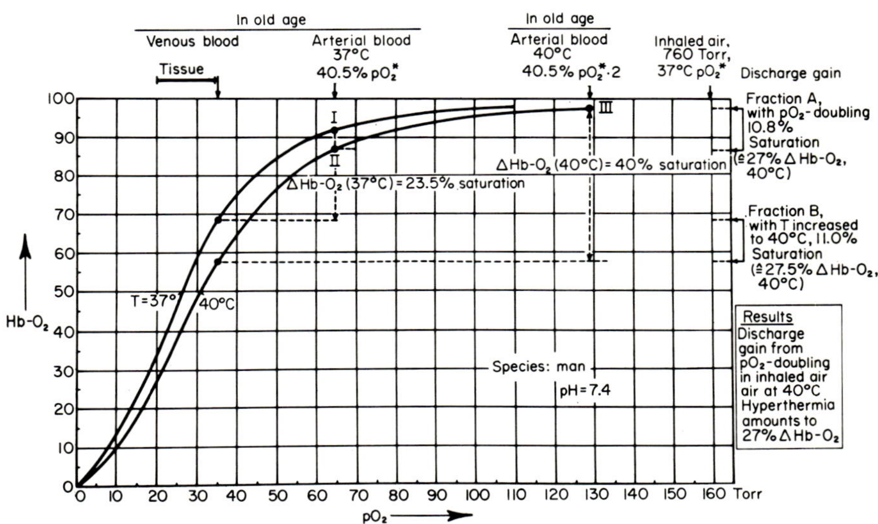

FIG. 19. Oxygen–hemoglobin dissociation curves for T = 37° and 40°C and extrapolation of *in vivo* data for humans of advanced age.

drops to $pO_2 \approx 65$ mm Hg due to decrease in pulmonary capacity. As is shown in Fig. 19, 40°C hyperthermia leads to a further loss of O_2 supply (Hb–O_2 saturation = 87%). By doubling the pO_2 of inhaled air from a normal pressure of 160 to 320 mm Hg, an Hb–O_2 saturation of ≈97.5% can be achieved upon 40°C hyperthermia for older persons. By this measure at 40°C, in the average case of a 65-year-old person, a gain of O_2 discharge of 27% of the total ΔHb–O_2 is achieved in accordance with Fig. 19, i.e., improvement of O_2 supply to all tissues. In middle age this gain is 15%, and at 80 years of age up to 50% of the total ΔHb–O_2. On the basis of measurements (von Ardenne and Lippmann, 1971) on time of increase in concentration of high-energy phosphates in rat brain after raising the pO_2 from 160 to 320 mm Hg, the pO_2 elevation should be started 90 minutes before beginning hyperthermia. In the interests of reduced mental stress for the patients, the O_2 is introduced through a flexible intranasal tube (von Ardenne and Lippmann, 1971).

A further way to increase tolerance of the process was by administering drugs, such as vitamin B_1 (Warburg *et al.*, 1970) (high doses of vitamin B

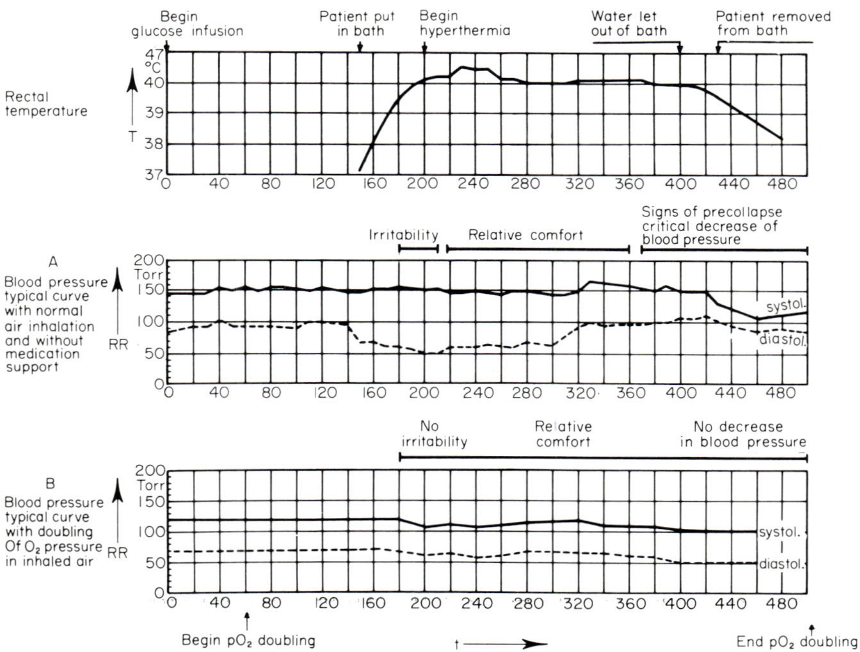

FIG. 20. Improvement of circulation, as referred to blood pressure, by doubling pO_2 of inhaled air during twofold approach (equivalent to 40°C for 280 minutes).

complex), dipyridamole (von Ardenne and Lippmann, 1971), vitamin B_{13} (orotic acid), and vitamin B_{15} (pangamic acid), which increase O_2 uptake by normal cells of the organism.

These measures, the common object of which is to increase markedly the energy reserves of normal cells (particularly the brain cells), led to a decisive advance. Whereas in earlier experiments with the twofold approach, a critical drop in blood pressure, as well as collapse and precollapse states were observed in the test persons toward the end of the process (Fig. 20A), these conditions did not develop with the new measures. An example of the improvement of the blood pressure curves is shown in Fig. 20B.

In the new concept, the hyperthermia time is reduced to only 150 minutes, because *in vitro* measurements showed that 40°C for this time period is sufficient for the liberation of the lysosomal enzymes (von Ardenne and Reitnauer, 1971).

Even older patients in a poor cardiac and circulatory states were able to tolerate the 40°C, 150 minute treatment without any crisis (von Ardenne and Lippmann, 1970). These results tie in with an increase in the universality and effectiveness of multiphase cancer therapy, because any increase in tolerance opens up the possibility of intensifying the treatment by longer duration of the twofold approach and higher dosages of the activating agents.

The experimental finding of the impressive increase in cardiac and circulatory reserves by simultaneous increase of the O_2 supply and O_2 utilization led to the observations summarized in the next section and to preliminary results in a new area.

J. Multivalent Effect and Integration of Combined Measures in Multiphase Cancer Therapy

One of the more trivial laws of physics states that in processes of separation the problem of selectivity is more easily solved the greater the difference between the (least) sizes to be separated. In 1965, with this concept in mind the augmentation of the fermentation metabolism of cancer cells (von Ardenne, 1965a) evolved into one of the principal steps in multiphase cancer therapy. Only at the end of 1969 did the author realize that in the problem of cancer therapy the augmentation of respiratory metabolism of normal cells was also comprised in the full interpretation of this law. Thus, the combined measures in the process of multiphase cancer therapy were developed as described in the following (see Table III).

It was soon found that the *in vivo* stimulation of respiratory metabolism of the cells, for instance by measures such as A3, A5, and A7 (Table III), according to the concepts of Warburg (1967), also led to damage of small cancer cell aggregates or even to a partial redifferentiation of cancer cells (Warburg *et al.*, 1970) in the organism. A few months before his death, Warburg told the author that he had embarked upon experiments on cancer prophylaxis with vitamin B_1 or with vitamins $B_1 + B_6 +$ nicotinic acid amine (Warburg, 1967). We then made such experiments under particularly well-controlled conditions on a metastasizing model (see Table IV) (von Ardenne and Chaplain, 1971a). Upon oral administration of vitamin B complex alone (Table III, A5) the frequency of metastases was reduced from 100 to 29%. A further reduction down to 5–10% was obtained when the measures were combined with an increase of the pO_2 in the inhaled air (Table III, A3). The combination of elevation of the O_2 supply to the cells and improvement of O_2 utilization in the cells (see Table III, A3 + A5 + possibly A6 + possibly A7), therefore, represents a highly effective multiphase prophylaxis of cancer or cancer metastases. This effect, according to Table III, occurs automatically, and when it has fulfilled its role (O_2 supply in readiness and large-scale production of vitamins), it should be further used alone for general health protection.

In the process of multiphase cancer therapy, augmentation of the respiratory metabolism by combination of measures A1, A2, A3, A5, A6, and A7 (Table III) brings about greater stabilization of the normal cells, together with a significant improvement of energy metabolism, an acceleration in the removal of waste, and acceleration of other cellular processes requiring energy. In the total system of the organism the cellular and supracellular phenomena elicited by augmentation of respiratory metabolism takes the form of an increase in cardiac and circulatory reserves (so that the main process can be extended over a period much longer than 200 minutes and could be repeated several times) and in the form of an increase in the rate of waste removal in the blood vessels (von Ardenne and Lippman, 1971; Warburg *et al.*, 1970). Thus patients who have undergone the process of multiphase cancer therapy also automatically go through a rapid waste disposal treatment, a kind of "tissue washing." At the same time a further field is opened for the multivalent utilization of the methods and techniques of multiphase cancer therapy against diseases involving O_2 deficiency states, for instance, many diseases of old age and many diseases involving high fever. This view is justified by a growing number of impressive observations of the normalization of the blood pressure in hypertonic subjects of the sclerotic type and dramatic improvement of weakened peripheral blood flow (extremities) after several repetitions of the procedure with 40°C hyperthermia, in combination with the measures to improve the energy supply which in some cases lead to improvements lasting more

TABLE III

MULTIVALENT ACTION OF THE COMBINED MEASURES OF MULTIPHASE CANCER THERAPY[a,b]

Therapeutic measure						
No.	Designation	Dose (for 75 kg body weight)	Day(s) of application	Time program	Measure combination	Effect of multiplication of energy metabolism
A1	Intravenous glucose (40%) infusion	$D \cdot t_A \approx 1.4$ g min^{-1} (400 mg/100 ml blood glucose conc.)	8th	From $t = 0$ to 390 min	A1 A2 A3 A5 A6 A7	*In normal cells and normal tissues:* Stabilization of normal cells; improvement of their energy situation; acceleration of purification of cells
A2	40°C hyperthermia	Total-body process in 2-chamber hyperthermia bath	8th	From $t = 200$ to 350 min		
A3	pO_2 increase of inhaled air	From 320 mm Hg in younger to <400 mm Hg in older patients	8th	From $t = 60$ to 500 min		Rapid cleansing of blood vessels (tissue washing)
A5	Vitamin B complex orally	$D = 60$ mg vitamin B_1, etc.	8th	Daily, divided into three doses		
A6	Vitamin C orally	$D = 1$–10 gm/day	8th	Daily, divided into three doses		
A7	Dipyrimadole orally (curantyl, Persantine)	$D = 75$ mg	8th	$t = 60$ min		Arrest of viral diseases (virus propagation and infectious diseases)
B1	BCG inoculation i.c.[c]	$D = 0.4$ mg distributed over 4 injection sites	0	(Beware of contraindications)		
B5	Vitamin A palmitate orally	$D = 10^6$/day	1st–7th	Daily	(A1) (A2) A3 A5 A6	*In as yet not irreversibly dedifferentiated cells with cancer metabolism:* In some cases redifferentiation of cancer cells under good
B6	Vitamin A palmitate orally	$D = 2 \times 10^6$	8th	120 Min before beginning main therapy		

C2	Cancerostatic, e.g., cyclophosphamide	$D = 30$–50 mg kg^{-1}	8th	From $t = 180$ to 200 min	A7 (B1)	supply conditions (return to respiratory metabolism)
C3	Ionizing radiation	$D = 300$–600 R (focal dose)	8th	From $t = 220$ to 230 min	(B5)	Multiphase prophylaxis of cancer or cancer metastases
C8	Detoxification of degradation products of regressing tumors		8th–20th			Stimulation of nonspecific immune defenses (increasing leukocyte number, etc.)
					A1 A2	*In cancer cells and cancer tissues:*
					A3 A5	Labilization and killing of cancer cells
					A6 B1 B5	Selective hyperacidification of all cancer tissues (pH $\approx$ 6.0–6.3)
					B6 C2 (C3) C8	Selective activation of lysosomal cytolytic chain reaction in all cancer tissues with numbers of cells $N_c > 10^6$

[a] Four-hour multiplication of the rate of energy metabolism of all cells of the organism (particularly in man at an advanced age). Smaller rise for cells of the nervous system because of blood–brain barrier and blood–nerve barrier.

[b] Effects of measures A1: ensuring adequate glucose supply
A2: nonspecific increase in metabolic rate (factor $\approx$ 1.75)
A3: excess O_2 supply, particularly in older patients with much reduced pulmonary capacity
A5, A6, A7: improvement of O_2 utilization of the cells
} Twofold approach

[c] BCG, Bacillus Calmette-Guérin; i.c., intracutaneously.

TABLE IV

EXPERIMENTAL RESULTS ON PROPHYLAXIS OF CANCER METASTASES BY MULTIPHASE PROCESS OF STRONG INTENSIFICATION OF O_2 METABOLISM OF ALL TISSUES[a]

Nature of step	Step	Application	Single dose	Time program	Frequency of metastases[b] (%)
0	Control	—	—	—	≈100
1. Increase of O_2 supply to the cells	Increase of the pO_2 of inhaled air to 400 mg Hg	O_2 tent	pO_2 = 400 mm Hg	From day of operation (1st day) to 14th day thereafter	80
2. Improvement of O_2 utilization in cells	Administration of vitamin B complex ($B_1 + B_6 +$ nicotinic acid amide, etc.) (VEB Jenapharm)	Oral	0.8 mg kg^{-1} 0.2 mg kg^{-1}	On 1st, 7th, and 14th day From 1st to 20th day	29
3. Combination of steps 1 and 2	Increase of pO_2 of inhaled air combined with vitamin B complex treatment	O_2 tent Oral	Same as steps 1 and 2	Same as steps 1 and 2	5–10
4. Proposed combination of steps 1 and 2 with stimulation of nonspecific defenses	Same as step 3, but with additional single BCG inoculation[c] (Institut fur Mikrobiologie, Jena)	i.c.[c] (Single dose divided over 4 injection sites)	0.4 mg	3 Days before operation	Possibly 0

[a] Metastasis model: CBA mice. Spontaneous mammary carcinoma Ma 2122 (No. 79). Surgical removal of primary tumor grown during 16 to 18 days to a diameter of 12 to 15 mm; 30–45 days thereafter frequency of metastases ≈ 100% (metastases in lungs and regional lymph nodes). Experiment on 80 animals.

[b] Step 1 and 2 are the only ones that do not yet decisively reduce the frequency of metastases, but combination of these steps leads to an extremely effective cancer or metastasis prophylaxis. We believe that this combination will have great significance for prophylactic combatting of cancer in the future.

[c] BCG, Bacillus Calmette-Guérin; i.c., intracutaneously.

than 6 months. Of course, when using the process against diseases other than cancer, measures of the C group and for the most part also of the B group from Table III are not applicable.

Another area for the multivalent utilization of measures from group A (Table III) is the arrest of virus propagation by 40°C hyperthermia (Eggers, 1970), for instance, in poliomyelitis, but without measure A1 which enhances inflammation. Important new possibilities are also present for the arrest of severe infectious diseases.

K. Reducing the Stress Situation Due to Products of Tumor Disintegration Following Multiphase Cancer Therapy: Perspectives

The transfer of multiphase cancer therapy to clinical use must take place with considerable caution to avoid accidents and to avoid as far as possible giving any grounds for discrediting the process. For this reason, despite impatience at home and abroad, we first carried out trials to ensure a high

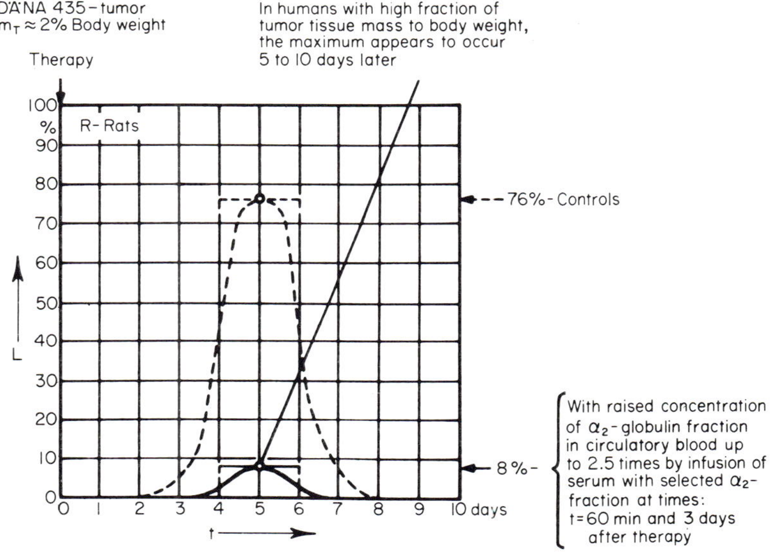

FIG. 21. Lowering by tumor decomposition products of lethality rate L from 76 to 8%, upon posttherapeutic infusion of serum with enriched α_2-globulin fraction (von Ardenne and Reitnauer, 1970d; von Ardenne and Chaplain, 1971b). Test animals, 50. m_T = tumor mass.

degree of tolerance of the therapy by human cancer patients (Section II, I). For the same reason, we are focusing our attention, preceding clinical application, on the formulation of combined measures to reduce stress emergencies which set in about 3 days after successful implementation of the main processes, due to products of tumor necrosis. The importance of avoiding fatalities, especially fatalities that may occur precisely because of the success of the therapy (regression of the tumor), is apparent from the experiments on laboratory animals summarized in Fig. 21 (von Ardenne and Reitnauer, 1970d; von Ardenne and Chaplain, 1971b).

The experiments show that, with the destruction of cancer tissue in rats by a single therapeutic thrust, between the third and seventh day, there frequently (76%) develops a fatal stress caused by the products of decomposition of the regressing cancer tissue, if the total mass of the cancer tissue (mI) on the day of treatment is about 2% of the total body mass. Animal experiments have further shown that the posttherapeutic death rate can be extraordinarily reduced (von Ardenne and Chaplain, 1971b) by infusion of serum with a highly concentrated α_2-globulin fraction to reduce the load after severe burns. According to Westphal (1968), the concentration of this fraction in the circulation is thereby increased 2.5-fold. Until serum of human origin with a highly concentrated α_2 fraction is available in sufficient quantity, other measures must be used for the reduction of the posttherapeutic stress situation caused by products of tumor decomposition. The following are examples of such measures, or combinations of measures according to (see Chapter A.21.3 in von Ardenne, 1971b): reducing the mass of decomposing tissue (treatment of the cancer patient at the earliest possible stage, surgical removal of the principal mass of the tumor), slowing down the accumulation of the products of decomposition [fractionation of multiphase cancer therapy (von Ardenne, 1970c) and protease inhibition], plasma exchange, enhancing the rate of energy metabolism of all cells of the organism (detoxification of organs) for instance by measures A1 (only orally in reduced doses), A3, A5, A6, A7 of Table III, from the first day of treatment to the twelfth day thereafter.

The pronounced decrease in the number of leukocytes observed when using cancerostatic agents, such as cyclophosphamide, during the posttherapeutic phase, intensifies the stress caused by products of decomposition of the tumor, due to a reduction in the rate of phagocytosis. In the classical chemotherapy of cancer used so far this presents a serious dilemma. In the posttherapeutic phase, precisely when endogenous defenses should be particularly active (involvement in the process of detoxification and destruction of cancer cells that have survived the therapy), they fail. For this reason we have attempted for some time to replace the activating cancerostatic treatment by procedures by which the cell poison is attached to a high-molecular vehicle (for instances albumin) forming a very stable chemical bond (von Ardenne and Reitnauer, 1969b; von Ardenne and Krüger, 1970). Such a loaded vehicle leaves the blood circulation at an accelerated rate in the tissue of the optimally hyperacidified tumor, because in this tissue, the capillaries, in their inflammatory function, are more permeable. The vehicles then reach the cancer cells by pinocytosis, where they are dissolved after their encounter with lysosomes, and liberate the cell poison [transformation of mode of action at the target site (von Ardenne, 1970d)]. According to the new concept, the immunological approach is effective after early beginning of glucose infusion, i.e., many hours before the cancerostatic action is stated. It seems that, in this manner, damage of endogenous defenses will be avoided.

III. Conclusion

This summarizing report is published at a time when there is every hope that the successful clinical application of multiphase cancer therapy can be implemented. Quite recently the number of experimental findings that it is really possible to create a highly selective and, therefore, universal whole-body therapy against cancer in humans have increased considerably. In order to give to the flow of information, which is now of such importance, greater depth and width, our original works (Nos. 1 to 107) have been published roughly simultaneously in a comprehensive version (von Ardenne, 1971b). How to implement quick testing, clinical use of the principles discovered and of the highly selected methods evolved, as well as application of the experiences of a decade of research aimed at a specific target, are only superficially touched upon in this report. It will, therefore, be necessary for the appropriate medical forums to study the contents of our original investigations and subject them to critical evaluation and, possibly, then be able to use them as a starting point for their own research.

References

Ashby, B. S. (1966). *Lancet* **2**, 312.

Bekierkunst, A., Levij, I. S., Yarkoni, E., Vilkas, E., and Lederer, E. (1971). *Science* **174**, 1242.

Cavaliere, R., Ciocatto, E. C., Giovanella, B. C., Heidelberger, Ch., Johnson, R. O., Margottini, M., Mondovi, B., Moricca, G., and Rossi-Fanelli, A. A. (1967). *Cancer* **20**, 1351.

de Duve, Ch. (1959). *In* "Subcellular Particles," p. 127. Ronald Press, New York.

de Duve, Ch. (1961). *In* "Biological Approaches to Cancer Chemotherapy" (R. J. C. Harris, ed.), p. 101. Academic Press, New York.

Druckrey, H., Schmähl, D., Steinhoff, D., Rajewsky, M., Bannasch, P., and Flaschenträger, Th. (1959). *Z. Krebsforsch.* **63,** 28.

Eggers, H. J. (1970). *Deut. Med. Wochschr.* **95,** 473.

Friedman, F. L. (1952). *In* "Introduction to Pile Theory," p. 111. Addison-Wesley, Cambridge, Massachusetts.

Lampert, H. (1948). "Überwärmung als Heilmittel." Hippokrates-Verlag, Stuttgart.

Mathé, G., Amiel, J. L., Schwarzenberg, L., Schneider, M., Cattan, A., Schlumberger, J. R., Hayat, M., and de Vassal, F. (1969). *Lancet* **1,** 697.

Morton, D., Eilber, F. R., Malmgren, R. A., and Wood, W. (1970). *Surgery* **68,** 158.

Quadbeck, G. (1967). *Hippokrates* **38,** 45.

Rauen, H. M., and Norpoth, K. (1967). *Arch. Pharm.* (*Weinheim*) **37,** 38.

Rieger, F. (1970). *Studio Biophys.* **21/22,** 133.

Shaw, J. G. (1966). *Arch. Biochem. Biophys.* **117,** 1.

Simmons, R. L., and Rios, A. (1971). *Science* **174,** 591.

Thomas, M., and Aldridge, W. N. (1966). *Biochem. J.* **98,** 94.

von Ardenne, M. (1965a). *Lecture Heidelberger Krebsforschungszentrum*; see von Ardenne (1971b). Chapter 18.

von Ardenne, M. (1965b). *Naturwissenschaften* **52,** 645; see also von Ardenne (1971b), Chapter 16.

von Ardenne, M. (1970a). *Z. Naturforsch. B* **25,** 1492; see also von Ardenne (1971b), Chapter 103.

von Ardenne, M. (1970b). *Naturwissenschaften* **57,** 43; see also von Ardenne (1971b), Chapter 81.

von Ardenne, M. (1970c). *Naturwissenschaften* **57,** 360; see also von Ardenne (1971b), Chapter 97.

von Ardenne, M. (1970d). *Z. Naturforsch. B* **25,** 897; see also von Ardenne (1971b) Chapter 98.

von Ardenne, M. (1971a). *Panminerva med.* **13,** 509; see also von Ardenne (1971b), Chapter 80.

von Ardenne, M. (1971b). "Theoretische und experimentelle Grundlagen der Krebs-Mehrschritt-Therapie," 2nd Ed., Vols. I and II. VEB Verlag Volk und Gesundheit, Berlin.

von Ardenne, M., and Chaplain, R. A. (1968). *Naturwissenschaften* **55,** 448; see also von Ardenne (1971b), Chapter 60.

von Ardenne, M., and Chaplain, R. A. (1969a). *Z. Gesamte Inn. Med.* **24,** 609; see also von Ardenne (1971b), Chapter 71.

von Ardenne, M., and Chaplain, R. A. (1969b). *Naturwissenschaften* **56,** 464; see also von Ardenne (1971b), Chapter 77.

von Ardenne, M., and Chaplain, R. A. (1970). *Deut. Gesundheitsw.* **25,** 861; see also von Ardenne (1971b), Chapter 79.

von Ardenne, M., and Chaplain, R. A. (1971a). *Naturwissenschaften* **58,** 221, 1971. see also von Ardenne (1971b), Chapter 105.

von Ardenne, M., and Chaplain, R. A. (1971b). *Z. Gesamte Inn. Med.* **26,** 175; see also von Ardenne (1971b), Chapter 100.

von Ardenne, M., and Krüger, W. (1970). *Arzneim. Forsch.* **20,** 65; see also von Ardenne (1970), Chapter 90.

von Ardenne, M., and Lippmann, H. G. (1970). *Deut. Gesundheitsw.* **25,** 1685; see also von Ardenne (1971b), Chapter 89.

von Ardenne, M., and Lippmann, H. G. (1971). *Z. Gesamte Inn. Med.* **26,** 149; see also von Ardenne (1971b), Chapter 95.

von Ardenne, M., and Reitnauer, P. G. (1968a). *Deut. Gesundheitsw.* **23,** 1681, 1739; see also von Ardenne (1971b), Chapter 57.

von Ardenne, M., and Reitnauer, P. G. (1968b). *Deut. Gesundheitsw.* **23,** 1681, 1739; see also von Ardenne (1971b), Chapter 54.

von Ardenne, M., and Reitnauer, P. G. (1968c). *Arzneim.-Forsch.* **18,** 666; see also von Ardenne (1971b), Chapter 54.

von Ardenne, M., and Reitnauer, P. G. (1969a). *Radiobiol. Radiother.* **10,** 145; see also von Ardenne (1971b), Chapter 65.

von Ardenne, M., and Reitnauer, P. G. (1969b). *Z. Aerztl. Fortbild.* **63,** 965; see also von Ardenne (1971b), Chapter 73.

von Ardenne, M., and Reitnauer, P. G. (1970a). *Klin. Wochschr.* **48,** 658; see also von Ardenne (1971b), Chapter 86.

von Ardenne, M., and Reitnauer, P. G. (1970b). *Acta Biol. Med. Ger.* **23,** 483; see also von Ardenne (1971b), Chapter 82.

von Ardenne, M., and Reitnauer, P. G. (1970c). *Z. Naturforsch. B* **25,** 872; see also von Ardenne (1970), Chapter 91.

von Ardenne, M., and Reitnauer, P. G. (1970d). *Z. Krebsforsch.* **74,** 99; see also von Ardenne (1971b), Chapter 92.

von Ardenne, M., and Reitnauer, P. G. (1970e). *Arch. Geschwulstforsch.* **36,** 319; see also von Ardenne (1970e), Chapter 101.

von Ardenne, M., and Reitnauer, P. G. (1971). *Arch. Geschwulstforsch.* **38,** 264.

von Ardenne, M., and Rieger, F. (1966). *Z. Naturforsch. B* **21,** 472; see also von Ardenne (1971b), Chapter 23.

von Ardenne, M., and Rieger, F. (1967). *Z. Naturforsch. B* **22,** 958; see also von Ardenne (1971b), Chapter 43.

von Ardenne, M., Krüger, W., and Rieger, F. (1967a). *Arch. Geschwulstforsch.* **29,** 36; see also von Ardenne (1971b), Chapter 32.

von Ardenne, M., Reitnauer, P. G., and Rieger, F. (1967b). *Naturwiss. Rundsch.* **20,** 155; see also von Ardenne (1971b), Chapter 37.

von Ardenne, M., Chaplain, R. A., and Prokop, O. (1969a). *Deut. Gesundheitsw.* **24,** 1589; see also von Ardenne (1971b), Chapter 72.

von Ardenne, M., Chaplain, R. A., and Reitnauer, P. G. (1969b). *Deut. Gesundheitsw.* **24,** 924; see also von Ardenne (1971b), Chapter 69.

von Ardenne, M., Chaplain, R. A., and Reitnauer, P. G. (1969c). *Deut. Gesundheitsw.* **24,** 1781; see also von Ardenne (1971b), Chapter 74.

von Ardenne, M., Chaplain, R. A., and Rieger, F. (1969d). *Z. Krebsforsch.* **72,** 258; see also von Ardenne (1971b), Chapter 58.

von Ardenne, M., Krüger, W., Prokop, O., and Schnitzler, St. (1969e). *Deut. Gesundheitsw.* **24,** 588; see also von Ardenne (1971b), Chapter 68.

von Ardenne, M., Reitnauer, P. G., Rohde, K., and Westmeyer, H. (1969f). *Z. Naturforsch. B* **24,** 1610; see also von Ardenne (1971b), Chapter 78.

von Ardenne, M., Reitnauer, P. G., and Schmidt, D. (1969g). *Acta Biol. Med. Ger.* **22,** 35; see also von Ardenne (1971b), Chapter 59.

von Ardenne, M., Chaplain, R. A., Reitnauer, P. G., and Rohde, K. (1970a). *Acta Biol. Med. Ger.* **23,** 671; see also von Ardenne (1971b), Chapter 85.

von Ardenne, M., Prokop, O., Fleischer, J., Schnitzler, St., Krüger, W., Lapin, B. A., Annenkow, H. A., Assanow, N. S., and Kolodin, V. J. (1970b). *Deut. Gesundheitsw* **25,** 813; see also von Ardenne (1971b), Chapter 83.

von Ardenne, M., Reitnauer, P. G., and Rohde, K. (1970c). *Deut. Gesundheitsw.* **25,** 1677; see also von Ardenne (1971b), Chapter 87.

von Ardenne, M., Röhner, H. U., Braun, W., Buchholz, W., Barth, J., Schmoranzer, H., Hartmann, H., Kipping, D., Ludewig, R., Nitzschner, H., and Standau, H. (1970d). *Deut. Gesundheitsw.* **25,** 333; see also von Ardenne (1971b), Chapter 76.

von Ardenne, M., Reitnauer, P. G., and Rohde, K. (1971). *Arch. Geschwulstforsch.* **38,** 15; see also von Ardenne (1971b), Chapter 104.

Waddel, W. J., and Bates, R. G. (1969). *Physiol. Rev.* **49,** 285.

Warburg, O. (1930). "The Metabolism of Tumours." Constable, London.

Warburg, O. (1962). "Weiterentwicklung der zellphysiologischen Methoden," p. 525. Thieme, Stuttgart.

Warburg, O. (1967). Ursache und Verhütung des Krebses. (Lecture 30. 6. 1966, Lindau.) Triltsch-Verlag, Würzburg.

Warburg, O., Geissler, A. W., and Lorenz, S. (1970). *Z. Naturforsch. B* **25,** 559.

Westphal, O. (1968). Personal communication.

Zbar, B., and Tanaka, T. (1971). *Science* **172,** 271.

Addendum

Recent experience has shown that glycolysis and increased oxygen pressure value (pO_2) beyond 320–400 mm Hg are more effective if started in an earlier stage of the treatment schedule, namely 24 hours before hyperemia. The resulting acidification can accelerate a phenomenon of tumor cell proliferation increasing their therapeutic susceptibility by a factor near 3.

Clinical experience with multiphase therapy in incurable female cancer patients has been reported (GDR-Gynecologists' Congress, Halle [DDR] 1972) by a team directed by Dr. E. Krauszold of the Gynecological Clinic of the University of Greifswald. An analysis of the therapeutic results showed total regression of large ovarian and cervical cancers and also of their metastases in liver, kidney, and brain.

The Application of Anthelmintics in the Feedlot

JOHN R. EGERTON

Merck Institute for Therapeutic Research
Rahway, New Jersey

I. Introduction

Mass prophylactic and therapeutic programs for prevention and control of disease are not recent developments in human and veterinary medicine. The concept of providing medication in a dietary form has been used extensively in veterinary medicine for prevention and control of protozoal and bacterial infections, particularly in poultry husbandry. In human medicine, cooking salt was used as a vehicle for administering daily doses of chloroquine in a malaria endemic area of Brazil as early as 1954 (cited in Anonymous, 1970). The more recent use of cooking-salt vehicle to treat a population for nematode infections of bancroftian filariasis was reviewed recently (Anonymous, 1970). In contrast, phenothiazine was in use as an additive to dietary salt for control of nematode disease of ruminants approximately 30 years earlier.

While not the earliest anthelmintic used in controlling nematode infections, phenothiazine was undoubtedly the most widely used compound up to the beginning of the last decade (1960). With the advent of thiabendazole* and several organophosphate anthelmintics, the field of chemotherapy of the helminth parasites of domestic animals blossomed. Reviews dealing generally with parasite chemotherapy (Gibson, 1965; Thompson, 1967) and more specifically with ruminant nematodes (Douglas and Baker, 1968) have recently appeared. In their review, Douglas and Baker state that complete interruption of the life cycles of the common ruminant nematode parasites can only be accomplished economically in "certain situations such as feedlots." It is this concept with which this presentation will deal.

* Thiabendazole = 2-(4-thiazolyl)benzimidazole.

The term "feedlot" has differing meanings in different parts of the world. As it applies to the United States cattle industry, the term is used to denote installations in which beef cattle to be fed to slaughter weight (usually 900–1100 lb liveweight) are grown and fattened in confined areas (pens) with an allowance of approximately 100–200 sq. ft per head. Water is piped into troughs in each pen, and feed is delivered, on a scheduled basis, to feeding troughs or "bunkers." A typical commercial installation would have 15,000–20,000 head of cattle on feed at any given time; many feedlots (farmer-feeders) have a capacity of only a few hundred head, while at least one commercial feedlot has the capacity to have approximately 100,000 head of cattle on feed at one time.

Depending on starting and finishing weights, the cattle are generally fed for about 150–180 days. The yearly turnover rate, at full capacity, is thus approximately 2–2.5 times the "on-feed" capacity of any given lot. In order to attain this rate of production, the cattle in the largest operation must cycle through the lots with roughly 5000 head per week being shipped for slaughter and being replaced in the pens with a similar number of incoming feeder calves. The incoming calves are grouped according to similarities which are anticipated to produce a reasonably uniform growth and finishing rate and initially fed a starter ration. Starter rations range from all long hay to all grain; however, grain in quantity is usually fed only after a period of acclimation to the feedlot. Shortly after arrival at the lot, the calves are subjected to vaccination against a number of infectious diseases, have their horns (if any) tipped, are castrated (if bull calves), may be implanted with estrogens, may be wormed by bolus or drench, and also receive other treatments as deemed necessary by the management. Cattle showing symptoms of illness are moved to a separate "sick pen" for specific treatment where they remain until they are returned to their feeding pen at the termination of treatment.

If the cattle are to be wormed through feed medication, it is usually done at the earliest time that the feeder feels the cattle have become accustomed to the feeding routine and are "on feed." Currently there are three anthelmintic compounds approved by the U. S. Food and Drug Administration for administration in the feed. Thiabendazole is usually fed at the rate of 3 gm/100 lb liveweight (67 mg/kg) but may be used as high as 5 gm/100 lb (110 mg/kg) as a single feeding in the form of top-dressing pellets or as a complete feed. One feed manufacturing company has approval from the FDA to use a multiple-dose feeding program in which 1 gm/100 lb (22 mg/kg) of thiabendazole is fed each day for 3 consecutive days. An organophosphate compound, coumaphos,* has recently

* Coumaphos = *o,o*-diethyl *o*-(3-chloro-4-methyl-7-coumarinyl)phosphorothioate.

been approved for feed administration to cattle as an anthelmintic agent. Coumaphos is to be fed at the rate of 0.091 gm/100 lb liveweight (2 mg/kg) for 6 consecutive days, the complete feed consisting of a mash containing not more than 0.0056% coumaphos. Another recently approved compound for use in the feed of cattle is levamisole.† It is to be fed in pelleted form at the rate of 0.1 lb of pellets containing 0.8% active ingredient/100 lb liveweight (8 mg/kg) as a single feeding.

II. Economic Losses

The latest available (U. S. Department of Agriculture, Agriculture Handbook 291) estimates of losses suffered by the cattle industry in the United States from gastrointestinal worm parasites are in excess of $100,000,000 annually. Approximately one fourth of these losses were attributed to direct loss through mortality; the remainder, a threefold greater loss, was attributed to morbidity. Losses from mortality have historically been well recognized, and treatment of affected animals has been attempted by veterinary practitioners and knowledgeable stockmen. Losses due to morbidity, particularly when intercurrent disease problems were present, have been less well recognized. Then, too, all too often when the disease problem was recognized as parasitic in origin, the available treatment was ineffective, hard on the animal ("setback") or even a combination of the two.

During the decade 1951–1960, while the losses in cattle which were attributable to gastrointestinal roundworms increased markedly over the losses from the previous decade, a concomitant sharp decline in losses from internal parasites occurred in hogs, horses, and sheep. The total numbers of cattle increased markedly, while stocking rates generally increased during the 1951–1960 period, thus reflecting the trend toward intensified husbandry practices which had been introduced to establish an increased production of cattle. With the progressive concentration of animals, the problems from internal parasites likewise intensified.

Most of the ruminant roundworms of economic importance have a direct life cycle involving egg, free-living larvae, infective larvae, parasitic preadult, and adult stages in their development. Cattle become infected by ingesting the infective forms with their feed and/or water and, less commonly, by direct penetration of the infective forms percutaneously. Grassland areas conducive to raising cattle are likewise conducive to the continued existence of their common internal roundworm parasites, particu-

† Levamisole = l-(−)-2,3,5,6-tetrahydro-6-phenylimidazo[2,1-*b*]thiazole hydrochloride.

larly under conditions of intensive husbandry. It is, therefore, not surprising that better methods of parasite control on a herd basis were urgently needed by 1960. The period 1961–1970 showed an even more prodigious situation. Although official U. S. Department of Agriculture loss figures for that decade are not yet available, some concept of the magnitude of the problems can be found in a report from the Cooperative Extension Service of the University of Arizona (Cable, 1971). Beef production increased 48% above the 1960 level. The 48% increase occurred with only a 12% increase in the total United States cow herd; the major portion of increase was accomplished by finishing cattle to heavier weights, switching from grass fattening to grain finishing, and by obtaining more rapid, efficient weight gains.

Approximately 70% of all beef cattle slaughtered in the United States today are finished in feedlots. It is reasonable to assume that by the end of the present decade the proportion of finished cattle coming from the feedlot will be greater than 70% of the total. If, as Cable (1971) indicates, beef consumption increases another 28% over the 1970 level, by the year 1980 the production problems faced by the cattle industry will indeed be formidable.

III. Preconditioning

Feedlots for growing and fattening cattle in the United States exist today for one reason: to produce the maximum possible meat in the shortest possible time at the lowest possible cost in the most efficient manner. At present, cattle entering feedlots are a motley population, originating in diverse geographical areas. Husbandry programs under which they were produced are equally diverse and in turn require that feedlot operators adjust and modify their programs to meet these varying conditions if their operations are to be efficient. Current efforts to alleviate some of these problems have developed into management systems termed "preconditioning."

An economic analysis of the potential benefits to dairy farmers from more comprehensive herd health programs was presented by Barfoot *et al.* (1971). Woods *et al.* (1970) reported that vaccination against IBR (infectious bovine rhinotracheitis), BVD (bovine viral diarrhea), blackleg, malignant edema, and leptospirosis plus anthelmintic treatment with thiabendazole significantly reduced the morbidity in Illinois calves and yearlings when they were placed into feedlots. Baker (1968) reviewed the role of enteric parasitism in preconditioning programs designed for California feedlot cattle. His remarks were directed specifically toward the problems of gastroenteric parasitism in the application of the most suitable preconditioning program predicated upon a sound knowledge of the health problems extant within any given herd of cattle.

Hjerpe (1971), in considering a program of preventive medicine for cattle in the feedlot, states that the aim of such a program "*is to determine and institute the level of control for each disease which is the most profitable for the individual feedlot.*" Under infectious diseases he lists six costs, other than death losses, which must be considered. They are: (*1*) cost of medicine for treatment; (*2*) cost of labor for care of sick and convalescent cattle; (*3*) loss of weight during sickness; (*4*) loss of time on feed during sickness and convalescence with (*5*) resulting reduction in rate of gain and feed efficiency; and (*6*) losses incurred with unthrifty and chronically sick cattle through condemnation or low sale price. Specifically mentioned as quite costly, though rarely fatal, was trichostrongylosis.

IV. Anthelmintics in Feedlots

Trichostrongylosis is a broad term connoting infection with one or more nematode parasites of the taxonomic group known as the Family Trichostrongylidae. Included in this group are some of the more pathogenic genera of ruminant parasites: *Ostertagia*, the medium brown stomach worm; *Haemonchus*, the large (barber pole) stomach worm; *Trichostrongylus*, small stomach worm and hair or bankrupt worm; *Cooperia*, cooper's worm; *Nematodirus*, thread-necked strongyle. Other important nematodes, not included in Hjerpe's designation, include the strongyle nodular worm, *Oesophagostomum*, the strongyle hookworm, *Bunostomum*, and the rhabditoid, *Strongyloides*, though the latter is probably most usually a problem in young calves.

As indicated above, it was a well-known fact that serious economic losses attributable to internal parasites were prevalent and increasing in the cattle industry by 1960. Factual information on the extent and severity of parasitism, where available, was mostly state or regionally oriented typified by that reported for South Carolina by Hitchcock (1956). More recently, Miller *et al.* (1966) reported the results of a survey based on fecal worm egg counts of cattle in the Midwest and Plains states. Ninety-four percent of the herds examined were roundworm positive. This does not imply that these herds were necessarily clinically affected by parasitism, however. Miller (1971), in updating these survey results, revised the estimated herd infection incidence downward slightly to 88% for the United States as a whole. Regionally the West and Northwest Pacific Coast revealed >99% incidence of herd infection, as did the Southeast. Midwestern (corn belt and upper central states) herd infections were 95%, Southwest and Mountain states 84%, and Northeast states had the lowest incidence with 78% of the sampled herds carrying nematode infections.

Prior to 1964, when thiabendazole was introduced to the feedlot, little data were available on the economic benefits attainable through the application of an anthelmintic to feeder cattle. The principle was not new; the practice had been attempted previously but with no noteworthy success. In fact, the introduction of this then new compound to cattle feeders may quite possibly have been hindered to some extent through lack of spectacular results, and even failures, following use of older available anthelmintics. With the removal of worms accomplished in varying degrees following treatment with the available compounds, the cattle feeders often obtained no better, and frequently obtained poorer, performance from treated stock. In retrospect, it is not too difficult to understand the feeders' early contention that worms did not generally detract from their operations. The "setback" encountered following these early treatments tended to discourage general use of the compounds in most animals in the lot and relegated their use, primarily, to animals in the "sick pen." Here those animals showing obvious symptoms of parasitism were treated in order to insure survival of the animal. Death losses were undoubtedly reduced, but just as surely the losses from the other causes stated by Hjerpe (1971) detracted from profitability under those conditions.

Other popular lore among cattlemen and feedlot operators was (is) that, though cattle coming off pasture may be "wormy," it would not matter once they went onto a full-feed, high-energy ration in the lot because the worms could be "flushed" out. In a study reported by Goldberg (1965), uninfected calves on a high-feeding level outgained those on a low-feeding level by 11.5 lb/100 lb of total digestible nutrients (TDN). However, parasitized calves on high-level feeding converted their feed less efficiently than their nonparasitized controls by 9.2 lb/100 lb of TDN consumed; parasitized calves on a low-level feeding were less efficient than similarly fed nonparasitized calves by 12.2 lb/100 lb of TDN. Further, he stated that moderate infection reduced feed efficiency more than mild infection, and that the *establishment of worms was not affected by the feeding level.* In a similar study, Leland *et al.* (1966) reported that grain supplementation to pastured calves prevented clinical signs of parasitism but did not completely counterbalance the influence of helminth infection on resulting hypoproteinemia, reduced packed cell volume, and parasite-induced changes in blood proteins. There remains little doubt today that parasites can interfere with the efficient utilization of feed and production of meat in feedlot operations. What is not as clear is the determination of when parasitism begins to cost the producer. Many "rules of thumb" have been promulgated in the past, e.g., worm the cattle if the average fecal egg count exceeds x eggs per gram of feces. In a restricted environment, this may be suitable and practical. However, under present conditions of buying and selling, it may well be impossible to determine with reasonable accuracy the origin(s) of any given lot of cattle. The "rule" for Montana cattle may not preclude death and morbidity losses if applied to Georgia cattle. As noted by Baker (1967), the "breakpoint" at which clinical disease occurs is dependent on numerous factors, i.e., immune state, nutrition, age, number and kind of parasites, hormone balance and stress factors, heredity, and other factors. The same factors undoubtedly affect the precise point at which the "economic disease" breakpoint occurs. "Subclinical parasitism" has come under attack (Baker, 1968) when used to denote instances in the host–parasite relationship under which beneficial effects are obtained following anthelmintic therapy. The term "economic disease" is used here in place of the more usual "subclinical disease" inasmuch as it has been demonstrated in recent years that parasites can influence the profitability of feedlot operations even in the absence of frank parasitic (clinical) disease.

There is no question that the diagnosis of clinical parasitism will vary with the diagnostic abilities of the individuals concerned, and that economic benefits can follow the use of a safe, efficient anthelmintic in cattle for which no diagnosis of parasitism was made. Flack *et al.* (1967) reported the results of six feedlot trials in which "better-than-average" commercial feeder cattle were divided into two experimental groups. Of the 3739 cattle involved, approximately half were not treated with an anthelmintic (1840), and approximately half were treated with thiabendazole (1899) administered in the feed. Fecal worm egg counts on 10% or more of the cattle in each trial averaged 100 eggs per gram, or less, in all trials. The cattle were "heavy in weight and above average in appearance" when the trials were initiated. Thiabendazole was administered to the treated groups at an average rate of 3 gm/100 lb of body weight by spreading the commercial wormer feed in the feed bunker. Average daily gain of untreated cattle ranged from 2.50 to 3.08 lb vs. 2.70 to 3.11 lb for the treated animals. Overall, treated cattle gained 0.042 lb per day more than the untreated cattle, a rather small advantage. However, as reported by Flack *et al.* (1967) the cattle treated with thiabendazole were, in fact, converted to more efficient production units. Feed efficiency was materially affected: treated cattle required only 96% as much feed as untreated cattle to attain the same rate of gain. At the then cost of feed, it was reported that feed costs were reduced $0.80/100 lb of gain, and the return per dollar invested in anthelmintic treatment was $4.45 per head through the growing and fattening period. Translated into added profits for a 10,000-head feedlot, the net return would be $34,500, assuming that comparable cattle were started. The cost for labor to administer the treatment was nil, because the treatment consisted of routine feeding.

Not all trials of this nature have recorded positive benefits following the administration of anthelmintics. Ciordia and McCampbell (1971) reported three trials in which levamisole was used in feeder steers for which no advantage in overall weight gain was observed. Treatment was by drench and top dressing, but their data did not include observations on feed efficiency or cost per unit of gain for treated vs. control steers. Ames *et al.* (1969), reporting on a trial using experimental infections of *Ostertagia* and *Cooperia*, noted relatively large effects from parasitism in the postinfection, prefeedlot phase, but no great differences in feed efficiencies or rates of gain between parasitized-treated and parasitized-untreated calves during the feedlot phase. They stated, however, that their results showed that worm parasites can be a source of economic loss in feedlot cattle. They also cited 22 comparisons (including those of Flack *et al.*, 1967) made with naturally infected cattle, half treated and half not treated, in which economic advantages were demonstrated in 17 of the trials following the use of an anthelmintic.

Perhaps the small positive responses reported in the trials of Ames *et al.* (1969) and Ciordia and McCampbell (1971) for which statistical validity could not generally be demonstrated may best be explained by a comparison with the data reported on by Flack *et al.* (1967). As is well known, the smaller the differences in parameters measured the larger must be the sample size examined (assuming equal variability and experimental efficiency) in order to demonstrate statistical reliability at any given level of probability. In the former two reports, group size ranged from 6 to 25 steers, whereas the six trials of the latter report had group sizes of 180 to 505.

Positive benefits in 77% of cases as indicated by Ames *et al.* (1969) or 80% of cases (Miller, 1971) in which thiabendazole has been administered under controlled feedlot conditions constitutes relatively good odds ($\simeq$4:1) that the routine use of anthelmintic medication could be a reasonable monetary risk in heterogeneous lots of feeder cattle.

Some explanation of the immediately preceding comments seem appropriate. Douglas and Baker (1968) put forth an elegant plea for the "rational use of anthelmintics," with which this writer agrees. As noted above, these authors further said that the only practical point for disruption of the life cycle of gastrointestinal nematodes is at the feedlot. Baker (1968) has restated his opinion that not all animals entering feedlot will show an economic benefit from treatment with anthelmintics, an opinion with which this writer also agrees. In his supporting argument, Baker said that the problem is differentiating those that will benefit from those that will not benefit, and that the differential diagnosis cannot be determined from visual examination, fecal examination, animal history, or physical examination alone. Further, he stated that one is in position to make judgment on the need of anthelmintic therapy only after evaluation of (*a*) a complete history which included the potential infection rate at the origin, (*b*) quantitative parasite egg counts on a sufficient number of individual animals, (*c*) careful physical examination of individuals in addition to the group as a whole, and (*d*) a careful appraisal of acceptance of water and feed in the feed lot. What is missing in reducing this concept to practice is the first listed essential point (*a*) in many, or possibly most, instances. Can one eliminate point (*a*) and still obtain a reasonably correct diagnosis using points (*b*), (*c*), and (*d*)? Are other combinations and permutations of these four points, taken three, two, or one at a time, equally good estimators of the need for medication? More likely, efficiency and accuracy of the estimators will decrease with decreasing numbers of estimatable parameters available. Consideration must be given also to the cost of such a program to the producer. If it is compatible with other health programs and is economically feasible, it should be utilized where possible.

A plan which has been adopted by many large feedlot operators is based upon experience with the use of thiabendazole since its introduction for use in cattle. It consists basically of treating those cattle which they predict will most likely produce more efficiently following treatment. Their predictions are based on some years of experience, duly recorded, in addition to the advice of consulting or contract veterinarians; in many instances, all cattle entering feedlots are routinely fed anthelmintic medicated feed. In a sense, this type program is analogous to the use of medicated salt for the control of filariasis (as cited above), wherein all individuals in a closed population receive the medication as part of their regular diet. Adjacent areas without the infection do not necessarily receive the medication *en masse*.

The cost of medicating all steers via ingested feed vs. cost of diagnosis and treatment of all, or part, through individual handling must be balanced against anticipated returns for dollars invested. Costs must include, of course, labor, both technical and nontechnical, as well as materials. When, as often happens, the multiple movements of cattle from sale barn to sale barn is repeated sufficiently often and cattle of similar appearance are blended together between sales before they reach the feedlot, the history of any particular lot of cattle becomes confounded, to say the least. Should examination indicate problems from internal parasites, the operator must decide whether it will be economically more profitable for him to worm or not worm; if worming is indicated he must then decide upon the more profitable program to be used. If sufficient information is available and labor costs and consultation fees are reasonable, he may elect the "rational" application of an anthelmintic to those animals judged most likely to respond. If, on the other hand, information is scant and ancillary costs are judged to exceed the estimated increase in profitability from the consumption of less feed plus better rate of gain (less the cost of medication), the operator may elect mass anthelmintic therapy supported by individual follow-up where necessary.

Profitability per production unit is a primary concern of the producer; under intensified production programs in use in the livestock industry today, more animals are exposed to greater risk from parasitic disease. When cattle enter feedlots for growing and fattening, mere survival through the feeding period is not sufficient; the inefficient animals are a liability to the producer. In quest of this increased efficiency, new approaches to beef production in the future will be required. A direct method to increase production of beef would be the use of synchronized breeding through estrus control and artificial insemination with brood stock selected for multiple birth potential (Hodgson and Hodgson, 1970). The calf crop produced would then be grown through to market weight under more uniform conditions. The growth rate of the calf is of primary importance in increasing the efficiency of beef production, and these authors foresee maximization of growth and fattening rates from calving to market as minimizing that proportion of feed required for maintenance. That is, producing a market weight animal in 1 year would require *less than* one half the total feed required to produce the same weight animal in a 2-year period. In order to accomplish this feat, calves will have to go into specialized intensive programs: high stocking rates on high-quality pastures with supplemental feeding or dry lot confinement feeding.

In those areas of plentiful pasture, the former program can be anticipated to be used in conjunction with the conventional extensive cow-calf operations now operable. It would seem that in the area of the intensified utilization of improved pasture, one can anticipate striking advantages for the rational use of anthelmintics in future. Where grass and cattle exist together, gastrointestinal roundworms will survive and flourish. Mass treatment for gastrointestinal parasitosis in feedlot cattle has been demonstrated to contribute to more efficient production of beef. Consider the vastly greater potential increase in production efficiency that would be attainable should safe, effective anthelmintics be properly applied during the critical rapid growth stage of beef cattle.

Until the United States cattle industry undertakes, on a herd basis, a program for the prevention of parasitism, the use of anthelmintics in feedlots will be of benefit in maximizing the efficiency of beef production.

References

Ames, E. R., Rubin, R., and Matsushima, J. K. (1969). *J. Anim. Sci.* **28,** 698.

Anonymous (1970). *Lancet* **i,** 660.

Baker, N. F. (1967). *In* "Symposium on Animal Health and Nutrition," pp. 5–18. Colo. State Univer. Agr. Ext. Ser., Ft. Collins, Colorado.

Baker, N. F. (1968). *In* "Preconditioning Seminar" (D. R. Gill and G. Crenshaw, eds.), pp. 58–63. Okla. State Univer., Stillwater, Oklahoma.

Barfoot, L. W., Cote, J. F., Stone, J. B., and Wright, P. A. (1971). *Can. Vet. J.* **12,** 2.

Cable, C. C., Jr. (1971). *Progr. Agr. Ariz.* **23,** 14.

Ciordia, H., and McCampbell, H. C. (1971). *Amer. J. Vet. Res.* **32,** 545.

Douglas, J. R., and Baker, N. F. (1968). *In* "Annual Review of Pharmacology" (H. W. Elliott, W. C. Cutting, and R. H. Dreisbach, eds.), Volume 8, pp. 213–228. Annual Reviews, Inc., Palo Alto, California.

Flack, D. E., Frank, B. N., Easterbrooks, H. L., and Brown, G. E. (1967). *Vet. Med. Small Anim. Clin.* **62,** 565.

Gibson, T. E. (1965). "Veterinary Anthelmintic Medication" (2nd Ed.). Commonwealth Agr. Bur., Farnham Royal, Bucks, England.

Goldberg, A. (1965). *J. Parasitol.* **51,** 948.

Hitchcock, D. J. (1956). *J. Amer. Vet. Med. Ass.* **129,** 34.

Hjerpe, C. A. (1971). *Vet. Med. Small Anim. Clin.* **66,** 60.

Hodgson, H. J., and Hodgson, R. E. (1970). *Agr. Sci. Rev.* **8,** 16.

Leland, S. E., Jr., Drudge, J. H., and Dillard, A. B. (1966). *Amer. J. Vet. Res.* **27,** 1555.

Miller, R. F. (1971). Personal communication.

Miller, R. F., Easterbrooks, H. L., and Brutsman, F. E. (1966). *Mod. Vet. Pract.* **47,** 52.

Thompson, P. E. (1967). *In* "Annual Review of Pharmacology" (H. W. Elliott, W. C. Cutting, and R. H. Dreisbach, eds.), Volume 7, pp. 77–100. Annual Reviews, Inc., Palo Alto, California.

Woods, G. T., Meyer, R. C., and Mansfield, M. E. (1970). *Mod. Vet. Pract.* **51,** 46.

AUTHOR INDEX

Numbers in italics refer to pages on which the complete references are listed.

C

D

E

H

I

J

K

L

M

N

O

S

T

U

V

W

SUBJECT INDEX

CUMULATIVE TITLE INDEX*

Boldface numbers indicate the volume numbers. (C) indicates titles from *Advances in Chemotherapy.*

* This index includes *Advances in Pharmacology,* Volumes 1–6 B, *Advances in Chemotherapy,* Volumes 1–3, and the combined series *Advances in Pharmacology and Chemotherapy,* Volumes 7–10.

D

E

F

G

H

I

K

L

M

N

O

P

Q

R

S

T

U

V